.30

A Medical Doctor's Home Guide for
ARTHRITIS, MUSCLE AND BONE AILMENTS

Also by the Author

A Country Doctor's Common Sense Health Manual
Doctor Hurdle's Program to Retain Youthfulness
Low Blood Sugar: A Doctor's Guide to Its Effective Control
The Biofeedback Diet: A Doctor's Revolutionary Approach

A Medical Doctor's Home Guide for
ARTHRITIS, MUSCLE AND BONE AILMENTS

J. Frank Hurdle, M.D.

ILLUSTRATIONS BY CLAUDIA ROULIER

Parker Publishing Company, Inc.
West Nyack, New York

©1980, *by*

PARKER PUBLISHING COMPANY, INC.

West Nyack, N.Y.

All rights reserved. No part of this
book may be reproduced in any form
or by any means, without permission
in writing from the publisher.

This book is a reference work based on research by
the author. The opinions expressed herein are not
necessarily those of or endorsed by the publisher.
The directions stated in this book are in no way
to be considered as a substitute for consultation
with a duly licensed doctor.

Library of Congress Cataloging in Publication Data

```
Hurdle, J    Frank
  A medical doctor's home guide for arthritis, muscle
and bone ailments.

   Includes index.
   1. Musculoskeletal system--Diseases. 2. Medicine,
Popular. I. Title. II. Title: Arthritis, muscle
and bone ailments. [DNLM: 1. Arthristis--Popular
works. 2. Bone diseases--Popular works. 3. Mus-
cular diseases--Popular works.  WE344 H962m]
RC925.H87    616.7'2         79-22618
ISBN 0-13-572636-0
```

Printed in the United States of America

What This Book Can Do for You

In this day and age of fast-paced living, people are constantly overdoing, and certainly among the first parts of your anatomy to feel the effects of this rushing around to get things done are your joints, bones and muscles.

Sometimes these amazing structures need just a little temporary attention. At other times, however, you may find that they need more than just a rest—they need tender loving care. This book is for the young, the middle-aged, and the elderly from all walks of life who find that their bones, muscles and joints need attention.

You may ask—and you should—why is this so important? There are many reasons. First, in properly caring for your "organs of toil," as muscles and bones are often called, you can head off untold trouble in the future. You may actually prevent your skeletal supports from becoming withered and stiff and useless!

Secondly, there are many infirmities that in the ordinary course of life get you down anyway. If you're to survive these ordeals, the better the condition of your muscles and joints when you have to be laid up temporarily, the more quickly and easily you'll recover. This book will show you how to keep bones, muscles and joints in top shape.

Did you ever consider how really tough it is to help yourself recover from a stroke, or from surgery, or from any illness when those muscles and bones and joints aren't working properly? Believe me, it's tough! This book is written to show you how to keep the moving parts of your body machinery well-oiled and functioning smoothly so that you'll feel better when you're well, and you'll be a mile ahead of the pack if something comes along to slow you down for a while. Why? Because you'll have every moving part in top running order right off the bat, and you won't have to spend weeks or months just getting yourself in form to recover—you'll be two-thirds of the way there already!

Ponder for a minute the several kinds of arthritis. This group of diseases afflicts millions every year—some lightly, some moderately, and some quite severely. Medical science has been struggling with this disease for hundreds of years and, frankly, we are no closer to really curing this enigmatic process than we were when it first appeared to plague mankind.

Does this mean we need to throw in the towel when it strikes? Give up in the face of what seems like overwhelming odds? Absolutely not! This book will explain how to cope with all the common types of arthritis—how to relieve pain, how to increase mobility and range of motion, how to prevent damage. Yes, and how to readjust your lives so that you can control this miserable pest rather than succumb and have it control you.

I don't suppose there is one of you who hasn't at one time or another had trouble in one or more muscles in your body. They can be bruised, pinched, pounded, overstretched, strained, and crushed, and they're affected when the nerves that make them work are on the blink.

This book will make you a better person if you will only follow its suggestions and learn from the experience of others with similar muscle problems. And it will add a bonus: It will show you how to prevent a lot of damage to your muscles from now on, even though you must put them through almost unbelievable activity and stress during the course of your daily work.

And what of aging joints? Or even those that aren't so aged? When they reach a state of rusty stiffness, is there hope? Of course there is! This book will show you how to lubricate that sticky machinery again and get those joints back to efficient function; how to get along quite well even though damage to one or more joints has already taken place; and what to do when you are in that dejected frame of mind and feel that you have to tell your friends you have one foot in the grave already. My friends, that is giving up, and if there's one thing this book will show you, it's that giving up the ghost with such problems is hardly even worth considering. You may think it's too late. It's *not* too late—read on and find out what you can do to live your life fully and actively again.

Finally, let me assure you that in three decades in medicine, I've seen people who have resigned themselves to their bed or chair and have decided that nothing could be done with their "worn out carcasses." You will meet some of these people in the book and you'll see exactly how their minds were changed and what they did to change them.

With a little help from this book, even if you're alone at home, you will hopefully be able to help yourselves to overcome the stagnation that often results from afflictions of joints, bones and muscles. That is what this book is all about. That's why you should read it.

And that is why, when you do read it, I think you'll soon feel a new zest for life that perhaps has been lost, and you'll not only be a better person for it, you'll influence others through your success to reach out for help themselves.

Good health!

J. Frank Hurdle, M.D.

Contents

What This Book Can Do for You 5

1. Why You Need a Home Care Guide for Arthritis, Bone and Muscle Ailments 13

    The Working of Your Organism—13
    The Key to Arthritis, Bone and Muscle Health—17
    Why Muscle Tone and Nutrition?—19
    Why Attitude and Common Sense?—20
    Mobility—22
    How Louise and Fred P. Overcame a Serious Problem—24
    Summary—27

2. How to Start Activity in Flagging Muscles and Joints Even at Rest 28

    Activity: The Key to Mobility—28
    The Put-off: What It Gets You—31
    Making the Most of Being in a Chair—37
    Things You Can Do in a Chair—38
    Your Goal of Impairment: Full Ambulation—46
    Summary—48

3. How You Can Regain Full, Efficient Muscle and Joint Mobility Fast 50

    The ABC's of Home Care Principles—50
    Losing Flab and Retaining Tone—58
    When Will Surgery Help?—61
    Less Formidable Surgery—63
    Sometimes Exercise Cures—65
    Summary—68

4. How You Can Adjust Bone and Muscle to Stress 70

Arthritis: Yes or No?—70
Role of Stress—72
Biofeedback Can Help You—81
Stress Breeds Frustration—82
Summary—84

5. How You Can Relieve Pain and Manage Painful Muscles and Joints 85

Strains, Sprains and Fractures—85
Osteoporosis—90
The Problem of the Phantom Limb—96
Causalgia Pain—99
Summary—102

6. How You Can Use Helping Devices for Ailing Joint and Muscle Problems 103

Using Splints to Advantage—103
More Immobilization Methods—110
When Limbs Are Paralyzed—113
How to Use Walking Devices—115
Household Aids and Hints—121
Summary—123

7. Keeping Your Mind As Flexible As Your Muscles and Joints 125

Activity at Rest—125
Biofeedback Again—129
Too Much Attention—133
Using What's Left—135
Summary—136

8. How to Reverse the Weak Stiff Limb Syndrome 138

Arthritis: The Stiffener—138
Stroke: The Stiffener—146
Double Trouble for Mel W.—154
Sand: Still Versatile—155
The Benefits of Water—157
Summary—158

Contents

9. Keeping the Rest of Your Body in Top Shape............160

    Your Digestive Tract: Its Care and Feeding—160
    The Urinary Tract—167
    Cardiopulmonary Tract—170
    Summary—176

10. The Care and Feeding of Your Bones and Muscles......177

    Tone That Bone—177
    Healthy Bones and Muscles—181
    Care of Your Upper Limbs—186
    Arm—188
    Elbow—189
    Wrist and Fingers—189
    Tammy D. Uses What She Has Left—189
    Lower Extremity—191
    Hip—191
    Knee—191
    Ankle—192
    Feet and Toes—192
    Vic McC. Goes the Route—192
    Summary—193

11. Coping with Problems of Nerve Damage to Muscles.....194

    Spinal Cord Injuries and Disease—194
    Limb Nerve Damage—198
    Toning Your Nervous System—206
    Summary—209

12. How to Manage a Problem Back......................210

    Your Back and Its Contents—210
    The Disc Syndrome—215
    The Whiplash—220
    Some Special Back Problems—223
    Summary—226

13. How You Can Get Back to Work **228**

    State Agencies—228
    National Agencies—233
    Work in Your Home—234
    Why Work?—235
    Summary—235

**14. Special Help with Special Bone,
Muscle and Joint Problems** **237**

    Special Exercises—237
    General Conditioning—247
    Special Skin Problems—252
    Bowel and Bladder—254
    Diet—258
    Biofeedback—264

Index **267**

A Medical Doctor's Home Guide for

ARTHRITIS, MUSCLE AND BONE AILMENTS

1

Why You Need a Home Care Guide for Arthritis, Bone and Muscle Ailments

Everyone at one time or another has some kind of trouble with the mechanical supports, levers and hinges of his or her body. With some people, this is because of the kind of work they do; with others, it's caused by injury or accident; and with still others, it's because disease or just plain wear and tear take their toll. We'll take a look at some of the causes and what's to be done about them in this first chapter.

There is no doubt in my mind that, in addition to the many and varied causes of joint, bone and muscle problems, your frame of mind has much to do with how you react to having something go wrong with, for example, a major joint; how you cope with it; and how, if you're not careful, this kind of infirmity can drag you to the depths of despair. I want to point out a few of these problems and discuss their control.

Finally, since your physical activity depends on the use of your limbs and joints and the muscles that move them, and since daily physical activity is the essence of good health and a keen mind (as those of you who have read my other books have come to see), I want you to discover why this is so and what you can do to vastly improve your mobility, as well as your total health and well-being.

THE WORKING OF YOUR ORGANISM

Your body is amazing. Its limbs are composed of muscle and tendon that are, under your brain's control, responsible for every move you make from threading a needle to swinging a sledge hammer. Tendons attach muscle to bone, bones are held in place by ligaments, and bones glide over each other on cushions of cartilage in joints. More important than this, however, is the fact that nothing can happen in bone, joint or muscle without blood to carry oxygen, nervous tissue to carry messages to and from your brain, and connective tissue—the basic cement of your body—to hold it all compactly together in compartments. Take away any one of these vital elements and none of the rest can function properly. Figure 1-1 shows how these elements all come together in a normal knuckle joint.

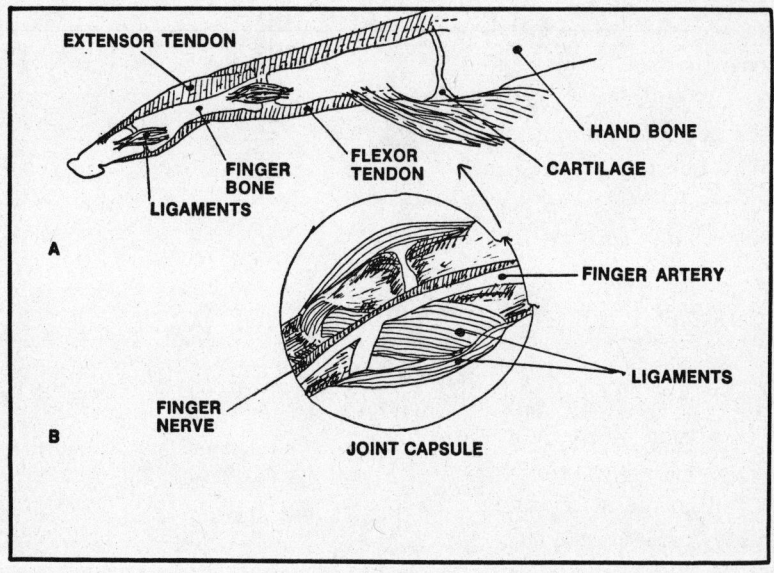

Figure 1-1

Muscles

Muscles are the work horses of your body. They move you from place to place and perform the work once you get there. They can be soft and flabby or firm and taut, depending on how you've taken care of them and what you put them through every day.

Your muscles are the "force" that moves the "levers" of your body—your bones. I'll be talking further about what muscles do and don't do under a variety of conditions and how they affect the other structures with which they work to keep you lively. Suffice it to say now that muscles must be kept toned if they are to do their job—if *you're* to do the jobs *you* want to do. Even in the face of joint ailments and bone disorders, muscles have to be toned correctly. If they are, you can overcome many troublesome problems that would otherwise be impossible to surmount—you can even learn to

Why You Need a Home Care Guide 15

"override" muscles that have been made useless by nerve damage and injuries in many cases.

Tendons

The tendons of your body are fixed ropes and pulleys—the guy wires that span the working gap between muscle and bone. They're hard, gristly, flexible cables that operate inside their own sheaths of automatically lubricated shells.

Tendons are not easily damaged or injured, but when they are, they can really raise Cain. We'll be looking at how to cope with damaged tendons later on, but look at them this way for the moment: Tendons gain strength and vigor from being used—they attach themselves to bone so that bones move when muscles contract. Moving bones at this attachment has many beneficial effects besides the motion produced. Use makes bones and tendons alike stronger and less vulnerable to disease and overstretching.

Ligaments

Ligaments are much like tendons, except that they take different shapes and perform a different function: They hold the ends of bones together and keep their alignment true. Both ends of a ligament are anchored in bone, unlike tendons which are anchored in bone at one end and in muscle at the other. Because joints are subject to much physical stress, ligaments are more susceptible to damage than tendons are.

A good way of looking at ligaments is to consider them as a joint's stabilizing and steadying guides, keeping in place the bony levers that help you move from place to place. Put one or more ligaments out of commission, and you have wobbly, floppy joints, as you'll see further along in this book.

Cartilage

Cartilage looks as if it consists of the same substance ligaments and tendons are made of, but here the similarity ends. Cartilage forms the cushions in every joint of your body—firm, flexible, tough layers on the ends of bones—that take the brunt of every movement, every weight-bearing force exerted on bones.

And like tendons, cartilage has a layer of lubricating sheathing over its surface to further protect it from the pounding it takes. In fact, this lubricating sheath covers not only the cartilage in joints, but usually surrounds the entire space of a joint so that if you could strip away the tissues and look at any joint, it would appear somewhat like a peanut shell—a thin layer of tissue enclosing the joint space and lubricating it constantly with joint fluid. Figure 1-2 shows the cartilage of a knee joint. I'll have many occasions to speak further about this joint membrane and the cartilage it contains as we go along.

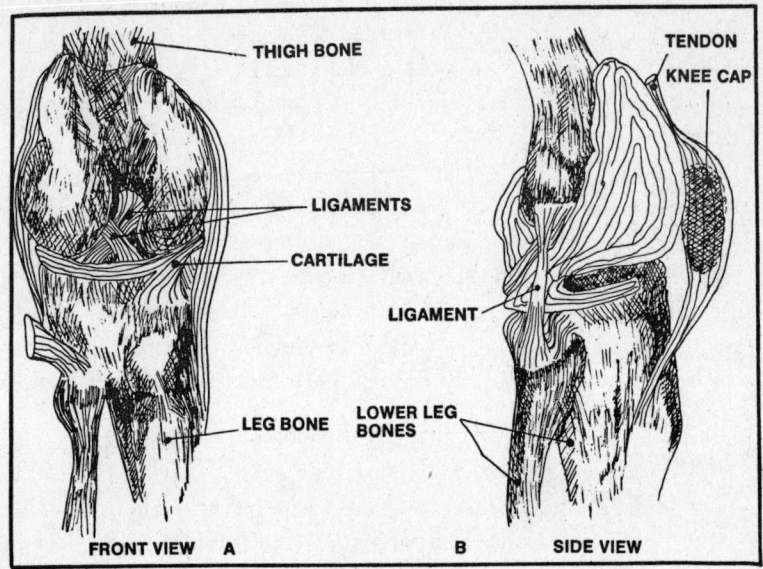

Figure 1-2

The power and fuel

So there you have it: the elements of your locomotion system—the prime movers in your day to day activities—the body's "anti-gravity" mechanism, for these structures do indeed constantly work against gravity to keep you upright. But we have two other ingredients to consider. First the power, the battery or dynamo or generator—whatever you may call it—that runs your locomotion system. This is your body's ignition: the nervous system. Every muscle in your body has one or more major nerves running to it that come directly from your brain—the part of this remarkable organ that has to do with willful motion. Without nerves of this kind muscles can't work.

It is well and good to speak of muscle, bone and joint disorders, but without nerves going to muscles, there isn't any movement. I'll talk further along, as I show you a variety of things that happen to slow you down, about nerves and how, in instances of nerve damage, you can still overcome much difficulty.

The fuel for the locomotion system is its blood supply, the vital tissue (and it *is* a tissue rather than just another liquid) that flows along in miles

Why You Need a Home Care Guide 17

and miles of tiny blood vessels in muscles, tendons, ligaments, and joints, bringing not only nutrition but also vital oxygen to burn the nutrients and convert them to energy.

This fuel source, like the ignition system, is essential to the smooth-working locomotion of your body. I'll be talking later about how problems with this fuel system can be solved when they arise.

THE KEY TO ARTHRITIS, BONE AND MUSCLE HEALTH

1. Muscle Tone	P
2. Nutrition	R
3. Attitude	E
4. Common Sense	V
5. Recuperation from Injury	E
6. Mobility	N
	TREATMENT
	I
	O
	N

Betty M. fails to heed key

Betty M., a patient who represents dozens of similar incidents in which prevention of trouble would have saved untold grief, was at a dead stop in her car at a traffic signal when she was struck from behind by another driver who was careless—he wasn't watching traffic patterns and his mind was miles away. Betty got her neck snapped back sharply and thereby sustained a "whiplash" injury. Betty went to her doctor and he prescribed three drugs designed to relieve pain, relax the muscles, and "calm her down." He also put her into a cervical collar, which is a simple device used to keep the neck from flexing and extending and limit its turning from side to side.

The only trouble was that four weeks later Betty felt more miserable than she had to begin with. When I saw her, there were several things wrong.

In the first place, this kind of injury does require that the neck be put at rest—for a time. A week or ten days is quite enough; then the cervical collar should be discarded, unless you are trying to impress someone, as Betty was. The insurance settlement wasn't as much as Betty thought it should be, so she was demonstrating to all who would look that she was still "hurting" from the injury. I told her when I first became involved with her case that unless any thought of further lawsuits was immediately put to the side, I could not help her, nor could anyone. She hesitated for a few days and then agreed. You can't possibly help yourself from the effects of this or any other injury if number 3 in the key, "Attitude," is neglected.

In the second place, Betty was about 30 pounds overweight and was flabby. I put her on a diet and got her to start a twice daily exercise routine. None of the exercises in any way placed undue strain on her neck muscles. Betty thus got control, in about six months, of key elements 1 and 2: "Muscle Tone" and "Nutrition."

Her doctor had prescribed daily go-arounds with traction about a week after her accident. Traction was administered by having Betty sit in a chair and applying a head halter with a rope, attached to overhead pulleys, which had a 10-pound weight on the end of it. The third thing I did was to stop the traction treatments. This got us to key number 4: "Common Sense." If muscles are overstretched and their attachments to bone (tendons) are irritated, how could one expect anything but more problems by further stretching the muscles involved? Traction in this situation was actually making Betty feel worse rather than better!

The next step was to stop Betty's drugs—that's right, all of them. In the first place, both the muscle relaxant drug and the sedative were causing Betty to become slothful. She couldn't even do her routine household chores without getting tired! The pain killer was too strong—all she needed was aspirin taken in doses of two tablets three or four times a day. And that's all she got.

Within three weeks, 80 percent of Betty's discomfort and distress was gone, and within another ten days she felt perfectly well.

Your job at this point

Taking a clue from Betty's case, if you have neglected any part of the key—no matter what your particular problem may be with arthritis, bone or muscle ailments—make a decision now! Make a decision that you'll take each one in turn and start on its correction today. Stop feeling like the woman in Figure 1-3!

If you're overweight (a very common problem in people with arthritis, but not necessarily a condition for having it) make a vow to yourself that you'll get that weight down to within normal range. If your muscles are weak and flabby, make another vow at this moment that you'll take time each day to tone them up. If you have a poor attitude toward your problem—whether you are blue and sad that you have to suffer through what you have, or whether you're angry at everybody because of your plight—resolve now to

Why You Need a Home Care Guide

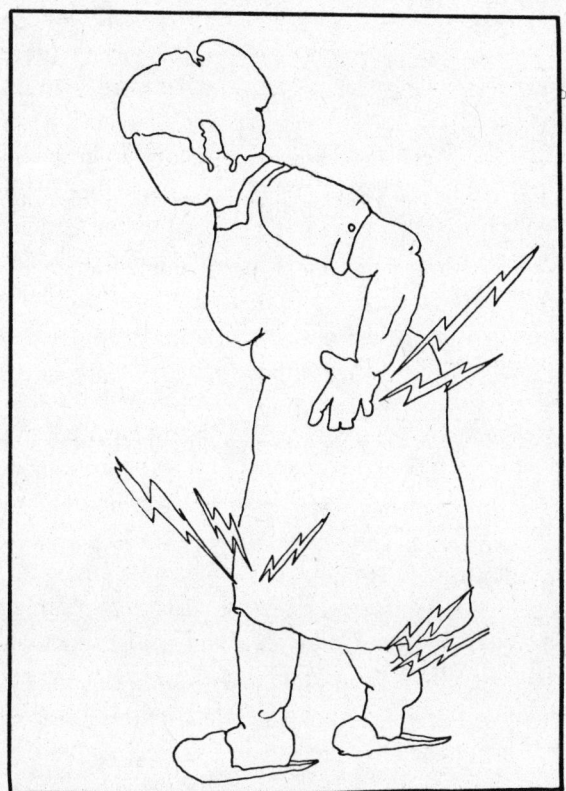

Figure 1-3

change your attitude. And if you have recently been injured or hurt for any reason, just calm down and remember that you have to give your body a reasonable chance to heal the damage before you can get started on helping yourself.

For help with diet, muscle toning, and attitude, I suggest you read either *The Biofeedback Diet: A Doctor's Revolutionary Approach*, or *A Country Doctor's Common Sense Health Manual*, two of my previous books.

WHY MUSCLE TONE AND NUTRITION?

Let's say you're 30 pounds overweight. Consider for a minute what you're asking your levers and joints to do: You're compelling your locomotion system to exert about 79,200 extra foot-pounds of work a day for every half mile you walk! (There are 2640 feet in a half mile, and you must move 30 extra pounds over this distance.) Secondly, when you shift about 30 extra pounds to, say, your right knee joint, you actually increase the forces exerted on that relatively small area of your knee joint by over tenfold! Is it any wonder you feel like just lazing around when you're overweight?

Bob D. discovers a key

Bob D., a young man I know, was born with a defect in his lower spine called spina bifida. It allowed certain parts of his lower spinal cord to protrude from inside the spinal canal and become subject to injury. His case required the attention of specialists and eventually his condition stabilized, but not before it had destroyed parts of the nerve supply to his legs. He found himself in a wheel chair by the time he was in his teens, even though he could walk with help as a child.

When I saw Bob, he was about 55 pounds overweight and was getting into a terrible state of mind because of his inability to get around like other people. The fact was, Bob hadn't studied the key. He had neglected his nutrition and he was well started on the path toward a permanent lousy attitude toward others, toward himself, and toward life in general.

When Bob first began to lose weight, he immediately felt so much better that he heeded the advice of his specialist and had leg braces fitted on both legs. This enabled him to stand with crutches and at least get out of his wheel chair once in a while. As his weight continued to go down, he was able to make his diminished muscle capacity in his legs move him forward a little bit.

Finally, at the end of a year, Bob's weight was within normal range for his height and bone structure, and he found that he could walk with the best of them with crutches any time he wanted. His wheel chair became rusty with disuse. When I next saw Bob two years later, he'd managed to restore enough tone to what remained of his diminished leg muscles that he was able to store his crutches in the closet. Today, Bob walks without aids, except of course the braces, and uses a cane only when he is extremely tired. If he hadn't decided to change his attitude and nutrition and had allowed what muscle power he had left to deteriorate completely, he'd still be in a wheel chair today. So you see, you can both prevent and deal with trouble if you only recognize the key elements and are willing to do something about them, now as well as after the trouble starts.

WHY ATTITUDE AND COMMON SENSE?

Dirk T., a brash young man who thought he could hasten Nature's process, fell during a skiing accident and sustained a rather serious fracture of his right main lower leg bone. His doctor was able to reduce it without

Why You Need a Home Care Guide

surgery and placed the leg in a cast and Dirk on crutches, stating that he definitely didn't want Dirk to put any weight whatsoever on his injured right leg until the bones had knit together. Dirk thought he knew better, and became quite bored and disgusted at having to walk around on crutches. Finally, he lost control, removed the cast himself, and began to walk on the recovering, but not completely healed right leg. He threw down his crutches and, since he didn't feel any pain, he felt he would be as good as new.

Unfortunately for Dirk, the soft callus of bone that had surrounded his fractured right lower leg bones, but had not yet had time to solidify, bent with his weight bearing and finally parted completely, refracturing the leg and causing Dirk no end of pain and discomfort.

Dirk's doctor was not pleased. He had to operate on the leg and plate the two fractured ends of bone together with metal and screws in order to insure its healing.

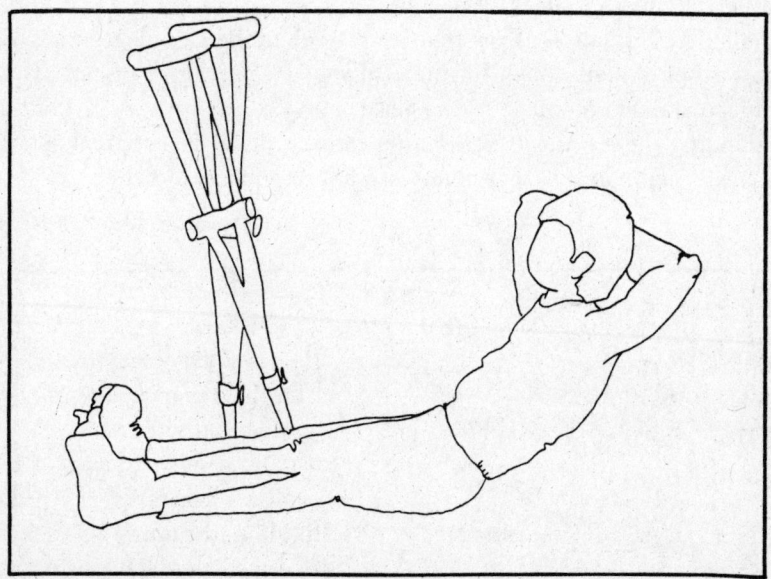

Figure 1-4

But once again, Dirk thought he knew more than his doctor did. He removed the cast long before it was ready and again started walking on his bettered leg. This time he wasn't so lucky. The bone became infected from the irritation of the bent metal plate and unhealed fracture site and his doctor in desperation re-operated on the leg and had to transplant a bone graft to the fractured site from Dirk's hip.

Finally, after 12 months, Dirk's fractured leg healed. He wasn't able to return to his job as a telephone lineman for another six months and took the heavy risk of being without a functional right leg for life.

The lesson from Dirk's case (see Figure 1-4) is that, first and foremost, you must take the advice of your medical counselor and allow the process, whatever it may be, time to rest when rest is indicated, and then get to work on restoration when that time comes along. In the meantime, you can put your spare time to good use by getting your nutrition, your weight, and the tone of all the rest of those muscles you've been letting get flabby, back into shape *even though you have to avoid using one limb or another part of your anatomy* while the injured or diseased part heals.

MOBILITY

The goal in any plan of home and self care is to become as mobile as possible, and if you can say now that you're mobile, then your goal should be to become more efficiently mobile.

Mobility is relative. If you're in a wheel chair, being able to stand with support is better than just sitting there. If you can stand with support, being able to move from one place to another a short distance away is better than just standing there. And if you master moving about in confined spaces, then mastering mobility anywhere you want to go is even better.

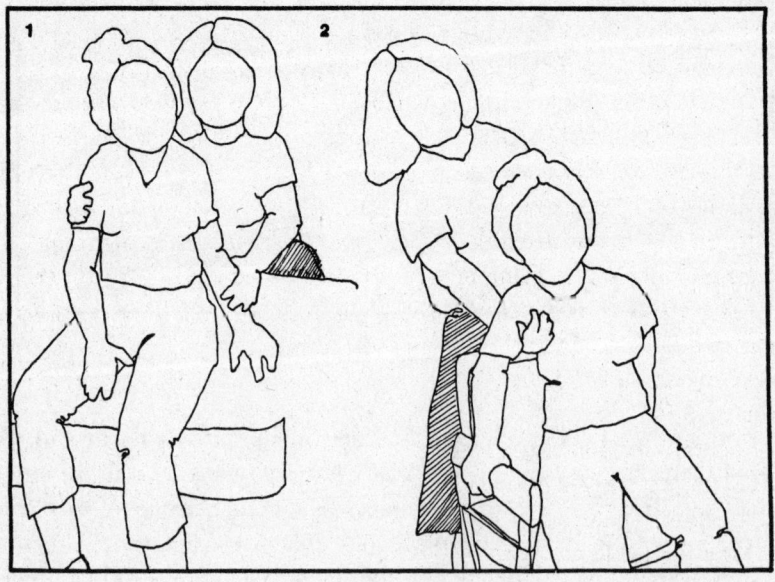

Figure 1-5

Why You Need a Home Care Guide

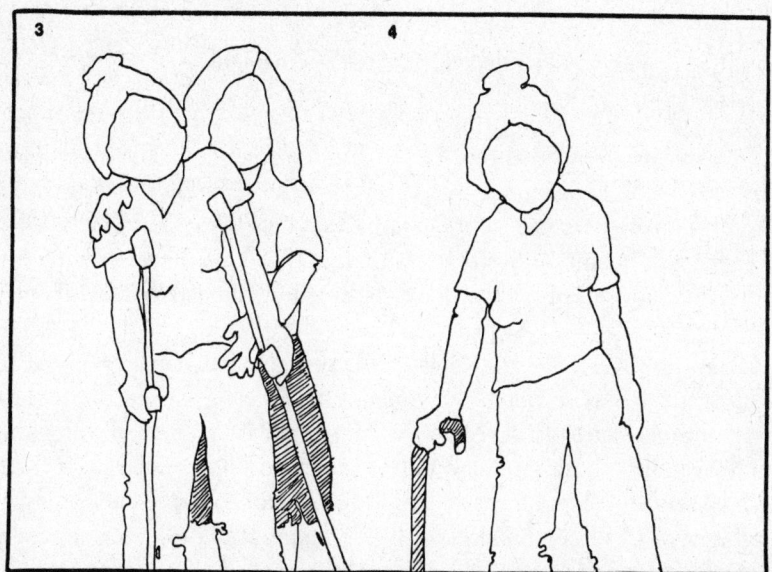

Figure 1-5 (continued)

If you have arthritis in, for example, your hands and fingers, being able to flex (bend) your fingers is better than not using them for anything. Once you are able to bend them, then being able to use them to grasp and hold onto objects is better than just bending them. Mastering the techniques of letting go of objects and picking up others is even better.

The point is that you should proceed with one step at a time, and that's what this book is all about—to show you the steps, and to point out that the fact that you reach one goal doesn't mean you should sit around and daydream about the price you had to pay for advancing. You should be thinking of how you're going to accomplish the *next* step, and start doing it!

There will be some of you who must do this by and large on your own because there's no one else around most of the time to help. Much can be done by yourself at home. You need guidance for this. That's why this book is for you.

There are other times when you need help from anybody who can be around for just a short period of time. There is usually help to be had in this regard. (See Figure 1-5.)

The following are possible sources:

1. Husband or wife
2. Friend or neighbor

3. City or county Visiting Nurse Service
4. Local hospital Physical Medicine Department
5. Local Social Services Department

The city or county Visiting Nurse Service where you live is probably run by the local department of Public Health. Even if you live in the country, this agency has an office nearby that can help you if you need it.

Your local hospital Physical Medicine Department can be counted on for help. You can call directly or have your medical advisor contact them for you.

It pays to investigate the social services agencies. Sometimes the red tape involved seems a bit much, but eventually you can get help either directly through one of several divisions in the agency or through a community group directly concerned with your particular problem (e.g., the National Arthritis Foundation, the Multiple Sclerosis Society, or the Department of Developmental Disabilities, generally a part of one of your state government departments).

If you believe that you're still capable of productive work in spite of what may be looked upon by most as a handicap, contact your State Department of Vocational Rehabilitation—the agency in your state government that helps disabled people get back to work. There are offices throughout your state, and you can get in touch with the one closest to your home.

HOW LOUISE AND FRED P. OVERCAME A SERIOUS PROBLEM

One of the best examples I recall of people who have helped themselves was a married couple who lived on a small farm not far from the town where I practiced. They were in their mid 50's, hard-working, self-reliant, and had a good deal of common sense. I was summoned to their house one morning by Louise, who told me that her husband was unable to move from his bed. She explained that her regular doctor wasn't available at the time and she was worried.

When I arrived at their place, I found Fred in his bed, unable to talk, and unable to move his right arm or leg, though he was conscious of what was going on around him. He was quite agitated and restless and kept pointing to his lower abdomen with his left hand. It was apparent from my examination that he'd had a stroke involving the left side of his brain. This was why Fred couldn't move his right arm or leg—the nerve fibers that control your right arm and leg originate in the left side of your brain; the

Why You Need a Home Care Guide

nerves that control your left arm and leg originate in the right side of your brain.

It also happens that in people who are right-handed, the speech control center is located in the left side of the brain—the so-called dominant side. That's why Fred was also having trouble with his speech.

In talking over the problem with Fred and Louise, I advised them that the best thing for Fred was to be taken to the hospital. But Louise disagreed and Fred shook his head. They wanted no part of going to the hospital.

I explained that it would be tough, but not impossible, to take care of Fred at home because of the physical therapy he'd need. This would accomplish two things. It would keep his paralyzed muscles in tone so that if and when some of them came back again, they would be strong enough to function; and it would ensure that Fred's left side didn't grow weak from disuse, even though it wasn't paralyzed. I explained further that there would be feeding problems, toilet problems, and the like, but Louise and Fred remained undaunted.

"I can take care of him myself," Louise said, "better than someone who doesn't know him." And she was probably right, but I was still skeptical.

"How are you going to take care of him," I asked, "if you also have chores and other things around the farm and the house to do?"

"We'll get our friends and our neighbors and our kids to help us," she replied without hesitation. "And, of course, you'll be around to supervise, won't you, Doctor?"

How could I answer anything but yes? I couldn't help but admire the will of these two and their determination to "take care of their own" even though there was perfectly adequate hospitalization available in town.

The first thing I did was to catheterize Fred—his full bladder was the thing that made him restless and agitated. As soon as his bladder was empty, he calmed down and smiled from one side of his mouth (the other was paralyzed). The next thing I did was to build up the head of Fred's mattress, with the aid of Louise, using some old bed clothing she had found. This had the same effect as cranking up a hospital bed: It raised Fred's entire torso upward from the level without having to pile a lot of pillows under his head, which serves only to crick the patient's neck and cause it to get sore and stiff, not helping breathing or comfort a bit.

The feeding problem had to be dealt with next. Fred couldn't swallow very well, and until he regained this facility, if he was going to regain it, he would need help. I brought an intravenous feeding stand to the house with a supply of fluids and taught Louise some nursing: how to hook up the tubes to the bottle, how to invert it on the hook of the stand, and how to put a needle into Fred's arm and connect the tubing to it. She caught on amazingly fast, and after two attempts could do it as expertly as anyone.

Then came the tough part, teaching Louise how to become a physical therapist of sorts. I showed her how to start with the paralyzed side and put each of Fred's joints through its full range of motion; how to do it sometimes with spasm in the muscles so that moving the joints was quite difficult; how to keep Fred's paralyzed right leg slightly pulled out at the thigh and bent at the knee; and how to keep his right foot properly propped up near the foot of the bed so he wouldn't develop a "foot-drop," a condition common to paralyzed legs even when power returns. It causes the foot to drag when the patient tries to develop mobility later on.

Then there was skin care, and bathing in bed, and caring for the bowel and bladder functions. Fortunately, Fred had retained control of his bladder and rectum so that repeated catheterization wasn't necessary, but Louise did have to learn digital rectal emptying because constipation is usually a problem even when rectal control remains.

Louise took to it all as though she'd worked in a hospital all her life! And I always knew what I'd find when I went to their home two or three times a week: a stroke patient in as good a shape as he would be if he were in a hospital. Perhaps even better.

Fortunately, Fred regained enough swallow reflex so that he could tolerate taking liquids and soft foods by the end of three days, and intravenous feedings didn't have to continue beyond this critical third day.

Their friends and youngsters helped Fred get to the bathroom and get out of bed into a chair, and they even helped Louise in giving him his three times daily physical exercises.

The net result was that Fred was up and walking with crutches within three weeks, with braces within six weeks, and with a cane as his only support within three months.

Amazing? Yes, it was, and more so when you stop to consider all that had to be learned by Louise and her friends and all that had to be done by Fred himself. In this book, I'll be getting into detail about the techniques of helping a person like Fred in the home, as well as hundreds of other useful things to do at home to help with dozens of other arthritis, muscle and bone disorders. You'll learn to be your own best therapist, your own best tutor, and your own best innovator for better ways of doing things.

I realize that you don't have to be laid up quite as drastically as Fred, but even if you're not, you'll come out ahead by learning what you can do in a variety of situations and disorders. If you're mobile, you'll be more mobile. If you're bed-fast, you'll learn how to leave that bed, at least for periods consistent with your general health. And if you're confined to one,

Why You Need a Home Care Guide

you'll learn how to make a wheel chair work for you rather than against everything you want to do.

Will I tell you to disregard everything you may already have done to help, ignore the advice of your medical counsel and forget all he's told you? Absolutely not! I'll just advise you to add this help to that already at hand. And be better off for it!

SUMMARY

1. Disorders of joints, bones and muscles also involve the care and feeding of nerve and blood supplies to the areas involved. If you properly care for all of the various parts that make up your mobility units, you'll be far ahead of the game, both in preventing trouble and dealing with it when it arises.

2. The key, both in prevention and treatment of arthritis, bone and muscle disorders involves attention to: *Muscle Tone, Nutrition, Attitude, Common Sense, Proper Recuperation from Injury, and the Goal of Most Efficient Mobility.*

3. There are times in everybody's life when certain activities require temporary help and assistance from others. There are a host of others to help. These include: your spouse, your youngsters, the city/county Visiting Nurse Service, your local hospital's Department of Physical Medicine, and your local Social Service Agency and its many departments. Most often, if an agency can't offer direct help, they can put you in touch with someone who can. Ask for names and numbers.

4. By reading this book, you will be able to do many things that perhaps you hadn't thought of before that will help you help yourself to better mobility and a better outlook on life in general, and may even help you to help others with similar problems!

2

How to Start Activity in Flagging Muscles and Joints Even at Rest

In this chapter I'm going to start to show you how and when to start getting yourself and your joints and muscles back in shape following a variety of afflictions. I will assume that you're back home now, either from a stint in the hospital or perhaps just over an acute bout with one of many disabilities that plague bones, joints and muscles. And I will assume that you have recently had medical supervision of some kind, you've checked with your advisor to make certain he agrees that you may start getting back to the land of the well and able again.

Next, I'm going to talk about how you can begin to make life a little easier even if you're confined to a chair. You're going to balk a little at first, but I want you to vow that you'll make a commitment to hang in there with me at least until you've given it a whirl.

Finally, I'm going to show you a little trick I introduced in my previous book on low blood sugar and enlarged upon in my most recent book on biofeedback diet: some ways to use your mind to help you help yourself out of bed and chair and back to useful life again.

ACTIVITY: THE KEY TO MOBILITY

I want you to pause a bit and think. Think about the illustrations in the first chapter showing a typical joint and its components. Recall that a joint consists of a junction of two or more bones with cartilage cushioning them, ligaments stabilizing this junction, and tendons spanning over, behind, and at the sides of the joint, smoothly gliding over bony surfaces because they have their own lubrication mechanisms.

How to Start Activity in Flagging Muscles and Joints 29

Now I want you to consider a general property of muscles: If they're not used, for whatever reason, they get weak and flabby. You've had this experience before many times, I'm sure. You went to the hospital and had to stay in bed for a few days. Or you got the flu and had to be inactive even if only for a day or two. Remember what happened when you first got out of bed in the hospital, or started to feel better from the flu and got up and around again? You looked, felt, and were indeed weak! Why? Because your muscles, those machines that move your levers of locomotion, were given just a short time off ... and they got weak.

This is a property of any muscle in your body: If they're not used, even for a day or two, they begin to lose their power to contract vigorously and efficiently. Some muscles show this "fatigue factor" much sooner than others, as we shall see, and in general the larger the muscle that's not being used, the sooner it begins to weaken. Figure 2-1 shows this effect a bit more graphically in a perfectly normal leg.

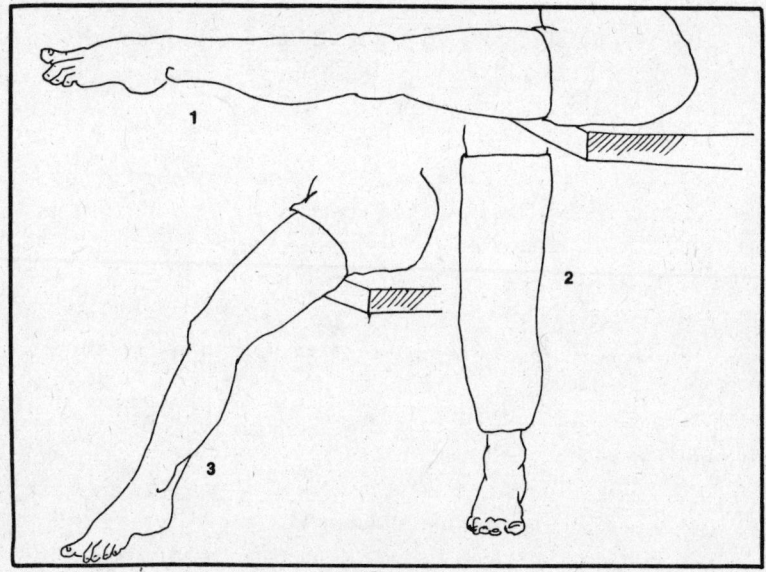

Figure 2-1

"But what can I do?" you ask, recalling how you felt when you were last bedfast or ill for any reason. What can anyone do if they're too sick or infirm in bed or in a chair to stop this from happening? Well, there are several things you can do, things you *must* do if you're going to keep those muscles from weakening.

Ray S. becomes a believer

Let me show you, through a case I once cared for, the extent to which what I've just been talking about actually occurs.

Ray S. was a young man in his 30's who injured his left knee in a machine shop where he worked as a lathe operator. He was bent over one day, lifting a moderately heavy metal blank up to his lathe, when he turned his foot and knee on a piece of scrap on the floor and threw all his weight (including the chunk of metal) on his left leg while at the same time twisting his left knee to the right. The result was that he tore his left knee cartilage, causing him much pain and disability.

He was taken to the hospital, following his doctor's examination, where his torn cartilage was removed surgically by an orthopedic surgeon. I happen to know this surgeon very well. I know he's a stickler for physical conditioning just as soon as it's practical following surgery. I know he instructed Ray to start exercises at home like those the hospital Physical Medicine Department started before he went home, only more vigorously than even the physical therapists did it in the hospital. But Ray wasn't listening or paid no attention. He didn't do as his surgeon advised but, instead, lollygagged around when he got home just doing what he wanted and enjoying all the attention from his wife and youngsters while he "recovered" from his surgery.

I was called to Ray's home because of illness among the youngsters about three weeks following Ray's surgery. His cast was off and I knew, of course, what had happened and was surprised to find Ray still hobbling around the house on crutches when I got there. I asked Ray how the recovery was coming along. He replied, "Well, it's slow, Doc. Can't seem to get the bum leg to work very good." I examined the kids, who had minor problems, and then asked Ray to sit down in a chair and take off his pants. What I saw amazed me and, I think, amazed Ray and his wife as well. His left thigh muscle, usually a muscle that's tight and bulges to the sides and front quite prominently, was really a sad sight. It was wasted, limp, and flabbily hanging off its thigh bone attachment.

I measured the muscle with a tape measure, and it was a full two inches smaller than the right thigh muscle! Think of it: After only three weeks of inactivity, this essential muscle for walking (it moves the lower leg up and down, and stabilizes the knee joint when the lower leg is thrust upward—straightened when walking) had lost that much of its vital mass in just three weeks! No wonder Ray was complaining. No wonder I really landed on Ray's back for slighting his toning exercises!

By the time I was through chewing Ray out for his neglect, I think he got the point: *You've got to keep those big muscles in action if you expect to*

How to Start Activity in Flagging Muscles and Joints

recover from the effects of injury and surgery. He started in on the relatively simple routine for restoring tone to the thigh muscle after it has been inactive: fixing a light weight (an ordinary electric iron) to his left foot, sitting on a high stool or counter, and making his thigh muscle pull his lower leg up even with the chair or counter top as illustrated in Figure 2-2.

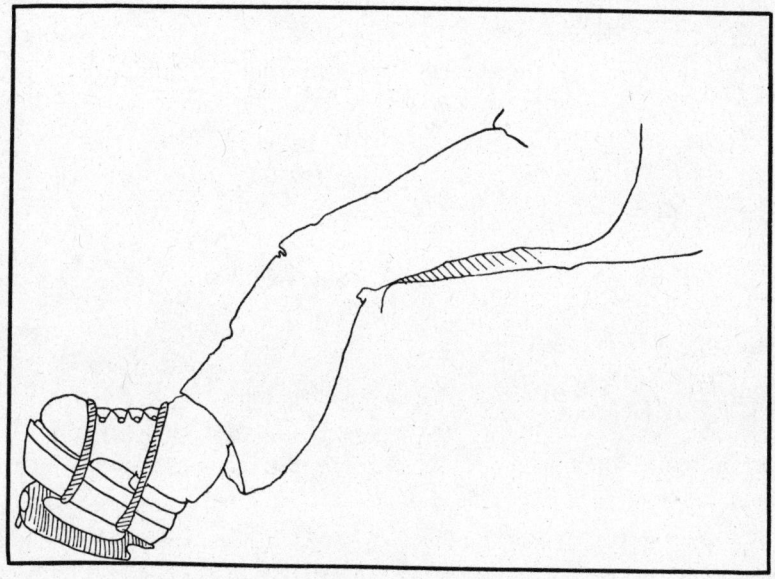

Figure 2-2

Ray also learned another important point: If you let your toning exercises go for too long, it takes *three times as long* to restore power to the muscles!

Ray did recover his thigh muscle power, but it took him eight weeks to do it. And he kept it up only because I rode him continuously about doing the exercises. He didn't like it because it was boring to him. But boring or not, he kept it up until the measurement around the middle of his left thigh was equal to that around the middle of his good right thigh.

THE PUT-OFF: WHAT IT GETS YOU

Most people don't realize it, but if today you were to put either of your perfectly strong legs into a plaster cast or brace, and leave it on just for 10 to 14 days, when the cast or brace came off, the thigh muscle on your leg would have shrunken from one to two inches! Remember, there isn't anything whatsoever wrong with this leg that we're putting into cast or brace—we're just doing it to prove a point. The thigh muscle really gets weak quickly when put out of commission for any reason at all.

And this thigh muscle, so vital to walking and climbing stairs and the like, isn't the only one that behaves in this apparently perverse way.

I can recall literally dozens of cases of shoulder disorders, for example, in a variety of people of all ages and sizes, disorders where the shoulder had to be kept at rest for a few days to a few weeks. What happened? Incredibly, the shoulder joint stiffened so much in some of the cases that it literally took months to restore their former usual motion again. And in a few of them, the motion at this vital joint never did return!

We see again an example of what happens to muscle and ligament when inactivity supervenes: *The stiffening that takes place by reason of not paying attention to the principles of mobility and toning at the proper time may be disastrous.*

Finger joints are another example, as are neck joints and elbow joints.

Arlene A. overcomes arthritis

Arlene was 51 years old when I first met her. She had noticed that slowly over the past three or four years, her "joints were wearing out," as she put it to me when we met in the office. Actually, the joints she referred to were her low back, her left shoulder and her right ankle. She would notice after a particularly active day that sometimes her ankle would swell and be painful, and that her back would hurt and her shoulder would limit the motion of her left arm because it was stiff and painful at times.

Further questioning revealed that these stiff and painful episodes didn't occur especially on any time sequence—it might happen after any day of heavy housework, or after a long walk. The most significant thing about Arlene's joint problem was that it was always "worse in the morning when I first wake up," and that "it seems to get better as the day wears on, if I don't overstrain."

What Arlene was describing was rather typical behavior of osteoarthritis, a form of joint disorder mostly caused by the gradual wearing down of those cartilage cushions we had a look at in Chapter 1, rather than the rheumatoid type we'll have a closer look at later on.

The trouble was that Arlene took too literally the well-intended advice to put her involved extremities at rest when they were bothering her. When her ankle bothered her, she put the entire right leg to rest; when her shoulder bothered her, she put her entire left arm at rest; and when her back hurt, she tended to put her whole body at rest on the couch or bed.

The net result of all this rest was that Arlene's joint problem was getting steadily worse instead of better. She had allowed the muscles,

How to Start Activity in Flagging Muscles and Joints 33

tendons, ligaments, and bones that weren't involved with the arthritis to get flabby and out of tone, and this triggered off all sorts of problems. Let's look at them in a little more detail and see what happened when she corrected them.

1. *Weight gain*
   Arlene had put on about 35 pounds of excess weight with all of her "rest." Her appetite was excellent, but she wasn't burning off those extra calories.

2. *Poor tone*
   Arlene had forgotten that in getting so much rest, the muscles and joints in the rest of her body got soft and lax. Soon Arlene was having pain and stiffness in other joints simply because their supports and levers lay fallow.

3. *Disuse effect*
   Arlene didn't take the cue that was clearly in front of her each morning: Although she normally felt stiff and aching when she first got out of bed in the mornings, most of it melted away as the day progressed, including her shoulder, ankle and back. The more rest she got, the sorer and stiffer her joints and muscles became.

4. *Mental blues*
   A vicious circle now developed: The more rest she got, the stiffer and sorer she felt; the more pain and distress she had, the more depressed she became, until she began to snap at her husband and children and grandchildren and was a regular bear to get along with. Any chance she had to utilize techniques like biofeedback to help her feel better soon disappeared.

Breaking the cycle of indolence

I asked Arlene when I first saw her and examined her joints if she truly wanted to feel better. She looked rather funny, paused a bit, then finally answered, "Of course I want to feel better! I want you to give me one of those new drugs that are supposed to cure arthritis!"

Arlene hit the ceiling when I replied that not only was I *not* going to give her any new drugs, but I was going to stop her from taking three others, including a popular tranquilizer prescribed for her "nervousness and being upset" all the time.

Arlene finally came down to earth when I explained the possible trouble she would soon have from taking one of the new drugs—what she had in mind was one of several cortisone derivatives. Here is a list of exercises Arlene started:

How to Start Activity in Flagging Muscles and Joints

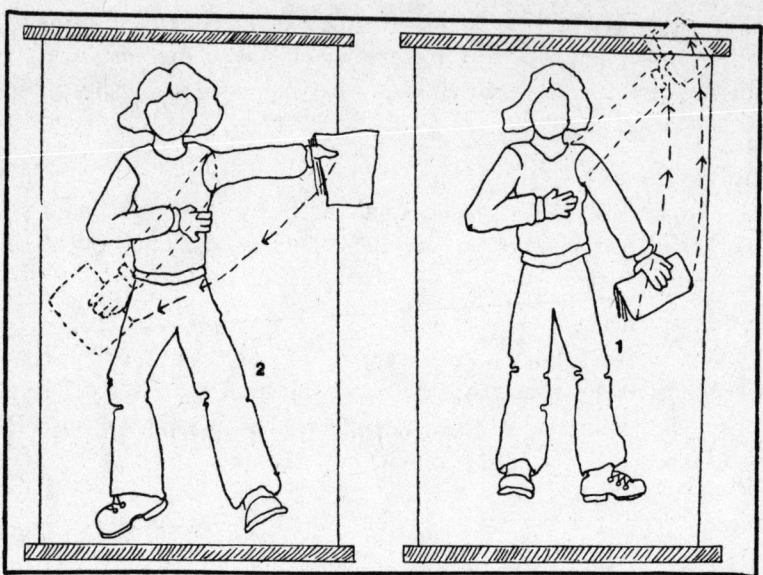

Figure 2-3

1. Although Arlene's left shoulder was often stiff in the morning, she learned how to exercise it while in bed or on the floor—*both of which positions relieved the added drag of gravity*! Figure 2-3 shows Arlene exercising her shoulder, holding on to an ordinary book.

2. Figure 2-4 shows Arlene exercising her ankle—*again in bed to relieve the effect of weight bearing which would make it the more difficult were she exercising this joint standing up.*

3. There was nothing wrong with Arlene's abdominal muscles! So she started on sit-ups and scissor-kicks, slowly at first because she was out of shape, and *gradually* increasing the number by two or three every two weeks or so until she could do 20 of each. The sit-ups carry an extra bonus for people like Arlene who have pain and stiffness in their backs: On the return swing back to the floor, *it's your back muscles that splint and are contracted, thereby exercising your back as well.* Figure 2-5 shows how Arlene helped her abdomen and back at the same time.

In short, Arlene went from being a slothful person to being an active person. Besides her exercise routines, which she did twice a day (if she was too uncomfortable first thing in the morning, she waited until mid-morning to start), I had her do much more walking—walking just for the fun of it, walking to the store, or walking to a neighborhood school to pick up her

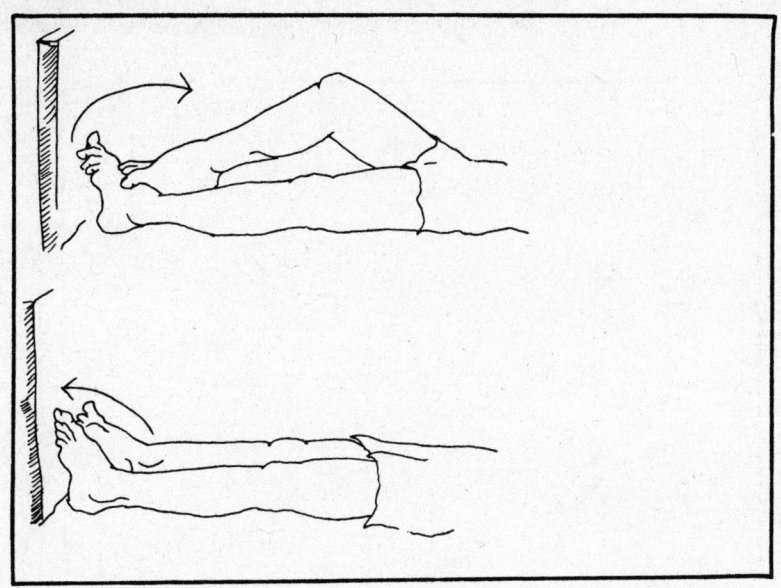

Figure 2-4

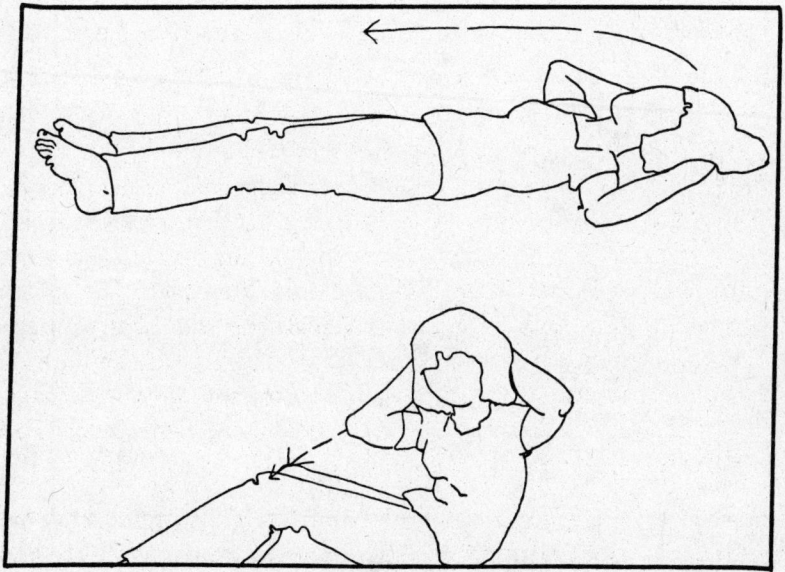

Figure 2-5

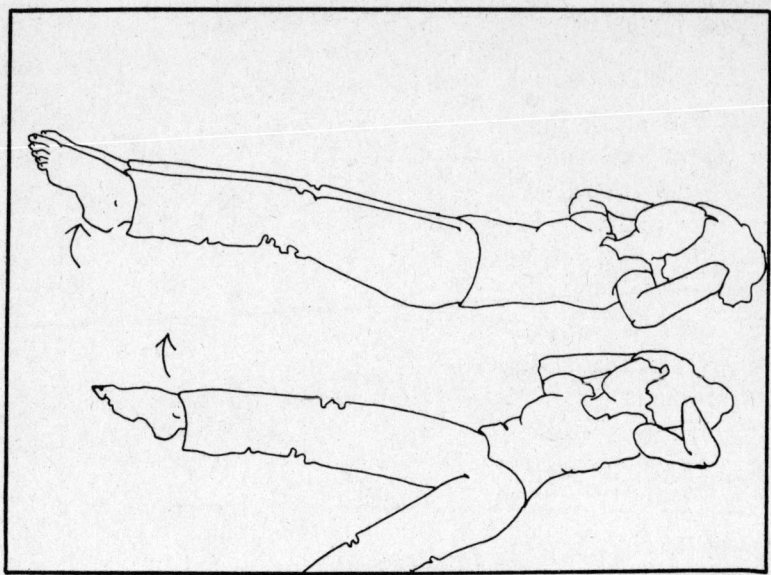

Figure 2-5 (continued)

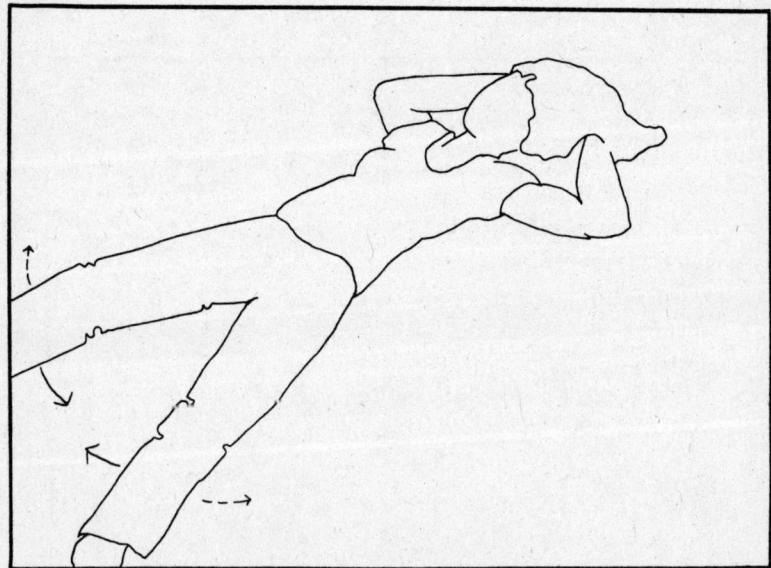

Figure 2-5 (continued)

small grandson. At least one good walk a day; two if possible when weather permitted. At first Arlene found that two blocks was about her limit, but

How to Start Activity in Flagging Muscles and Joints

after only three months of a systematic exercise program with weight loss, she got up to a mile and a half a day! She has since taken up bicycle riding during good weather.

Arlene's diet was a fairly easy 1200 calorie balanced diet. In Chapter 14, I've constructed some easy tables to help you follow a diet tailored to your individual needs. The diets are all specially formulated so that you will get maximum nutrition while losing weight.

With her toning and weight reduction and the vast improvement in her ability to use her afflicted joints again, coupled with withdrawal from the drugs she was taking, Arlene's blue, grouchy, bearish mood gradually melted away and she became the most enthusiastic member of her family, especially when it came time for outings and going places.

MAKING THE MOST OF BEING IN A CHAIR

There are times when it is necessary to limit your activity because injury or disease temporarily or permanently places one or both legs out of commission. As I have said before, being confined in a chair should be regarded as another phase in reaching total mobility, if it is humanly possible.

Fred P., whose case we looked at in Chapter 1, was confined for a time in bed, then to a chair, then to using walking assists, and finally to walking by himself. Not everyone is as fortunate as Fred but certainly there is always hope and good reason for expecting improvement over "just being stuck in a chair."

The reasons for moving to a chair from a bed are that you immediately increase your own mobility range of movement dozens of times over. Secondly, there are many things you can do sitting in a chair that you can't do lying down or sitting in bed. Finally, it is even possible to learn to drive a car with both legs completely paralyzed! The steering mechanisms can be revised for this purpose.

I've seen a good many people confined to chairs, just sitting all day long, asking for and receiving help with their every move and change of position and having to be pushed in a wheel chair every place they go, whether outside or inside the house.

If you have even one good arm and hand, and have control of your chest and abdominal muscles, there is no reason whatever why you can't help yourself to get around most of the time. In fact, I've also seen people confined to chairs who have taken pains to over-develop their necks, shoulders, chests, and torso muscles to the point where their arms function about as well as their legs used to!

THINGS YOU CAN DO IN A CHAIR

1. Tone up face, neck, shoulders, upper and lower arms, hands, chest, and upper back. If you've neglected any of these parts, all of which go into the vitality of your health and mobility functions, then it's time to get busy. Having two good arms, or even one, makes it possible for you to move your own wheel chair without any assistance except on rare occasions on outings when an incline or decline may be steep.

2. You may need help at first in getting from bed to chair and back again, but your goal is to master these transfers on your own. You can do it. It may take a little time and patience on your part, but you can. As the toning restores strength to your shoulders, chest and arms, it becomes easier with each passing day. Figure 2-6 shows the proper way to get from bed to chair and back again, with or without help.

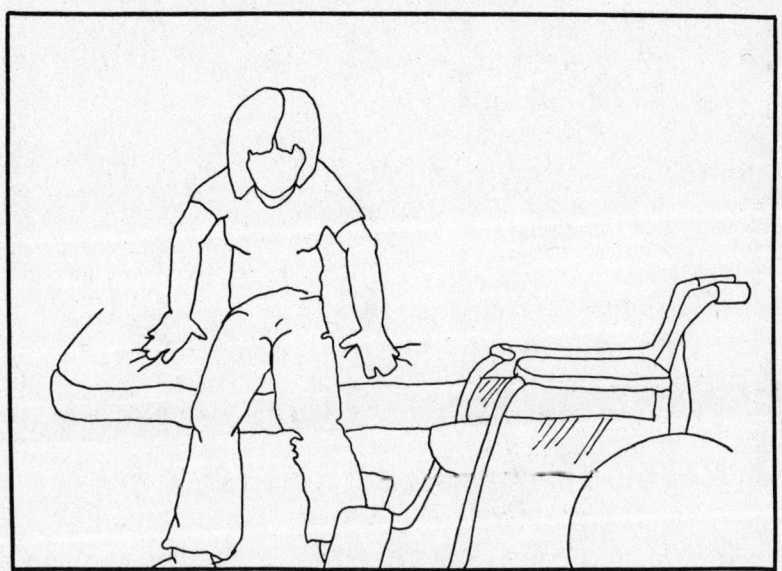

Figure 2-6

3. With further practice, you'll be able to get from chair to bath tub and to toilet and back. We'll see how this is done by a man who lost the function of both his legs a little further on in this chapter. Mastering this step allows you even more independence and mobility.

How to Start Activity in Flagging Muscles and Joints 39

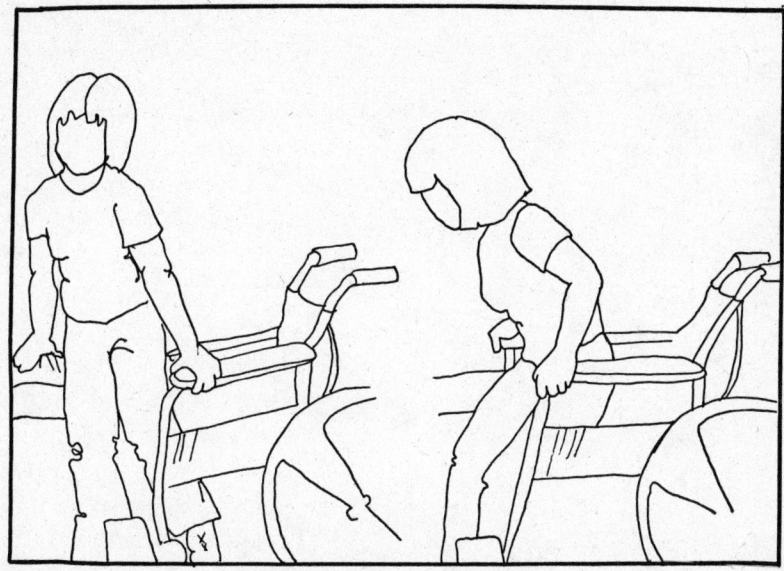

Figure 2-6 (continued)

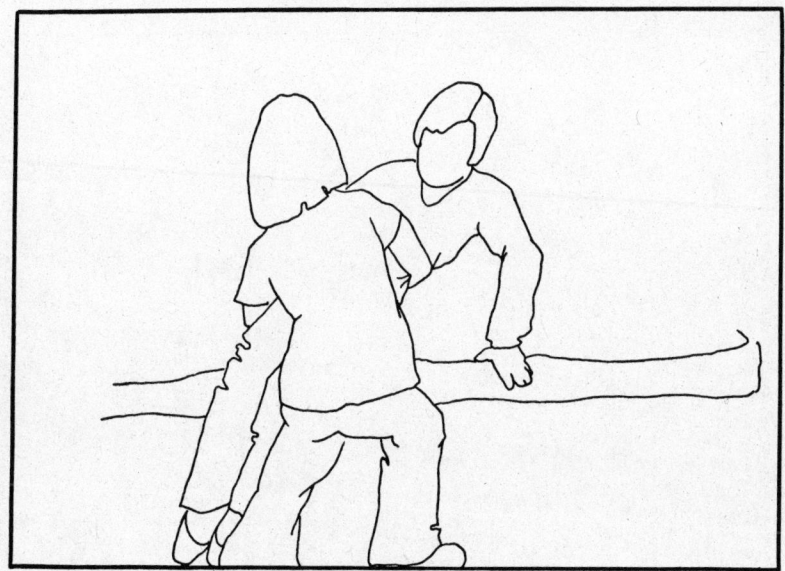

Figure 2-6 (continued)

4. Read, study and learn. These functions will help improve your mind and your skills and will restore confidence in your abilities to be useful and helpful. Reading and taking courses or classes are best done while sitting in a chair as opposed to trying all this from a

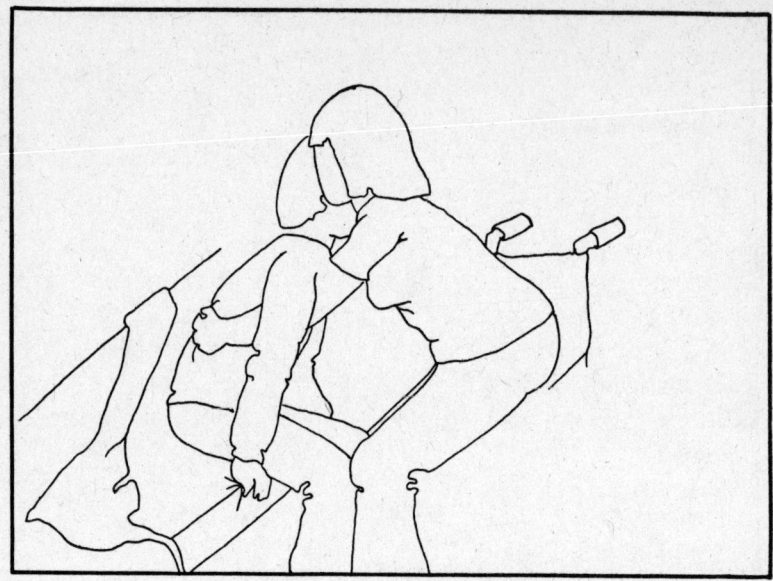

Figure 2-6 (continued)

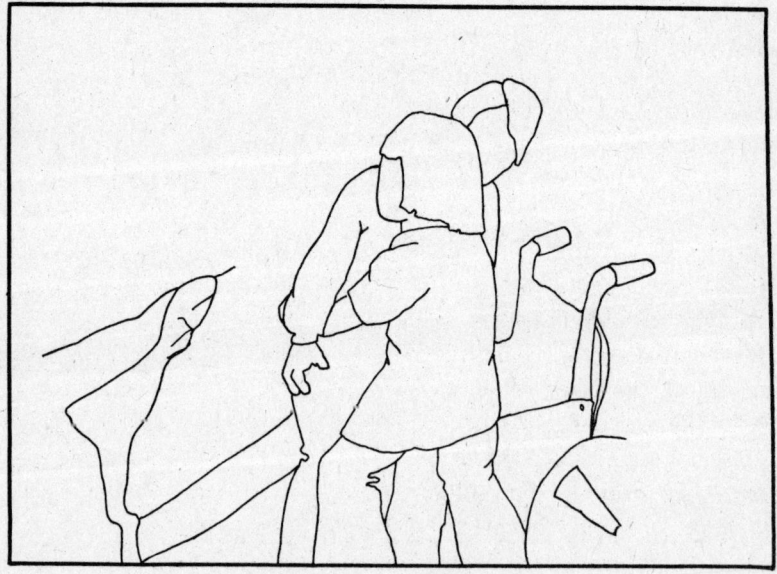

Figure 2-6 (continued)

bed. You don't tire as easily and you can learn to concentrate better from a chair. And of course you can attend distant classes and courses by means of a wheel chair that you couldn't if you were lying in bed.

How to Start Activity in Flagging Muscles and Joints 41

5. When you've mastered muscle toning and transfers, and are sharpening your mind by adding to your knowledge, you may be ready to see how you might master standing—even ambulating—with assistant devices for short distances!

How George V. overcame two-leg paralysis

George V., a young man I first knew many years ago when he was only a teenager, was one of many unlucky people of his generation—there had been no polio vaccine available when he was young and he acquired the disease. It left him without the use of both his legs. Fortunately, as is the case with most such victims, his bladder and bowel functions were left intact. But he was depressed and resigned to the "life of a cripple" from then on.

George was listless and had allowed himself to get soft and flabby, preferring to remain in bed where his devoted family had become used to waiting on him hand and foot.

George and I had some long talks after I made a call on him at home one day because of a urinary tract infection. This is a frequently seen side effect of being inactive from any cause.

I couldn't believe what I saw—a young man in his physical prime in the process of wasting away. At this rate, I told him, he'd have troubles and medical complications coming out his ears by the time he was 25, and he might not be around at all to see his 30th birthday. He thought this over for a few days, and when I returned again for a check on the progress of his infection, he casually asked how he might do better with himself and his life.

Among other things, I impressed him with the idea of being persistent and patient, and using biofeedback techniques to strengthen his capacity to tone his muscles from the waist up and to enlarge the scope of his interests.

He started with isometrics for his chest, shoulders and arms. Isometrics are exercises you can do while sitting in a chair. They involve pitting one set of your own muscles against the opposite set. For example, with one arm flat on a padded chair armrest, hold your wrist with your opposite hand while forcing your flat arm to curl upward at the elbow joint. This flexes your biceps muscle, the one in front of your upper arm, pulling your forearm upward toward your shoulder against the resistance of your opposite hand and arm.

Figure 2-7 shows how George took advantage of objects in his home to begin his toning. He usually *kept the wheel on his chair locked* while doing these exercises.

I don't recall ever seeing such a change in a person as the one that took place in George over the next two-year period. It had been some time since

I'd last seen him, and I was at one of the local high schools where some friends' youngsters were competing in sports events. Much to my amazement, George was entered in the weight-lifting contest, and he won, sitting in his wheel chair! Later I had a chance to visit again with George. He had

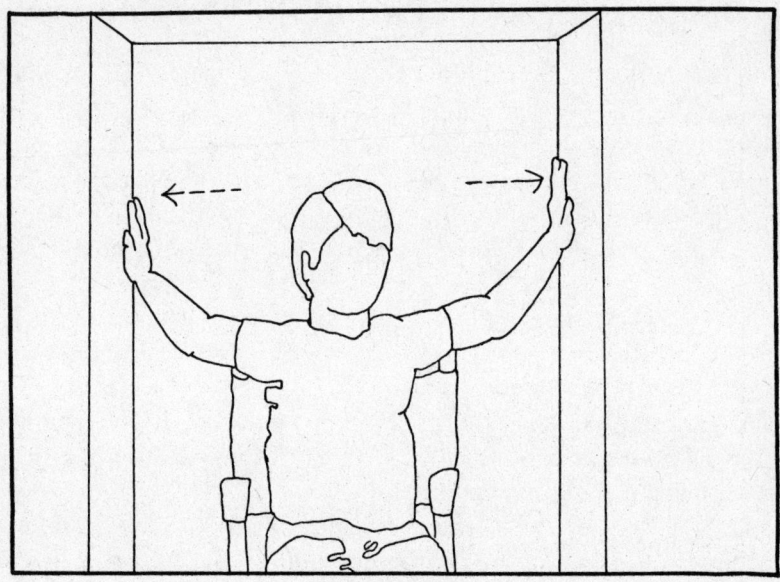

Figure 2-7

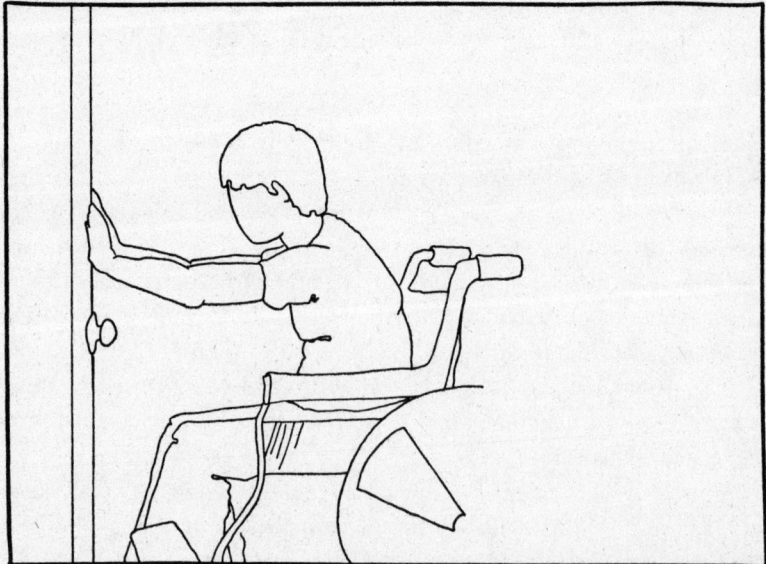

Figure 2-7 (continued)

How to Start Activity in Flagging Muscles and Joints 43

the most beautifully developed physique from his waist up that I've ever seen. It seems he'd developed his muscles as well as he could by using things around the house and decided to take up weights. He then took up swimming and even learned to bowl, having acquired a wheel chair with

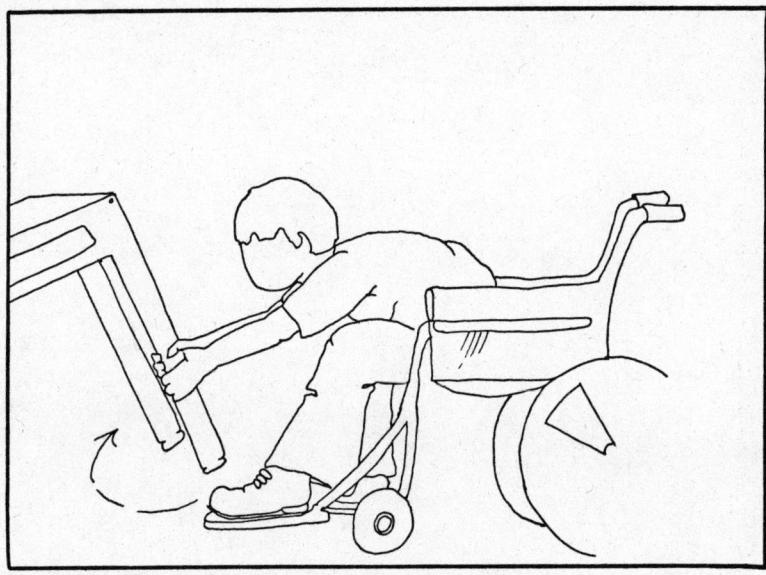

Figure 2-7 (continued)

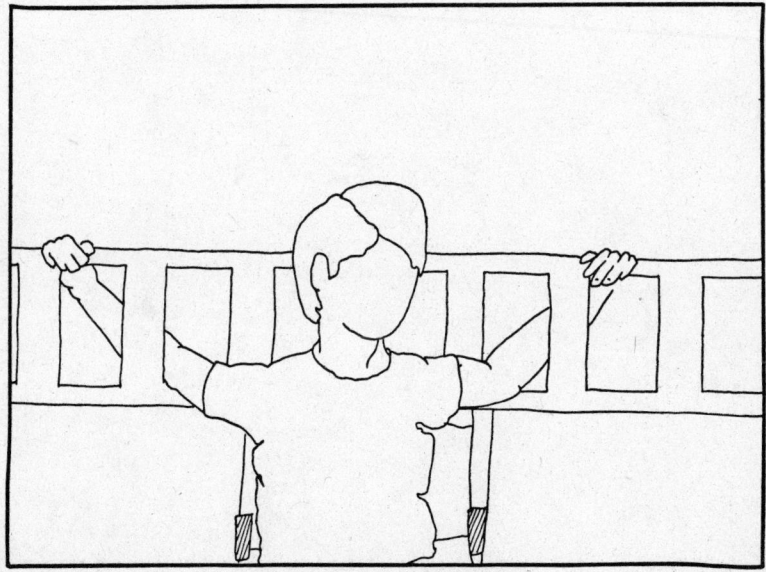

Figure 2-7 (continued)

fold-down arms. He got hold of a pair of Lofstrand crutches (these are held with weight bearing on the forearm, the hand grip in front, and can be obtained with tripod floor supports—see Chapter 6) and even learned to ambulate over short distances using his highly developed arm and chest

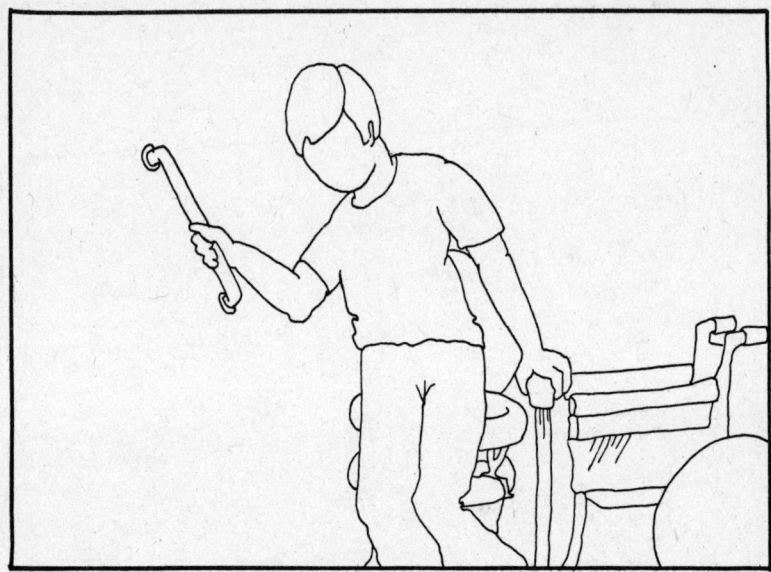

Figure 2-7 (continued)

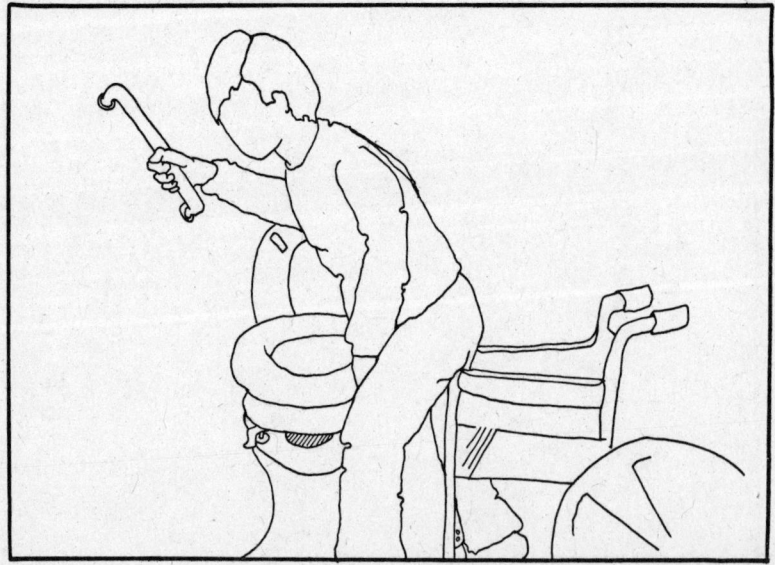

Figure 2-7 (continued)

How to Start Activity in Flagging Muscles and Joints 45

muscles to "carry" his legs along, using the crutches even though his legs couldn't support any weight.

George showed me an adaptation for the shower that he and his father had made after he mastered the bathtub in their bathroom. It consisted of

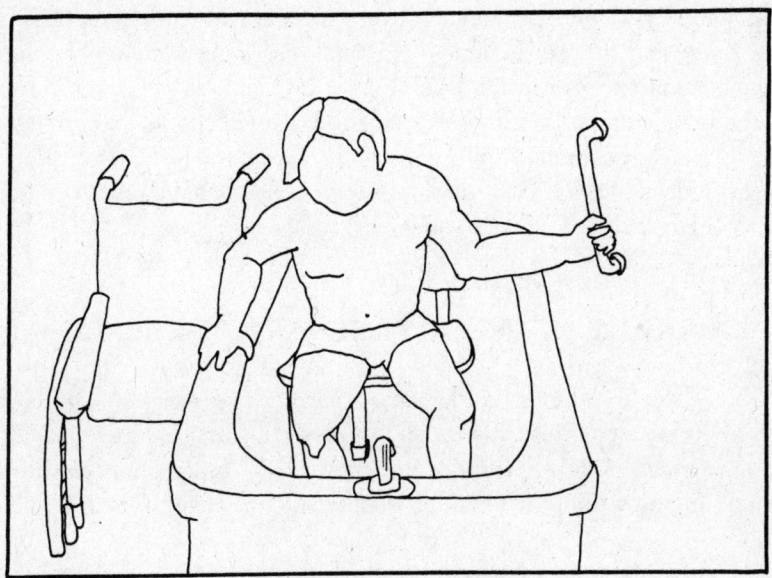

Figure 2-7 (continued)

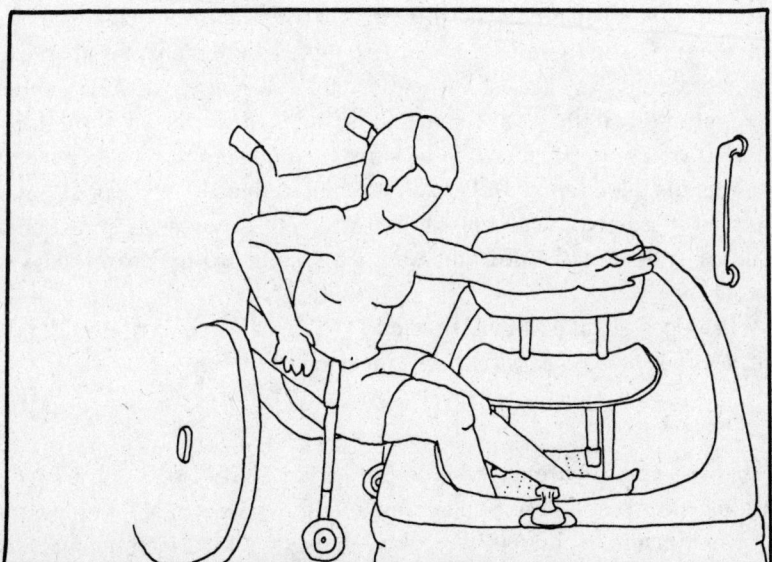

Figure 2-7 (continued)

two vertical grab bars, one on either side just inside of the shower stall, and a horizontal bar that was padded in the center, extending from one side of the stall to the other. George was strong enough to go from his wheel chair to an upright position by using the vertical bars; then, switching to the horizontal bar, he was able to support his body while showering.

Eventually, George became a physical education instructor at the high school level, and he can do almost anything his young students can do in the gymnasium except run the track. What he lacks in leg power, he has more than made up for in arm power. Not everyone, of course, can expect to get to George's position, but I thought his case was worth mentioning because it does show what is possible—even when things aren't in your favor to begin with—if you set your mind to it.

YOUR GOAL OF IMPAIRMENT: FULL AMBULATION

One of the first things I'd like you to learn before going on in this book is the difference in definition between two words: impairment and disability.

Impairment is an interruption in usual bodily function. It can result from anything that hinders function, whether it be a finger or both legs and arms.

Disability is your allowing any impairment to make you unable to function. It results from giving up when an impairment enters the picture.

What we're trying to do in this book is to see how you can prevent impairment from becoming disability, how to overcome obstacles that seem like mountains. The three cases we've examined in this chapter all started with impairments. Ray almost let his become a disability. Both Arlene and George were well on their way to having full-fledged permanent disabilities. All three still have impairments to be sure, but none of them would consider themselves disabled today. In fact, if you hinted that George was disabled, he'd probably grab you with one of his extremely strong arms and squeeze you like a rubber doll until you would be quite willing to retract your statement.

What does it take, then, first and foremost to convert disability to impairment? It takes *determination*. Sheer unadulterated *drive*.

How you get drive

To overcome anything, whether it be adversity, weakness, lack of motivation, laziness, flabbiness, or character flaws, you must first recognize it as a problem and begin to think of ways to deal with it. Anything that must be done by *you* has to start *inside you*. Analyze, compare, add up good

How to Start Activity in Flagging Muscles and Joints

points and subtract bad ones, *think* about what you can do. This is the intellectual side of the first step.

The emotional side is more difficult. It requires you to *accept* the idea that you're going to help yourself. Doing this requires *reinforcement*, going over the problems again and again, concentrating all the while on the mental commands: *I will* and *I can*.

When you have seized on this method and have begun to use it like Arlene and George did, you have mastered the secret of *biofeedback*, a technique many medical advisors and non-medical people have been using for years, but have only recently called it biofeedback. It is a technique I've used for years to help people help themselves, and I have incorporated it into a book titled *The Biofeedback Diet: A Doctor's Revolutionary Approach*, to show people how they can lose weight easily.

Lois makes a biofeedback switch

I took care of Lois B., a lady in her late 30's. She was a woman who, as a youth, contracted rheumatic fever, an acute disease of the joints, often involving impairment of the heart as well. By the time she was in her early 20's, open heart surgery had been perfected to the point where her severely damaged heart valves could be successfully repaired—and they were. This miracle of skill and technique made quite a new woman of Lois, and for five years she literally learned to live again. There was almost no activity she could not engage in with full vigor and physical exertion.

Think of it: A woman is suddenly able to count herself among the living again after over 25 years of invalidism and confinement, in the latter part of her young life, to a wheel chair.

But fate wasn't done with Lois. Suddenly, one day, out of a clear blue sky, she formed a blood clot on the replaced artificial valve in her heart. It was pumped to the left side of her brain where it caused a major stroke on her good right side. For a time her right arm and leg were paralyzed and she couldn't speak. Slowly, over time and with patience and help, Lois regained her ability to speak, the use of her right leg and foot, and the use of her right upper arm. But the forearm muscles—the ones that move your hand and fingers—were useless. The nerves were gone for good.

Did Lois let this stand in her way, even though she was a right-handed person? Absolutely not! Lois's lifelong ambition was to be a drafting engineer. In order to accomplish this, Lois needed her right arm and hand ... or did she?

Lois actually learned to make her left hand, which was unaffected by the stroke, do everything her right hand used to do and in some ways, do it better!

How did she accomplish this? By using the following simple steps.

1. Three times every day at roughly the same hour, Lois sought a quiet, comfortable place and stretched out as if to take a nap. Then she concentrated, putting everything else out of her mind no matter what she'd been doing.
2. In her mind's eye she formed a picture of the right side of her brain—the side responsible for moving the muscles of the left side of her body. She got a picture of the nerves originating in this right side of her brain and traveling down her spinal cord into her left arm and hand.
3. Then she repeated ten times: "My left hand will take over the duties and functions of my right hand. The nerves to my left hand will raise their efficiency and conduct impulses rapidly and accurately. I will learn to use my left hand better than I used my right hand."

Does it sound unreasonable that such a simple routine could improve function? It shouldn't, because it worked! And it's the essence of what biofeedback is all about.

Within two months, Lois became a completely converted "lefty," enrolled in a drafting school and graduated two years later with one of the highest recommendations ever given by her instructors—*even though these same instructors had advised strongly against her enrolling in the school in the first place!*

Today, Lois is successfully employed as a draftsperson. She is married and has a family. She is impaired, but has no handicap. She has overcome two extremely serious insults to her organism. Think of what *you* can do if you apply yourself to those impairments *you* may have!

SUMMARY

1. Muscles, bones and joints need physical activity to keep their health, maintain their function and help unaffected muscles, bones and joints assist those that are unable to function their best.
2. Full mobility is the goal of any impairment, no matter how trivial or severe. To become mobile, you must start with muscle toning, if for no other reason than to enable your stronger limbs to assist the weaker ones.
3. Following surgery and/or an injury, you must pay particular

How to Start Activity in Flagging Muscles and Joints 49

attention to those toning and activity plans suggested by your medical advisor; then you must follow them religiously.

4. Toning starts to combat atrophy (shrinkage) of muscles, tendons and joints. It helps keep your good muscles from getting flabby. And toning starts you on your way to getting rid of those mental blues that set in after you've been inactive and feeling sorry for yourself.

5. You can start by figuring out what you can do in bed in the way of toning and exercise. Then you can switch this activity to a chair, then to the floor or to the upright position using objects in your home.

6. You can then utilize techniques like biofeedback to help you keep up your toning, to make you feel uncomfortable if you are physically inactive, and to expand your mind.

3

How You Can Regain Full, Efficient Muscle and Joint Mobility Fast

This chapter will present some home care principles and show you how you can apply them to your ailing skeletal supports. We'll have a look at a number of conditions, including gouty arthritis and stroke, and see how you may be able to help yourself at home should either of these two ailments intrude on your well-being. We will also examine an extremely important enemy of good health—one that brings on more ailments of joints, bones and muscles than all the rest put together, and one that causes more complications and prolonged illnesses once joints, bones and muscles are involved with disease than any I know: fat, flab, and untoned muscles.

We will take a look at what modern surgery has to offer you folks who may have been unfortunate enough to have very serious trouble with bones and joints. The field has made some rather surprising strides in the past 20 years, but there are some things to be considered before you decide that surgery is the route to go. I'll try to point out how you may better judge whether surgery will help, perhaps even cure, certain locomotion disorders.

THE ABC'S OF HOME CARE PRINCIPLES

The essentials for home care of ailing bones, joints and muscles may be listed as follows:

1. Rest and immobility during acute periods.
2. Activity as soon as possible.
3. Full mobility as soon as practicable.

Regain Muscle and Joint Mobility Fast

4. Proper application of heat and cold.
5. Pain relief.
6. Active prevention of further episodes.
7. Vigorous treatment of specific causes.

As I take you through each of these principles, I will use one case to illustrate all of the points. The case is that of Jerry M., a young man who had gout. This is a rather common form of arthritis, often overlooked as a cause for joint, muscle and bone trouble because of myths that have been built up around it, and because it isn't quite so common a cause of arthritis as the rheumatoid type (usually in younger people) and the osteoarthritic type (as in the case of Arlene's problem in Chapter 2—usually in middle age or senior life).

Rest and mobility

It is only common sense, and medically sound as well, that when any bone or joint or muscle is acutely inflamed (red and tender), has suddenly puffed up and is swollen and sore, or has just been acutely injured (pulled, strained, bruised, or broken) no matter what it is that caused it, you are well-advised during this "acute" stage to put the member at rest, at least for a time.

This doesn't mean you have to put your entire organism at rest, however! If you break an ankle, for example, and it's been put in a plaster cast or splint—whenever you're sitting at rest with your injured leg and foot propped up on a stool, on a chair, or on the couch beside you where you're sitting—you can start with that part of your leg that isn't involved in the cast or splint and begin toning the muscles there on the same day you suffered the injury. If your knee joint is free of the cast (and it will be except in more severe ankle fractures), begin to tone up your thigh muscle. You already have a weight on your foot and lower leg (your cast), and keeping it moving when you sit by moving your lower leg to a horizontal position and then letting it back down again, as Ray S. did in Chapter 2 with the steam iron strapped to his shoe, you are going to be well ahead of most others when that cast finally comes off. You're going to be able to get back to normal walking again three times as fast and five times as comfortably!

This was the stage at which Jerry found himself when he had his last attack of gout. The large toe joint on his right foot became acutely red, swollen and exquisitely tender, the pain radiating up his entire right foot into his ankle.

So, until the major part of the swelling and tenderness resolved as a result of taking specific drugs for his gout, Jerry simply walked around on crutches, and when he sat down he elevated his involved right foot onto a foot stool in front of his chair.

While he was sitting and reading or watching TV, he formed the habit of toning up other muscles; his neck, shoulders, arms, chest, and abdomen. He did this by using isometrics until the acute process in his foot was better. Figure 3-1 shows how he performed some of his exercises.

This got him in better shape to use his crutches, and it helped overcome some of the distress and pain caused by his ailing foot. It also provided a bonus in that when the attack of gout was finished he was prepared to go into the more vigorous activities of muscle and joint tone that were needed to keep him in top physical condition.

Activity—when?

You needn't ever become totally inactive from bone, joint and muscle disorders. Conditions like multiple sclerosis and stroke, for example, usually cause *only certain muscles* to be out of whack. If the muscle is weakened, there is all the more reason for starting to tone it, even though it won't do all the things the leg or arm on the other side (the uninvolved side) will do. Put weak muscles through whatever they'll take!

Activity of the involved limb or part of a limb, joint, or injured muscle should begin when it's reasonably comfortable for you to do so. And there's only one real way anyone can say when this time arrives: You can be the judge by *carefully* putting weight on your arthritic knee joint, or your injured ankle, by *carefully* and slowly bending and twisting your aching lower back, or by grasping objects with your arthritic fingers. If you can honestly say when doing these activities that it doesn't hurt nearly as much as when the condition first started, then it's time to get the involved member active again. It may be for only a few minutes at first, for 15 minutes in a couple of days, and then for a half hour. Finally, in a week or so, half a day or a full day's activity will be indicated.

In Jerry's case, as soon as the crucial first two or three days passed, he began gingerly to test weight on his gouty foot with the help of his crutches. He continued to bear weight on his crutches, but he dropped his foot to the floor and *carefully* shifted some weight slowly onto his right leg. He continued to use two crutches for a couple of days until he felt reasonably stable on his right leg, and then used a cane for another couple of days to take a little of the stress of weight bearing off his right leg. Finally, he could walk without aids of any kind. Figure 3-2 shows how Jerry progressed through these stages

Regain Muscle and Joint Mobility Fast

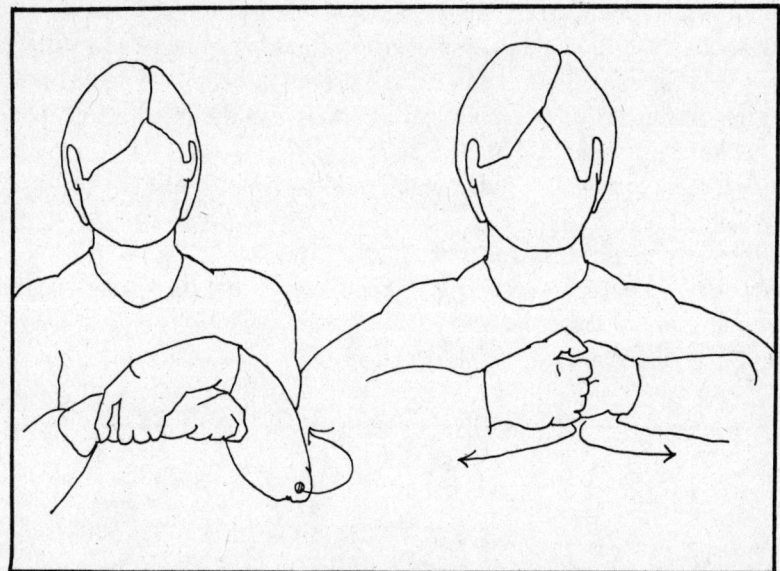

Figure 3-1

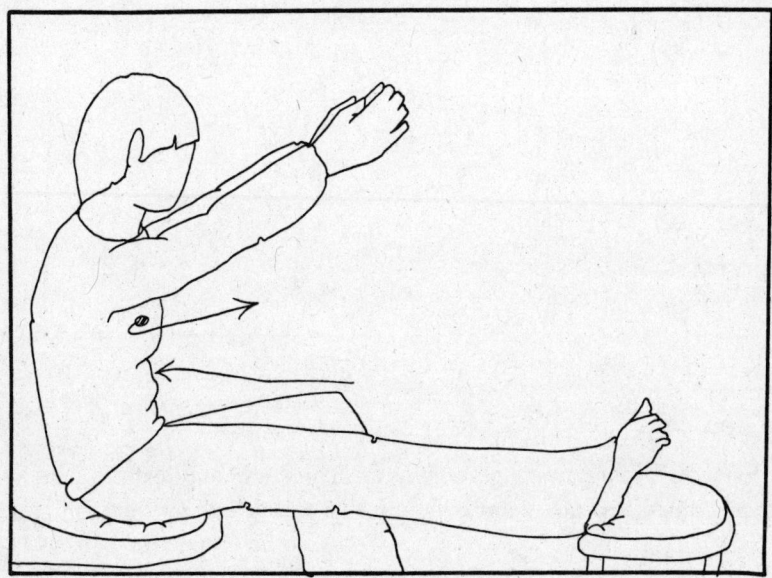

Figure 3-1 (continued)

Full mobility—how soon?

When the acute process—the extreme tenderness, pain and redness—is over and you've begun to use your ailing joints and muscles again full mobility or normal use should come along as quickly as you feel comfortable in so doing. In some arthritic conditions such as in your low back, you'll find that there is some distress even if there is no acute process going on. In this case, you must learn to overcome the discomfort of using your back in spite of a little pain. Set the goal for full use of an ailing part as soon as it feels reasonably stable and free of pain and swelling when you're using it.

Jerry's acute phase of gout subsided in about four days; he began to put some weight on his foot on the fifth day. By the eighth day, Jerry found he could pretty well do what he wanted on his ailing right foot, and do it safely without crutch or cane.

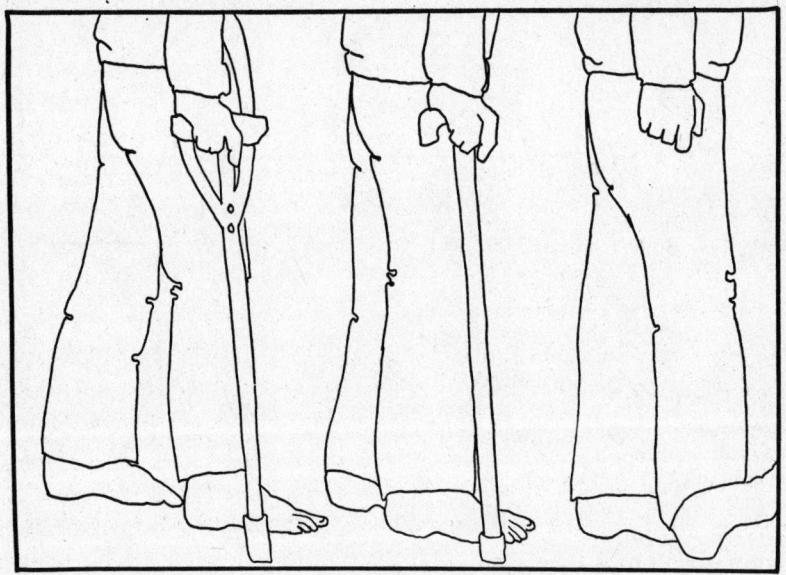

Figure 3-2

Heat and cold

We'll be talking much more about heat and cold applications, but here are some general principles about both that will stand you in good stead:

1. "Cold first; heat last" is a reasonably good memory tool to help you decide what to use with regard to muscle, bone and joint ailments. It's generally true that heat during any acute phase will only make the pain worse, the swelling increase, and the redness deepen.
2. For injuries, cold is best for the first two or three days; then properly applied heat will serve you well.

Regain Muscle and Joint Mobility Fast

3. For healing scars and bones (following surgery or fracture), heat should be *delayed* even longer so that normal healing may follow rapidly and completely.
4. Caution should always be used with heat and cold application. Heat increases the cells' need for oxygen in those tissues being heated. If the blood supply (veins and arteries) are healthy in the area, the increase (heat and cold) can be handled; if not, there are dangers and *caution is indicated*.

Jerry avoided applying heat to his gouty arthritic foot for the first few days; during the acute red, painful phase of his disease, heat only made things worse. The application of an ice pack to his foot, however, did relieve the pain quite well and it reduced the amount of swelling around his big toe joint.

Jerry found that leaving his foot bare—no socks and certainly no shoes or slippers—made for more comfort as well. The inflamed toe joint seemed not to tolerate even a whisper of anything touching it for the first day or so.

Even after the first couple of days, Jerry discovered that if he took an old pair of slippers and cut out the toe portion completely from the right one, it was helpful with the pain.

Pain relief

I've found that most people think they need strong narcotic drugs for their pain, regardless of what's causing it. The truth is, very often they are *not* needed. What is needed is proper use of the milder drugs that are still effective.

The mainstay of all such drugs is plain, ordinary aspirin—that's right, aspirin used properly. For arthritic and injury pain, aspirin can be taken three tablets at a time, and should be. Moreover, aspirin should be taken every three hours, if needed, *around the clock*.

The secret to lasting and continuous relief with aspirin is in building up a fairly high blood level of the drug and *maintaining it*, sometimes (as in the case of rheumatoid arthritis, osteoarthritis, and injuries) for as long as two, three, or even four weeks! Whether pain is or is not a problem after the first couple of days—especially with arthritis—aspirin needs to be kept up after the acute process has apparently died down.

There are two major exceptions to this rule. Jerry's affliction—gouty arthritis—is one of them. There are two main drugs that are used to treat acute gout and there are two or three others used to prevent the recurrence of gout attacks. Jerry's doctor had him take a drug called phenylbutazone for two or three days when an acute attack started; then he had him taper off over seven or eight days. Jerry started on the prevention drug—called allopurinol—a few years back, and he hasn't had another attack of gout since.

Aspirin interferes with the action of both phenylbutazone and allopurinol, and aspirin *is not indicated* if you're taking either of them for the treatment of gout.

The second major exception to the aspirin rule is that if you have to take one of the drugs that thin your blood to prevent it from clotting so easily, aspirin also interferes with most of these drugs. You should *not* use aspirin if you're on one of these drugs, so be certain to check with your medical advisor if there is a question. Figure 3-3 shows how to further avoid complications of aspirin therapy.

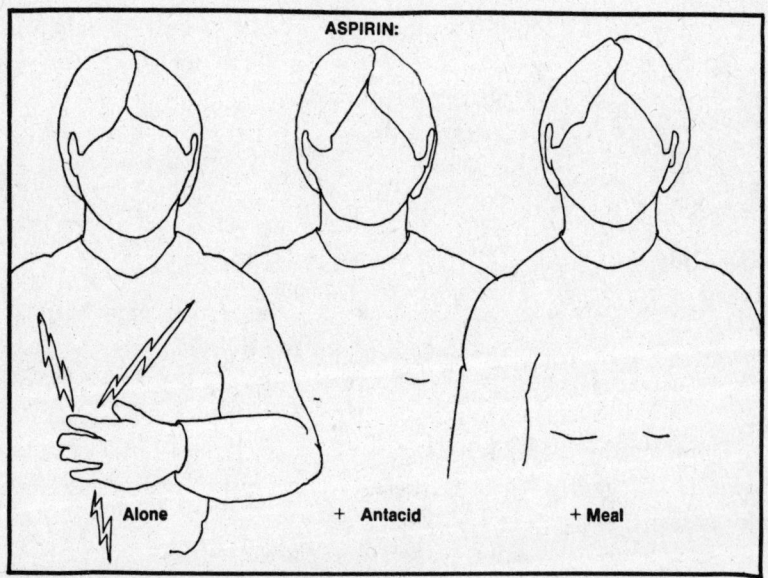

Figure 3-3

Prevention

Prevention of injury is based on the tenets we've discussed: the maintenance of good muscle tone. If you're a skier in winter, pay attention to your instructor, who will advise you first and foremost to get those legs and arms in shape *before* you go out onto the ski slopes. The same applies to hiking, tennis, volleyball, fishing, and virtually everything else you might like to do. In all major sports, the coach starts his team members on a

Regain Muscle and Joint Mobility Fast

conditioning program long before the season for the sport. This is what training camps are all about.

The same rule applies to arthritis—rheumatoid and osteoarthritis. Conditioning must be started during a quiet phase and *kept up* from that time on. Of course, you won't put a swollen, stiff elbow or shoulder through the same vigorous physical strain as you will your opposite elbow and shoulder, but put them through *some* toning—right up to the point where it *begins* to hurt, then stop. You'll find that slowly and gradually, the amount of toning even an involved rheumatic joint can take will increase.

The prevention of some ailments, like Jerry's gout, depends on the prescribing and long-term use of certain medicines. Jerry was lucky. He had an ailment which can now be controlled completely in most cases by the use of one of the newer preventive drugs. Jerry started taking the specific drug for gout prevention about six years ago. He hasn't had an acute attack of gout since, and probably won't. The drug doesn't work with other types of arthritis, however, but there's hope that we'll have a similar one for rheumatoid and osteoarthritis one of these days. Meanwhile, there is much you can do without drugs.

Figure 3-4 summarizes the preventive measures you need to take to ensure maximum protection against arthritis, bone and muscle ailments.

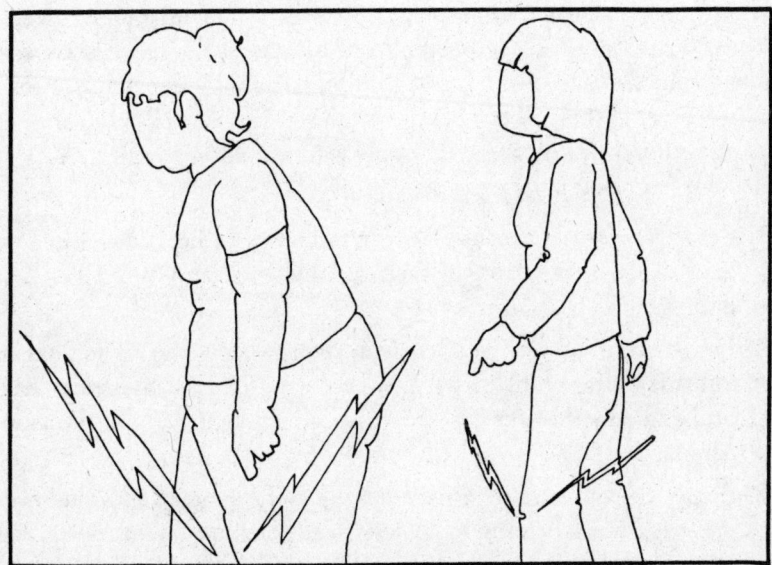

Figure 3-4

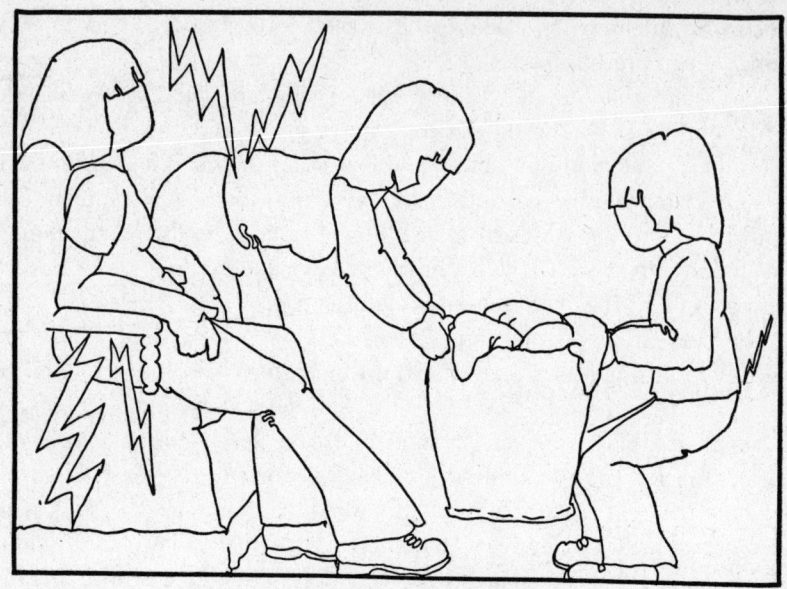

Figure 3-4 (continued)

LOSING FLAB AND RETAINING TONE

In my personal experience in 27 years as a general practitioner, a whopping 80 percent of all the people I saw as patients for all reasons were over ideal weight! Some of them just a little; a lot more dangerously so.

Why? What is there about being fat that's so terrible? I've been asked this question hundreds of times. To reply fully would take half a day, but consider the following points:

1. Being fat *contributes significantly* to increased heart disease, lung disease, abdominal organ disease, diabetes, stroke, cancer, and injuries.
2. Being overweight tremendously increases the chances for having arthritis, bone problems, flabby muscles (followed by strain, easy bruising and the like), accidents, and for being a very unhappy person.
3. Being flabby slows healing after injury or surgery and may even prevent normal healing in some cases. Being fat increases the risk for post-surgical complications by about five times!

Doesn't it make common sense, then, to reduce your chances as much as possible in view of all these problems? Of course it does!

Regain Muscle and Joint Mobility Fast

Diet and exercise

These two activities should never be thought of as anything but *joined together* with any weight problem, and in keeping yourself at ideal health potential after you've reached ideal weight. The closer you get to 40 years of age, the more important it is for you to start *both* if you've been fortunate enough thus far to have avoided arthritis, bone or muscle ailments.

If you've passed 40 and have discovered some problems, remember that it isn't too late to start. To do so now will not only hasten the clearing up of your problem, but will act to help prevent many other problems in the future.

On page 258 there is a height/weight/frame table. Consult it. Find your ideal weight according to your height and bone structure (frame). Set a goal today of reaching it through one of the diets given, and by starting on a toning routine involving at least ten minutes twice each day. And when you've reached your goal, resolve to stay with diet and toning routines from then on—you'll be healthier in the long run, and you'll be able to cope with your arthritis, bone and muscle problems so much more easily, you'll wonder why you hadn't started years ago!

The secret, if it can be called that, in losing weight is to take in *fewer* energy calories than you burn up during the course of a day. That's what the diets in the back of the book are designed to do. If you do this, and keep it up, you can't help losing weight. It's only when you hedge a little all the time that you'll fail. This fact is also why toning helps: Exercise helps burn up calories, makes you feel better (dieting isn't a bowl of cherries), and tones your metabolism, keeping those muscles, tendons, ligaments, joints, and bones up to snuff as far as their nutrition is concerned. And it sharpens your mind.

Clara discovers the truth

I recall a patient named Clara F. who had neglected her weight for most of the 48 years of her life. She had a stroke and it made her left side practically useless. She progressed during the post-stroke period to a wheel chair and crutches, but she simply had too much bulk to allow her left leg (only partially paralyzed) to bear weight on it so she could walk. In spite of this, something had to be devised to keep the tone she did have in her left leg at least from disappearing completely. Figure 3-5 shows how Clara managed this at home. Clara started on a reducing diet of 1200 calories and a regular toning program.

Clara lost ten pounds in the first three weeks, eight pounds in the next six weeks, six pounds over the next four weeks, and within three months lost

60 **Regain Muscle and Joint Mobility Fast**

the remaining 16 pounds to total the 40 pounds excess she'd been carrying around!

Clara now walks with only a short-leg brace on her left side, and gets around almost anywhere she desires without crutches or cane. She keeps

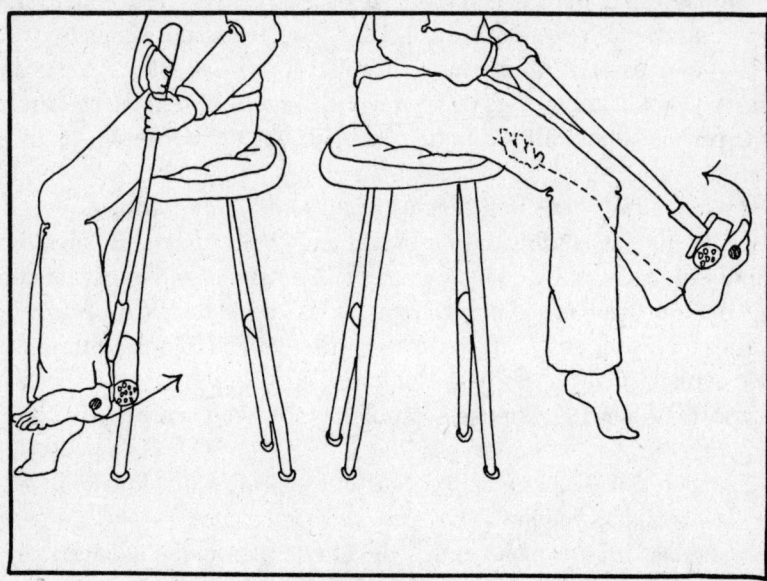

Figure 3-5

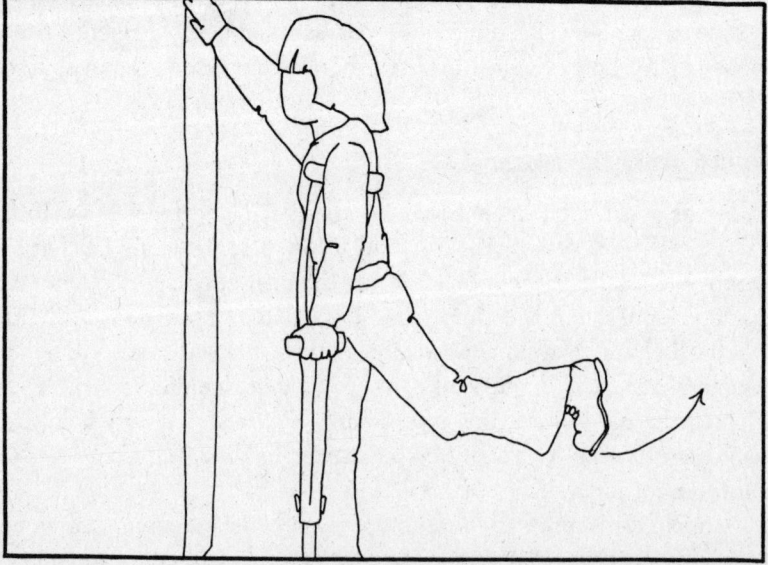

Figure 3-5 (continued)

Regain Muscle and Joint Mobility Fast

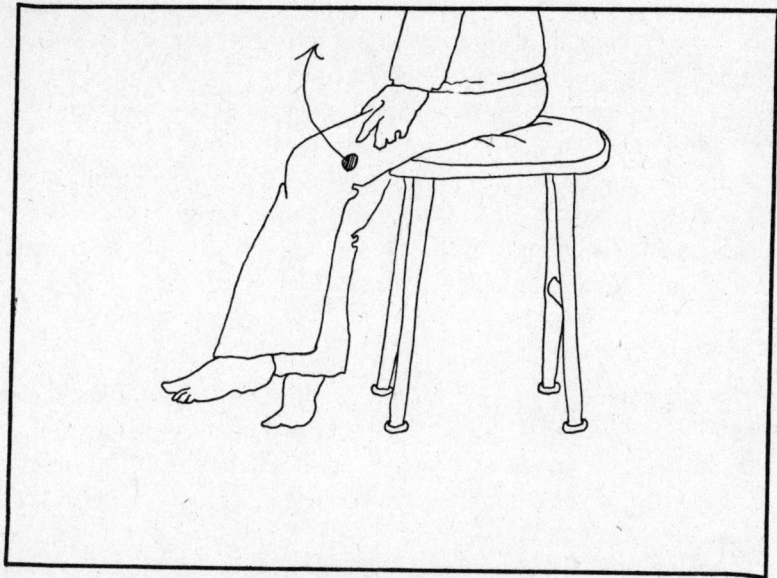

Figure 3-5 (continued)

her figure at a trim 140 pounds (about right for her five feet, nine inches) and the blood pressure problem she had before her stroke has been controlled with only one drug since she shed her flab.

WHEN WILL SURGERY HELP?

Orthopedic surgeons have developed some amazing techniques for ailing joints and bones over the past years. Among the more recent and well-known of these has been entire joint replacement for a variety of ailments.

Like all newer techniques, experience has shown some things about joint replacement that are often overlooked by sufferers of joint problems in their natural desire to be rid of what can be severe trouble. The following joints can be replaced with modern techniques:

1. Elbow joints
2. Hip joints
3. Knee joints

There are experimental techniques being devised at present which may make successful replacement of shoulder, wrist, finger, and ankle joints possible in the near future.

62   Regain Muscle and Joint Mobility Fast

One thing surgeons have learned about joint replacement is that for a patient to be a candidate for such surgery he must have *severe distress and deformity* before such surgery is considered wise. This sounds a little cruel, but there are dangers in any surgical replacement of an entire joint. If even the slightest infection should happen to enter the wound following surgery, the artificial joint might have to be removed. For this and other reasons, surgeons have learned that joint replacement can't be done simply to fix, for example, a shortened leg and limp from a bad hip. It must be a crippling and very painful ailment before such chances are taken.

Bill is lucky

An example of what I mean by the right time for joint replacement is the case of Bill W., who was born with a congenital dislocation of his left hip. Unfortunately, it wasn't detected until Bill had aged to three years (before this age, this condition can be corrected by proper casting of the hip and leg).

By the time Bill had progressed to his teens, his left leg had shortened by 3½ inches compared to his right leg, and he had to wear a lift on his left shoe. His hip joint was small and deformed, and caused a marked limp when he walked.

By the time he'd reached 35, Bill began to notice severe pain along with his marked limp. At 43, Bill got to the point where he couldn't bear

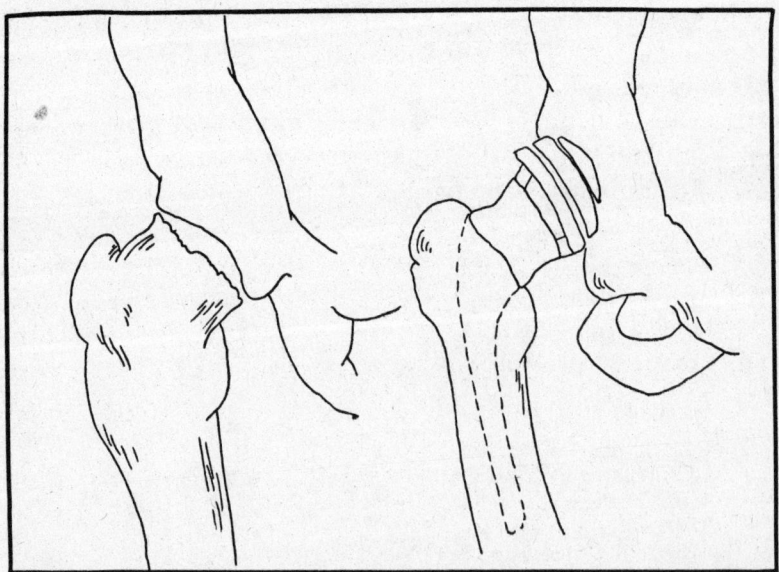

Figure 3-6

Regain Muscle and Joint Mobility Fast

weight on his left side any longer. This is when surgeons decided that the risks involved with joint replacement could reasonably be taken—his left leg was practically useless. (See Figure 3-6.)

Bill survived the surgery without untoward effects and today he has a perfectly normal left leg he can use to walk, run, ride a bicycle, and drive a car.

LESS FORMIDABLE SURGERY

Often, with joint and bone problems, there are things that can be done without quite the risky business associated with entire joint replacement. These procedures are done every day around the country, and are usually successful as well as free of a host of complications.

The following list shows situations in which these less troublesome procedures can be done safely at almost any age, and without waiting for severe trouble to supervene:

1. *Fusion of joints*
   This procedure involves scraping the bony parts of joints and packing their raw surface with bone "grafts"—bone chips removed from a place such as your hip bone. Fusion operations, when healed, prevent motion in one or more of the planes that the fused joint used to go through with ordinary action, thereby relieving a high percentage of pain.

2. *Osteotomy*
   This surgery involves removing parts of bones, usually at or near joint surfaces, to straighten a crooked joint, or to alter growth rates in a long bone so it will remain the same size as its counterpart on the opposite side.

3. *Release of tethered tendons and ligaments*
   With this type of surgery—very common, for example, in wrists and hands afflicted with arthritis—the scar tissue and the connective tissues that overgrow as a result of a long siege of rheumatoid arthritis with its profuse inflammation are removed, and the tendons are released from the binding effect such tissues produce. Surgeons who do a lot of work with hands can often turn a useless hand, crippled and deformed by arthritis, into a hand that is able to function again.

4. *Bone graft for ununited fractures*
   In this surgery, fractures that won't or can't heal, usually following an accident of severe nature, even though they might have been

plated and screwed together to hold them in good position, often can be made to unite by removing the "hardware" and packing the fracture site with bone chips, as in the joint fusion procedure mentioned previously. The packed chips of bone eventually heal as a solid bony strut to unite the injured bone.

5. *Muscle tendon transfer*

Very often in someone afflicted with cerebral palsy or polio at an early age, the legs end up being the most serious remaining locomotion disability. Usually starting in childhood, these weak, atrophied legs can be restructured to a certain extent by taking the tendons from leg muscles that do work, and attaching them to a crucial spot, such as at the ankle, so that the weak useless ankle can at least be made to flex up and down, where before it couldn't move at all.

A young lady I knew named Valerie G. was involved in an auto accident in which her right ankle was seriously crushed. She recovered from other less serious bumps and cuts, but the ankle bones protruded from her skin when she was first brought to the hospital (a so-called compound fracture). Surgeons plated the bones in position using three screws to hold the broken bony pieces together. Valerie got on well for a time following her release home, but the pain in this ankle even after it healed was so intense

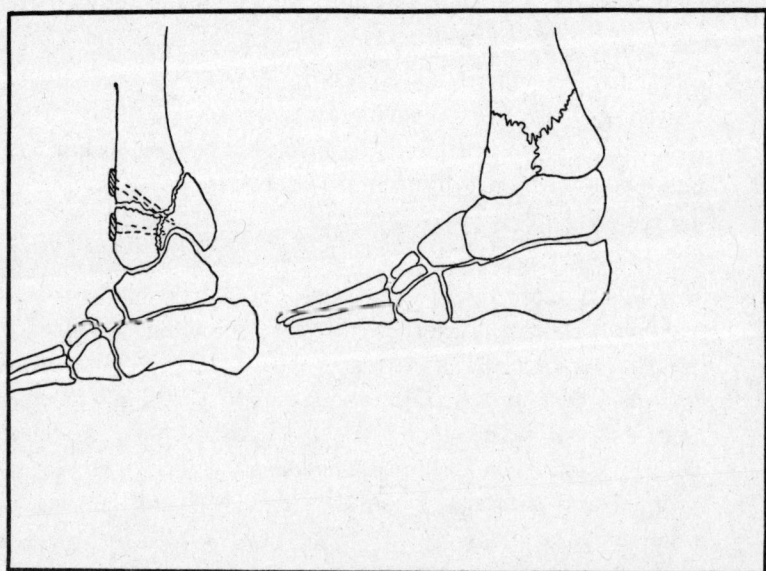

Figure 3-7

Regain Muscle and Joint Mobility Fast

that she had to continue using crutches long after the usual time of healing (two or three months).

Finally, surgeons readmitted her to the hospital and removed the screws completely. They scraped the ends of the main lower leg bone and the first large ankle bone, and packed the ends and sides of this joint with bone chips from her hip. Eventually, Valerie's ankle healed with the ankle about midway between full dorsal flexion (pulled all the way upward), and full plantar flexion (pulled all the way down toward the floor). But importantly, Valerie could bear weight and walk (though stiff-ankled) without pain and without crutches or cane. Figure 3-7 shows how Valerie's ankle looked before and after surgery. The sacrifice of normal motion at a joint for comfortable weight-bearing and ability to walk was thus achieved.

SOMETIMES EXERCISE CURES

Let's look for a minute at the things a good toning or exercise program can do for you.

Joints: Tones those ligaments that hold bones together. Tones cartilage that cushions bones as they push together. Tones tendons that cross joints and adds strength to their solid union.
Stimulates the membrane that secretes lubricating fluid in joints to increase the efficiency of the bones that glide over each other at the joint. Helps break up stiffening scar tissue in joints and helps free joints for increased motion.

Bones: Steps up calcium and protein metabolism in bones by increased pull and stress of tendons attached to them during exercises. Increases bone strength and resiliency.
Increases circulation inside bone—the marrow where blood elements are manufactured. Stimulates release of new red blood cells to carry oxygen and white blood cells that aid in your body's defense against infection.

Muscles: Hardens muscle masses and increases their tone, making all your body movements more efficient and easier to perform. Holds the bones that make up joints more snugly in place, since muscles span virtually every joint in your body. Makes seldom used muscles work, thereby building up your ability to move various joints far more efficiently, especially in the event that you may have lost part or all of one or more major muscles through injury or disease.

Increases coordination, allowing for more smoothly running joints.

John H. gets bonus

A patient of mine named John H. had complained for some time of chronic pain in his low back. A thorough work-up failed to show anything seriously wrong with his back, but he'd hurt it at work two years before and it was entrenched in his mind that he was doomed to suffer from the problem for the rest of his life.

One day John came in with an inguinal hernia, a bulge in his groin indicating that the tissues in this region had given way and had allowed part of his intestinal tract to protrude. This kind of hernia is quite common and is to a degree hereditary, which is to say it's often found occurring in one's family tree.

John had a big flabby belly which protruded over his belt. At age 39, he looked more like 49. He wanted to have his hernia repaired surgically, which is about the only way to do away with a hernia problem. I told him that before I'd allow the operation to proceed, he must lose at least 40 pounds—and even so, he wouldn't be within range of his ideal weight for his height and frame.

After much hemming and hawing and argument, John finally agreed. Over the next eight months, he lost 40 pounds by adhering to a 1000 calorie a day diet like the one in the back of this book. He had his surgery and came through it with flying colors, and the surgeon was able to do a very satisfactory repair by pulling in strong firm tissue from the surrounding area and sewing it in place over the defect that had caused John's hernia.

After two months had passed, John asked me what he might do to prevent further such trouble—either a recurrent hernia on the same side, or another hernia on the opposite side. I told him that among other things, he must keep his weight under control as he had started to do before his surgery, and that he must take measures to strengthen his belly muscles. To help with this, I had John do sit-ups and scissor kicks on a daily routine. He complained loudly at first but soon got used to it. When he could do 30 sit-ups and the same number of scissor kicks each day, I had him start doing them both at the same time! He really protested at this one, and I'm sure I was thoroughly cussed in the mornings and before bedtime on many an occasion as John struggled through these exercises. (See Figure 3-8.)

Regain Muscle and Joint Mobility Fast 67

But I had an ulterior motive in mind. Not only did John trim down to a flat well-toned belly with extra strength built into his groin areas to prevent future hernias, he also got rid of his chronic low back complaint. Why?

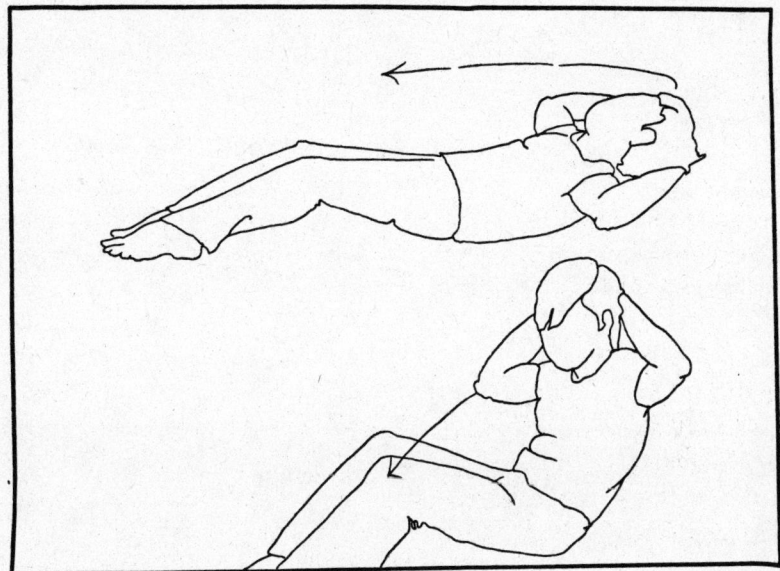

Figure 3-8

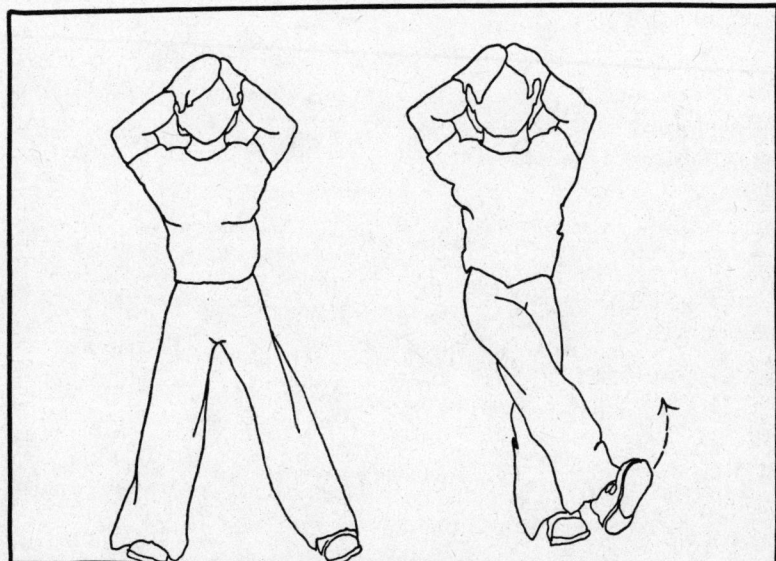

Figure 3-8 (continued)

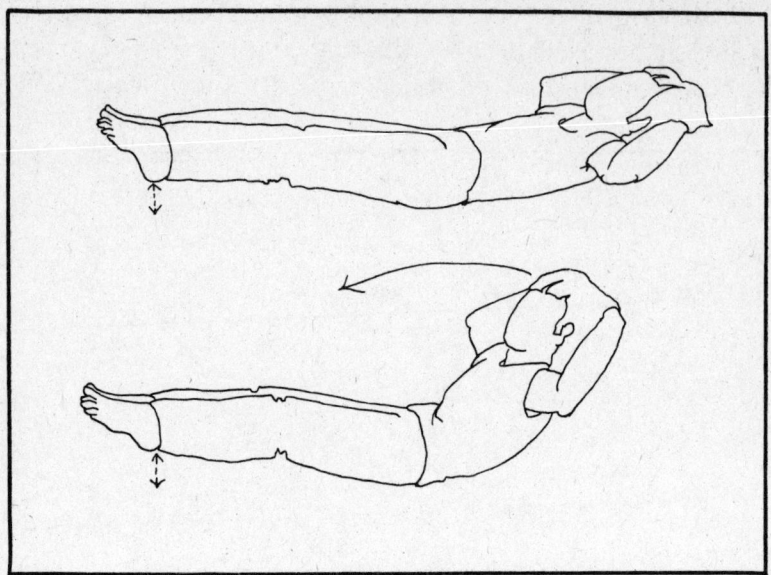

Figure 3-8 (continued)

Because in doing sit-ups you use your belly muscles to pull you up from a flat position on the floor, and you use your back muscles to let you back down to the floor. *The toning up of John's back muscles without his really realizing it had been responsible for the cure of his chronically sore low back.*

So don't underestimate what toning can do for you and your bones, muscles and joints. And don't neglect toning before or after you may have ailments involving these structures. John found out just how important toning can be.

SUMMARY

1. The seven keystones for care of your ailing bones, joints and muscles are: rest and immobility during acute phases, activity as soon as possible, full mobility as soon as possible, proper application of heat and cold, pain relief, and prevention of further episodes.
2. Shedding excess flab and fat and restoring tone to your soft muscles will aid immeasurably in the restoration of bones, muscles and joints.
3. There are times with bone, muscle and joint ailments when surgery is indicated, and there are other situations when surgery is not

feasible. If you think you may have a surgically correctable condition, you should consult your medical advisor.

4. When surgery may be indicated, you should always strive to reduce your weight to near ideal levels and should tone your muscle system as best you can. Following surgery, your medical advisor can tell you when you may reasonably start your toning program to promote the best recovery.

5. Both weight reduction and toning programs can be done right in your own home and needn't send you to a health spa or physical fitness class.

4

How You Can Adjust Bone and Muscle to Stress

In this section I'm going to discuss how you can cope with stress—physical and mental stress, I mean. Why stress? Because it's a common cause of bone, muscle and joint disorders, and if stress doesn't bring on the disorder, it often follows after the disorder and makes things a lot worse for you.

We'll see, for example, how stress acts to cause rheumatoid arthritis, and how you can take some measures today to head it off. I'll also show you how stress enters into the problem of gouty arthritis and osteoarthritis, and what you can do to minimize its effects.

Very often, stress actually brings on a chronic low back syndrome. I'm going to show you how, why, and what you can do about it. Stress often acts to aggravate other joint syndromes and ailments. I'll show you how you can temporarily overcome the pain and muscle spasm often associated with muscle and bone ailments, and in so doing control that ailment.

Finally, I want to show you how mental stress can act to turn you into an ogre, and how this can bring on many unwelcome conditions that will eventually get you down if you don't head it off. You'll learn how you can deal with it here.

ARTHRITIS: YES OR NO?

Throughout the ages arthritis has been a kind of smoldering scourge—it can strike the young as well as the elderly, it can cripple, it can deform and incapacitate. It hurts. What are the advances in treatment from medical science in the face of such a common malady? About the same as against the common cold—surprisingly little. This doesn't mean that nothing can be done with arthritis, or that things necessarily look bleak in the face of it.

How You Can Adjust Bone and Muscle to Stress

It means that the more we learn about the disease, the more we find out how subtle and complex are the mechanisms that set it in motion.

Rheumatoid arthritis

This is the kind of arthritis that comes on earlier in life, usually affects several joints at different times, may be ushered in by low grade fever and a feeling of general illness in addition to the joint problems, and is characterized at the joint by pain at rest, redness and swelling. Sometimes fluid may collect in the joint spaces involved, and both tendons and ligaments in and around the joints may be caught up in the process in addition to the joint surfaces themselves. Rheumatoid arthritis is also characterized by sudden flare-ups and relatively quiet periods in between.

Osteoarthritis

This is the type of arthritis that comes on later in life, usually affects the joints generally subjected to the most physical stress, and once started tends not to "migrate" about your body as does rheumatoid arthritis. Osteoarthritis is generally not so severe or sudden as rheumatoid, tends to be bothersome over long periods, getting better with physical activity and worse at rest, and usually isn't ushered in by redness and swelling of the joints involved (as with rheumatoid).

Gouty arthritis

One usually sees this type of arthritis (a less common type) come on at mid-life or beyond. It involves specifically the large toe joint of the foot (though other single joints can be involved) and is ushered in by redness, swelling and exquisite pain in the toe or other single joint that may be involved. Gout is characterized by a rather short acute course (because of the effectiveness of specific medicines to deal with it) and by more or less permanent cure (because of newer medicines developed to prevent recurrences).

Traumatic arthritis

With this type of arthritis, you see the onset in a specific joint only, one that has been seriously injured as with a severe ankle sprain with tearing of the ligaments, a ski injury in which one knee was badly twisted, or a fall from a high place in which the mid or lower back might have been injured. It is most apt to occur when a fracture involves a joint space, or when metal screws or plates must be used properly to repair such a fracture.

ROLE OF STRESS

In my opinion, the stress factor is one of the chief considerations in all kinds of arthritis even though it is accepted at present that gouty arthritis is caused by an inherited defect in protein metabolism, and usually responds to treatment for this defect.

Stress is especially important in rheumatoid arthritis. Over the years I've observed hundreds of cases of this affliction in patients, and in almost every one of them, close questioning about the time of the onset of their rheumatoid arthritis reveals emotional stress that began a short time *before* they started having trouble.

It would be simple if we knew all we could about the subtle reaction to stress in the human body. Some people seem capable of withstanding emotional stress all their lives without so much as a joint twinge. Still others react with arthritis after what seem to be only the usual stresses and strains of everyday living.

Emily F.'s experience

Emily F. illustrates what I mean by the stress factor influence in rheumatoid arthritis. Emily was a young woman of 32 when I first met her. She had two youngsters in grade school and had been healthy most of her life. Healthy, that is, until her husband died rather suddenly after a short illness. Within three months Emily began to notice soreness and stiffness in the finger joints in her right hand. Some time later, she had a sudden flare-up of swelling and pain in her left knee, and then swelling, pain and redness in her right shoulder joint. Emily had begun to contract rheumatoid arthritis.

Now certainly not every woman whose husband dies gets rheumatoid arthritis. But the depth of emotional shock must approach the same deep feeling of loss, loneliness, despair, frustration, anger, and depression. This is a normal reaction to the death of any loved one.

What was it in Emily's case that caused her arthritis to result so closely following her husband's death? She'd never been troubled with joint distress before at any time that she could recall. She was in good physical condition. Her weight was ideal for her height and frame, she enjoyed good health and had always been a physically active person, and she was happy with her life as a housewife and mother. The only thing I could uncover in Emily's background, and I'd seen it before and many, many times since then, was that in Emily's family history there were numerous instances of what probably was rheumatoid arthritis—generally among the female members

How You Can Adjust Bone and Muscle to Stress

I like to view rheumatoid arthritis as a train. The cars of the train represent some type of genetic (hereditary) abnormality that *by itself* isn't enough to cause the disorder. The engine represents stress, and this can be emotional and/or physical stress. Taken by themselves, neither the engine nor the cars are a complete train, but link them together, and you have a complete train: You have rheumatoid arthritis.

Figure 4-1 illustrates this concept.

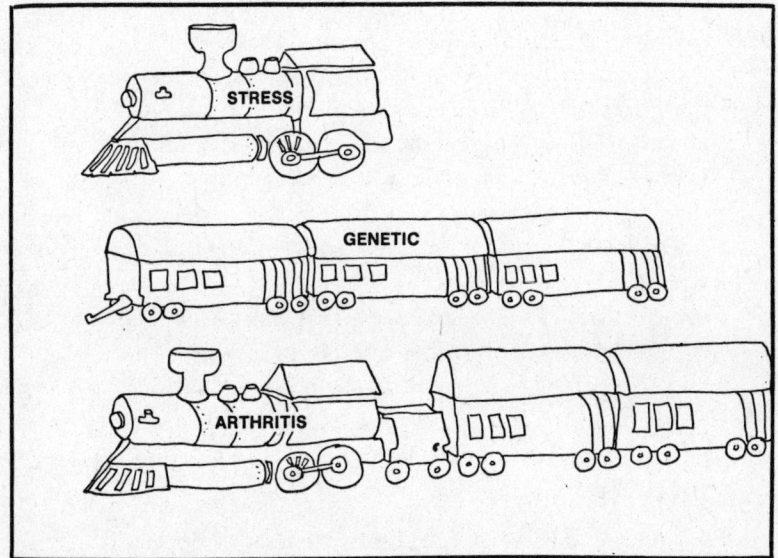

Figure 4-1

Medical evidence at the present time points quite strongly to the genetic problem having to do with the person's (family) immune system—the system that protects us all from the ravages of germs, viruses and other foreign invaders in the body. For some reason, the appearance of a stressful situation triggers a chain of chemical reactions which, because of something wrong in the body's normal response to such stress, causes "wild" antibodies to be formed (antibodies being the chemicals that destroy, for example, strep throat germs that attack the joints and joint structures). Why this happens isn't known at present, but medical researchers are looking for the answers.

Emily, in the meantime, discovered some important controls for her problem. I've listed them as follows:

1. Control of the acute joint attacks. She took aspirin in doses of three tablets four times a day at the first sign of joint trouble; then continued this level of aspirin intake for at least three or four weeks

even though her joint pain and stiffness disappeared within a few days or a week.

2. Increased use of her affected joints *when the acute phase subsided.* Emily started an exercise routine daily that involved her affected finger joints (squeezing a ball), her knee joint (deep knee bends—see Chapter 14 for method), and her right shoulder joint (push-ups—see Chapter 14). When she had a sudden flare-up, *only the joint or joints involved were exempt from the exercises.*

3. Learning to handle stress. Emily learned that whenever stress entered her life in any form, the first thing to do was to sit or lie down in a comfortable chair or in bed and take ten breaths. Then she focused her mind on the stressful situation, analyzed it, thought about it slowly and rationally, and reduced it to its basic terms. She learned to concentrate on dispelling the fear, the threat, the uncomfortable feeling that the stressful thing made her experience. She concentrated on an all-consuming feeling of calm and serenity—filled her mind with nothing but this feeling. Then she let the stressful situation enter into her mind slowly, a little at a time, and she "defused it" with her calm, serene attitude. She concentrated on the theme: "I will not let such a situation upset me again in the future." She repeated this 15 or 20 times, then put the matter out of her mind entirely.

In addition to this technique, Emily soon found out that in a few days, following the worst of the swelling and pain in her joints, she could use contrast packs with great benefit. This is the technique for such packs:

1. Apply an ice pack—made up of ice cubes wrapped in cloth or plastic—to the red, painful, or stiff joint. Allow it to chill the area for 10 or 15 minutes.

2. Have one or two fairly heavy wash cloths or clean rags soaking in a simmering saucepan of hot water on the stove while your ice pack is in place. (A hot water bottle on a moist cloth does as well.)

3. When the time is up, remove the ice pack and wring out the hot water soaked cloth slightly (don't burn your skin!) and apply the moist heat to the area for the same amount of time, replacing the wash cloth with a fresh one that has been soaking in the simmering hot water when the first cloth begins to cool.

4. After 10 or 15 minutes, replace the heat with the ice again. Then, use the moist heat once again. Keep up this alternating hot and cold

How You Can Adjust Bone and Muscle to Stress 75

packing for 45 minutes or an hour. You can repeat this routine two or more times during the day.

Figure 4-2 summarizes the use of heat and cold.

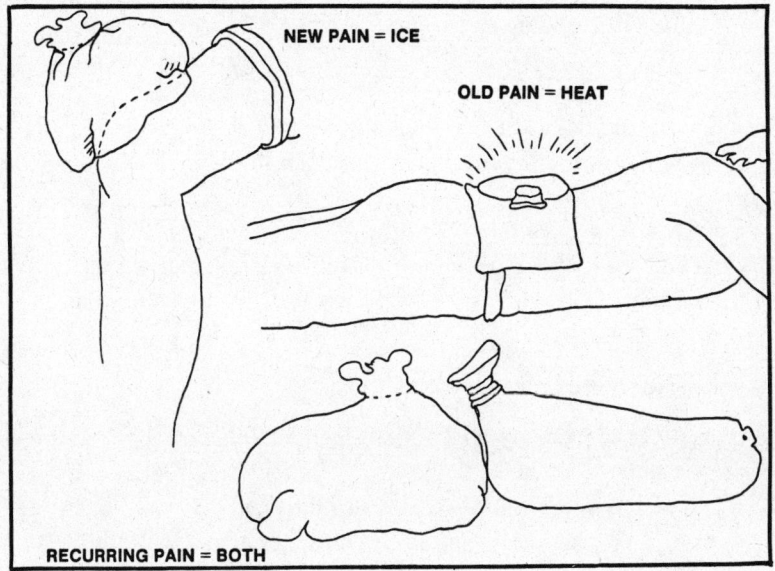

Figure 4-2

Jake P. finds stress point

Prior to the days of the medicines that control the recurrence of gouty arthritis attacks, I had occasion to treat a patient named Jake P. whose gouty attacks seemed to be occurring more and more frequently in spite of both our attempts to control them.

One day I was called to Jake's house to see him with yet another sudden bout of gout. I found him in his front room, his right foot up on a foot stool and his first toe joint swollen to three times its normal size. And it was red as a beet. Jake was in misery. As I checked him over, I noticed something I hadn't noticed before. Jake's breath smelled strongly of alcohol—he'd been drinking quite heavily, though I wouldn't call him an alcoholic.

Later on when Jake's gout began to subside, I quizzed him closely about his drinking and found that of the last ten attacks of gout he'd suffered, eight had followed an especially heavy bout of drinking—social drinking of the type that most people would call normal or usual. We had a long talk about it and finally Jake agreed not to have any alcohol for a period of six months. I made him promise faithfully and had his wife listen to the promise as well. Incredibly, Jake didn't have a single attack of gout during the next six months. This made a believer of him, and although he had an occasional glass of wine in the evening, the more heavy drinking stopped and so did about three quarters of his gouty arthritis.

Some time later, Jake, like so many others with gout, was lucky in that researchers came up with two potent and effective medicines for controlling the process in the body's protein metabolism that seems to cause gout. And like so many others, Jake hasn't had more than three mild attacks of gout in the past ten years.

But this is significant: All three of these milder attacks occurred following heavy drinking again—drinking because of the *stress* of work, family problems and the like. Gout, too, seems to be precipitated by stressful situations.

The many forms of stress

Stress comes in many packages. Emotional shock, as you've seen, is stressful for some people. But lesser mental strain over a long period of time can be just as stressful. And there are various physical types of stress—the sudden trauma of a broken elbow, for example, or a bout with influenza, or a surgical procedure, or the stress and strain of being overweight.

To help you counteract stress, I offer the following recipe:

1. Providing you have no physical handicaps that would prevent it, throw yourself into an exercise routine of some type when you feel high emotional stress building up. Swim, bicycle, jog, punch a bag, do sit-ups or push-ups, play tennis—anything to work up a really good sweat for 30 minutes or so.

2. Practice one of the forms of meditation. Do yoga, practice biofeedback, take up a musical instrument, develop an interest in an academic subject or hobby that interests you and that you really have to study to master—bury yourself in the depths of such an interest frequently during times of stress.

3. Plan to get away from the site of the stress, even if it's for only a short time. Do it frequently at times of high stress. Get out of the house. Visit friends, neighbors, relatives. Get involved in your community with anything entirely outside family ties. Spend some time helping others who appear to have problems of their own; you'll be surprised at how this melts away what appear to be "crushing responsibilities and demands" made on you by others.

How You Can Adjust Bone and Muscle to Stress 77

4. When you are able to foresee stress coming up, take steps to reduce its effects on you. If surgery is in the offing, talk to others who have had it. Get yourself in as good a physical shape as you can before surgery and practice deep breathing and isometric exercises that you can do in bed, as discussed further along in this book. Reduce your weight to reasonable levels if you're overweight, and adhere to principles of good nutrition.

5. If there has been a death of a loved one, someone close to you for whom you feel a great loss, grieve fully—let it all go; don't hold back anything you feel—let the depression that inevitably follows come, *but let it go in a reasonable time.* A good way to start lifting such a blue mood is to fasten your attention and your interest on others who need your help, get yourself moving physically, *get active.* And at the same time, think about how your lost one would like you to be were he or she still alive. Would he really be pleased if you continued to mope and drag yourself around? You can do yourself and the departed spirit the best favor by living your life to its fullest. After all, you too will someday depart from this world. Do you want those who remain to be immobilized from that point on because of it? Of course you don't.

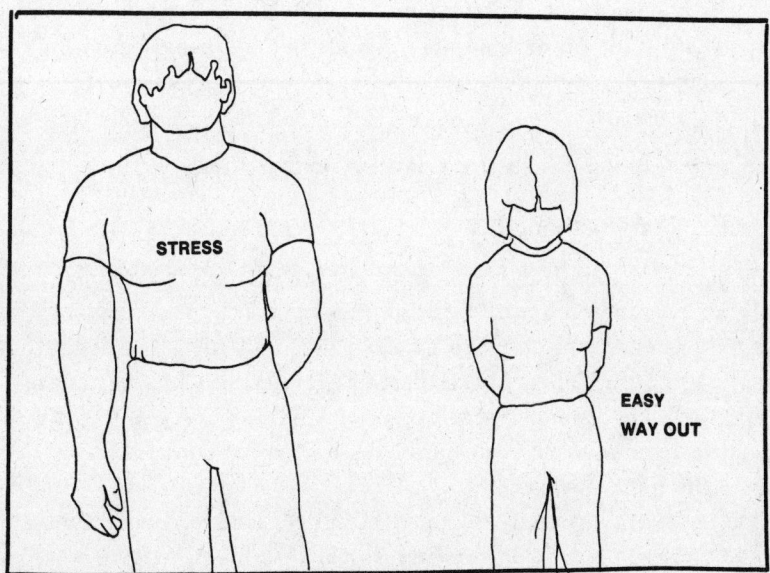

Figure 4-3

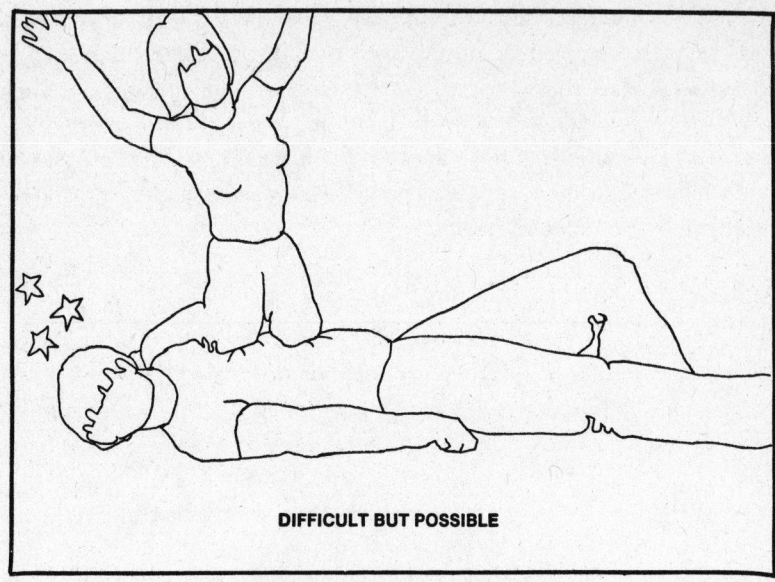

DIFFICULT BUT POSSIBLE

Figure 4-3 (continued)

6. Avoid taking tranquilizers and other potent medicines at times of stress if at all possible. They will only put road blocks in front of your recovery.
7. Finally, avoid self-pity at all costs. You're a mature human being fully capable of caring for your own needs and fulfilling your own destiny. If you have strong religious beliefs, use them to help you become strong—make your beliefs become a *positive* influence on your activities.

Figure 4-3 emphasizes your part in fighting stress.

Helen W. fights osteoarthritis

A patient named Helen W., a woman in her late 50's, was plagued by "lumbago," as she called it. What she meant was that her low back had been giving her trouble for five or six years, and it was getting steadily worse. In addition, Helen noticed that her left knee joint had started "acting up" and the pain was noticeably worse over the past two years. Helen also noticed the appearance of some hard bumps around the joints of some of her fingers—the joints just below her nails.

Helen didn't have redness about her knee, back or finger joints, and she didn't have a whole lot of swelling either. In addition, in spite of the long standing complaints, the joints involved weren't actually deformed and her pain was more or less steady, day in and day out, and didn't suddenly flare

How You Can Adjust Bone and Muscle to Stress

up. All this was in contrast to Emily's problem that I spoke of earlier in this chapter. What Helen had was yet another form of arthritis, a kind called osteoarthritis.

When I first examined Helen, she was suffering from a good deal more than arthritis—she was very blue and down on herself. "I'm wearing out," she told me. "I'm no good to anyone or for anything!" So I sat Helen down and pointed out a few things. First, I said that I thought she had a right to be mad at having her joints begin to wear down. After all, nobody likes to see parts of their body show signs of wear and tear. But I told her that I didn't think she had the right to start running herself into the ground because of it, nor did I think she had any right to extend such a mood to others.

Helen had a good husband and her three youngsters were grown and married. I asked her how she knew she "wasn't any good to anyone." She began to cry and shake her head. When she was a little more settled (a good cry is sometimes best let go until it's finished), I said, "Look, you have a good man for a husband and three perfectly normal and healthy children who are married. Your behaving like this isn't helping them much—and believe me, they will continue to welcome your help. So will your husband. And so will you. The first thing that we're going to do is to reduce some of the things that add stress to your joints; and by the way, just because some of your joints are showing signs of wear doesn't mean they're worn out. Take care of them, and they'll function for you until you're ninety."

Helen seemed ready for help. Here's what she did to awaken a new spark for her life:

1. Helen was about 30 pounds overweight, most of it around her abdomen and thighs. She started a 1500 calorie a day diet. The extra heft she carried around her middle wasn't helping her sore back one bit, and the added strain of extra weight above her knee joints added more stress than she needed on her sore knees.

2. Next, an exercise routine. This twice a day period included sit-ups for her weak, sagging belly (and remember, doing sit-ups also tones the back muscles). The routine also included the cradle rock (Figure 4-4) and the standing arch (Figure 4-5). One of her exercise sessions was to be done first thing on arising in the morning. Why? Because most osteoarthritis sufferers notice that they are stiffest when they first get out of bed in the morning. What better time to "unstiffen" and get yourself ready for the day? (Sure it hurts at first, but the pain soon lessens as the exercises progress!)

3. Two of Helen's daughters worked. I asked Helen to volunteer to house-watch or baby sit once or twice a week when her daughters

needed it. (The daughters actually over protected their mother in trying to help her with her "lumbago.") This took some doing, but in the end it worked in proving to Helen that she was an important person in many ways.

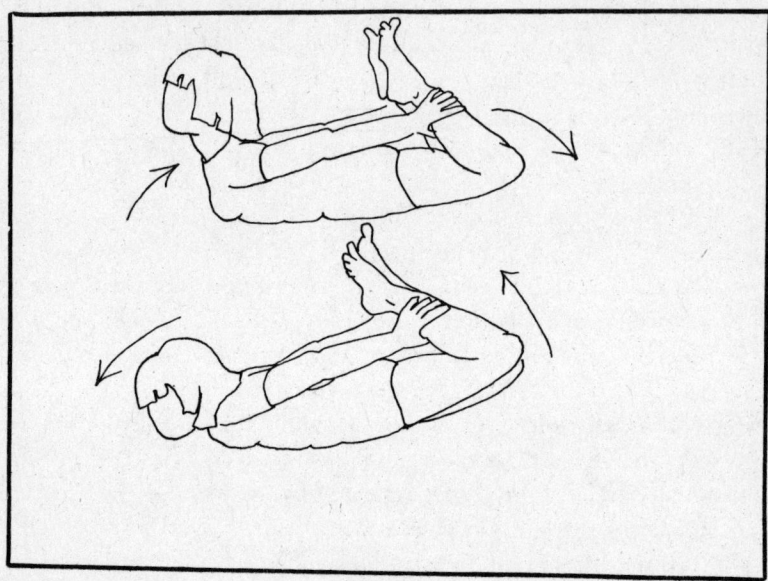

Figure 4-4

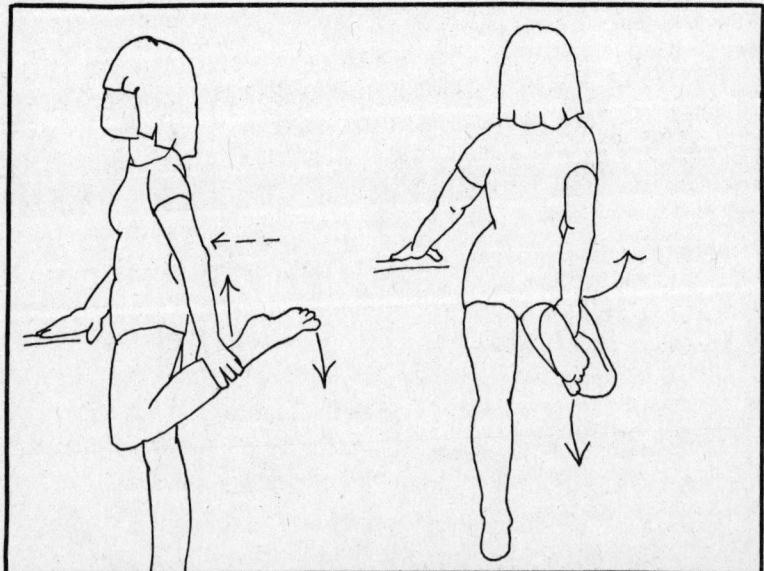

Figure 4-5

How You Can Adjust Bone and Muscle to Stress

4. I removed all of Helen's medicines (she took four different pills every day) and limited her to just two: aspirin as necessary, and a muscle spasm relaxer which helped her with her exercise routines. Later, Helen was able to give up this drug as well.
5. Helen, I learned some time later, had quite a talent for oil painting. With the help of her family, she was enticed to take some art lessons sponsored by the local YWCA. She enjoyed them, she enjoyed painting and is now painting and *selling* her work to this day. This had an extra bonus because painting was good for her stiff finger joints!

BIOFEEDBACK CAN HELP YOU

You've noticed that I've mentioned biofeedback several times thus far in the book. What is biofeedback? Isn't it something that requires expensive gadgetry and experts to teach you how to use it? Isn't it something that goes on in medical center laboratories? The answer in each case is yes, but neither gadgetry nor a laboratory are necessary.

Biofeedback has been used for years and years by city and country doctors alike to help their patients get better. The only difference between what they did (and still do) and what is called biofeedback in the fancy laboratories of today is that the old-fashioned docs didn't call it biofeedback, and they used it often without realizing they were using a very effective tool in combating the ills of human disease.

Elements of biofeedback

To utilize biofeedback for your problems, consider the following points, practice them, and adapt them to your particular situation:

1. Find a place that's quiet and free from all distractions. A good time and a good place for this setting is just after you climb into bed at night following your nightly exercise routine.
2. Reduce what you want to "feed back" to your body to the simplest terms—the bare necessities. For example, if you want to reduce pain, think of the painful area (such as your knee joint), visualize the sore knee joint in your mind's eye, and let no other thought intrude on the picture.
3. Your knee joint is sore—this is the message going to your brain from your knee joint. In your mind, accept the message of pain, concentrate on the nerves to your knee joint getting numb, repeat this "getting numb" message back to your sore knee joint over and over ("My right knee joint is sore. I'm aware that the pain is to tell

me there is something wrong in the joint. Now I want the pain to diminish—it will diminish," etc.) at least 20 times.

4. Then put the entire matter out of your mind. Purposely think of something else or simply drift off to sleep. It will take some practice, but once you've mastered the technique, you can actually cause such pain to be diminished by feeding back from your mind to your body that which you want your body to do.

Frank O'H. fights low back pain

Utilizing biofeedback techniques, a patient of mine named Frank O'H. helped his chronically aching low back pain, the result of an injury at work in a foundry, and was able to get back to the heavy work he used to do when his pain was controlled without further trouble. Here's how Frank did it.

1. Part of Frank's low back pain problem was muscle spasm—tightening of his low back muscles after very little stress or strain. He concentrated on his low back muscles being tight and then suggested that they relax. He fed back the message to relax over and over again each time he concentrated. Soon he could actually feel his back muscles loosen up.

2. Yet another part of Frank's low back pain was simple irritation of nerve endings that persisted after the muscle spasm was relieved (X-rays had shown nothing wrong with Frank's spinal discs, a subject I'll talk about in detail later on). For this, Frank concentrated on the area becoming numb. He repeated this over and over. Very soon, Frank was able to quiet down considerable back pain after two or three minutes of biofeedback concentration.

STRESS BREEDS FRUSTRATION

Another state that is provoked by stress is a mental attitude that invariably works against you if you let it go. Continued stress, in other words, can cause certain changes in your personality, and such changes can and do provoke a series of physical problems as a result.

Consider this series of events:

You're under stress from some cause. It begins to "get on your nerves." Soon, you muster emotional defenses against the continued unremitting stress, or chance losing control altogether. Your personality changes—you grow morose, grumpy, blue, even grouchy all the time.

After a while, all this grouchiness and blue mood builds up tension in your mind because it isn't like your usual self to behave this way. The tension has to be let out some way—it can occur as a bellyache, as cramps in your intestines, as a headache, as palpitations of your heart, and as pain in joints.

Julie V.'s interesting case

A good example of what unrelieved stress can do to you is illustrated by the case of a middle-aged woman I know named Julie V. Julie was in perfect physical health. She enjoyed good nutrition and kept her weight within normal bounds.

She had been married to a very difficult husband—difficult in the sense that he was completely without feeling for anyone but himself. He was inconsiderate, sloppy, lazy, and expected to be waited upon hand and foot. He was the typical spoiled brat who never grew up. During the raising of their two kids, it was Julie who got up each and every time there was a cry in the night. It was Julie who bought their clothes, took them to the park and to cub and girl scouts, drove them all over town as teenagers, and was their confidential listener when problems came up.

Julie was not only mother and father to the kids, she was also the main breadwinner in the family, having worked as a legal secretary for most of her married life. This she did even when hubby wasn't working, which was a good deal of the time, owing to his talent for not getting along with anyone with whom he worked.

Julie was the type to make the ultimate sacrifice. She kept up with this state of affairs through hell and high water. Julie was the long-suffering type who rarely complained, yet the lines of marital stress wore deep grooves in her makeup. She reacted to this situation by becoming a manipulator. That is, she unconsciously coped with her stress by causing people to feel sorry for her, by placing others in a position of being obligated to her, and by actually setting one person against another for no obvious reason. In short, Julie became a real shrew.

When I first met Julie, she complained of a pain in her low back area that seemed to radiate into both buttocks. It was generally worse at night when she came home from work. It was for some reason, I discovered in talking to her further, also worse during weekends and holidays, though she hadn't noticed this phenomenon until I'd asked her. A complete workup of Julie's case, including X-rays of her lower spine, revealed completely normal bones and joints. Examination was just as inconclusive: There were tender areas in her low back and buttocks, but on no two examinations were the painful areas in the same location. In describing the pain to me, Julie would term it "burning or stinging" or a feeling of "sharp tingling." Occasionally, the pain was "just a toothache located in my bottom."

None of the usual conservative therapy seemed to afford relief for Julie, and this only confirmed my original suspicions that Julie's problem was stress induced.

This turned out to be the sequence of Julie's problem:

Completely unhappy married life—stress reaction to it—stress relief through manipulating (setting up) others—pain in her buttocks. Why the pain? Because deep inside Julie knew what she was doing to others, but couldn't help it. She had a conscience but it wouldn't allow her to face the real problem: her irascible husband.

In other words, Julie's slobbish husband literally gave her a chronic pain in the rump! (See how the mind can take a common phrase and make a reality of it?)

When Julie was finally confronted with the evidence that she was manipulating others and then getting the pain afterwards, and when she was finally able to admit that her husband drove her up a wall, she proceeded to get rid of her pain. In Julie's case, it ended in a separation from her husband.

Not all stressful situations end up so drastically, but this case serves to show what can happen when stress is buried rather than defused.

SUMMARY

1. The causes of bone, muscle and arthritic disorders are numerous and many of them are not well understood at the present time. There are no miracle cures for this disease, but there is a great deal you can do to get it under control.
2. Good nutrition, ideal weight for your height and frame, proper rest, exercise, and the breaking up of stress are essential for keeping arthritis under control.
3. Proper application of ice, heat, and the specific medication, if needed, for the specific kind of joint and tendon problems are also necessary.
4. Stress takes many forms. It can't be avoided, but can be handled properly. One of the most important ways in which you can handle stress is to learn biofeedback techniques. In addition, proper muscle toning, getting away from the stress on occasion, proper grieving following the death of a loved one, and the avoidance of self-pity and unneeded drugs are essential.

5

How You Can Relieve Pain and Manage Painful Muscles and Joints

In this chapter I will describe the practical management of sprains, strains and fractures, how they occur, how you recognize them, and what you can do about them. I want to show you what you can do at home to help them heal and to keep things going smoothly when they do heal so you're ready to pick up and take off as always, and not be in such bad shape that it takes two months or more just to recover from inactivity.

There is a common affliction of bones that comes on with the natural process of aging, as well as being artificially caused by a variety of things. The disorder is called osteoporosis. We'll have a look at this ailment and see what can be done about it.

There are also a variety of painful conditions that don't involve injury directly, but are just as disabling nevertheless. One of these conditions is called phantom limb pain—the kind that comes on, for example, following amputation of any part of a limb. We'll examine this and other such ailments in this chapter and learn how you can apply useful therapy on your own to fight such maladies.

Included in these afflictions of limbs is another important, though fortunately rather unusual condition known as causalgia. We'll look at causalgia and deal with its control.

STRAINS, SPRAINS AND FRACTURES

The words strain, sprain and fracture represent progressive stages of injury to muscle, tendon and ligament—that is, a simple pull or excess tightening of one of your muscles may *strain* it. The injury is mild and usually clears in a couple of days. A wrenching or twisting injury, as in the severe in-turning of your ankle joint, for example, may *sprain* your ankle.

With a sprain there is overstretching—as with a strain—but there is also tearing of fibers of ankle ligaments, and there is usually a certain amount of bleeding as well, characterized by "black and blue marks" overlying the injured part that eventually gravitate downward toward the most distant part—the foot—and even the toes in the case of an ankle sprain. There is also considerable swelling around most sprains.

When a bone is *cracked* or *fractured*, the most severe of this group of injuries, there are all the signs of sprain that I've just mentioned, in addition to which there is so much pain that weight bearing or any use of the injured part is almost impossible. There may also be angulation along the injured site—that is, if your forearm is broken or fractured, there is an interruption in the usually straight line of your forearm.

It's very difficult to tell a moderately severe sprain from a fracture. Better put, it's difficult to tell if you've fractured your ankle joint in addition to having sprained it when swelling, black and blue signs, and severe pain are present.

Dealing with strains

Many people are particularly subject to straining muscles and joints. We all strain some muscles during our lifetime. Strains usually come on after a sudden jerking motion of a particular limb or the back during the course of routine chores or work. Occasionally, strains don't become obvious until the end of your working day when you sit down to relax—then the arm, shoulder, back or leg lets you know it's been pulled too hard in connection with something you did and may not have even noticed at the time.

The secret to dealing with strains is to put the member at rest for as long as it takes to heal it. This doesn't necessarily mean that you have to completely immobilize the part, but just rest it for most of the day.

Joyce P. learns a trick

A woman I know had a particular problem with her right hamstring muscle. This is the large muscle group in the back of your thigh that acts to bend your lower leg at the knee joint. Joyce worked in a hardware store and found herself having to squat down to reach floor level bins and counters to retrieve and replace certain items that her customers needed. Every once in a while, Joyce noticed that her right hamstring gave her fits after a particularly heavy day at work with a lot of squatting down. She noticed that the pain began about six inches above her knee joint and extended down to and including the large cords directly in back of her knee. To put things at

How You Can Relieve Pain 87

rest when this happened, Joyce fashioned a cylinder of cardboard (see Chapter 6 for this technique) extending from about mid-thigh to just above her ankle.

Then she learned a more aesthetic technique with the help of her husband who fashioned a piece of leather of the same length as the cardboard—a piece that was reasonably soft and supple rather than too stiff—and made holes at both sides of the leather where they met at the side of Joyce's leg, just like the holes in your shoes. He fashioned laces from leather thongs to lace them firmly in place. By padding the back of her knee with foam rubber about half an inch thick, Joyce found that this made an excellent cylinder brace for her ailing hamstring muscle. The brace simply prevented her from *bending her knee*, yet she could walk (stiff-legged) for the couple of days it took for her hamstring pull to heal. Figure 5-1 shows Joyce's splint.

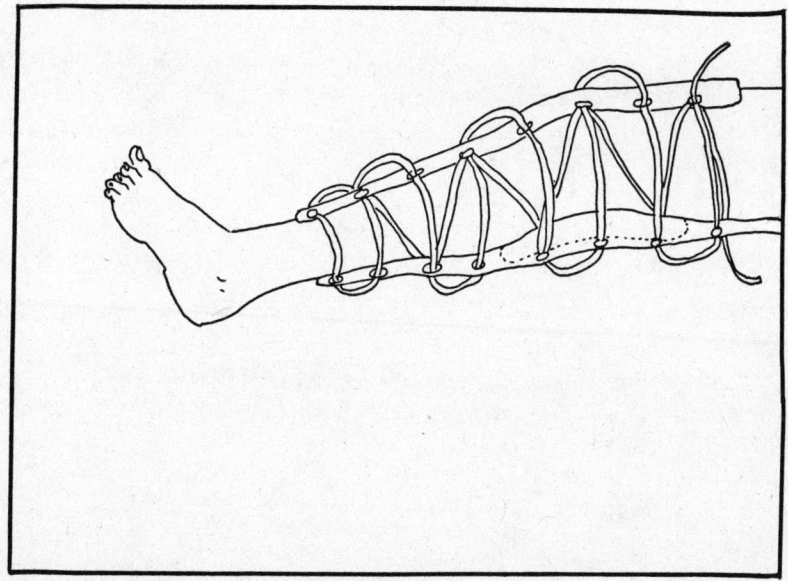

Figure 5-1

The caution here, as with splinting any joint, is to carefully pad the joint (in Joyce's case, the back of her knee joint) so that you don't put too much pressure on the blood vessels that are fairly near the surface at some points. This means you should make such splints *snug but not tight*. You can tell if you've got a splint too tight by a feeling of numbness and pain, usually below the area (for example in your foot if you're splinting a knee joint, or in your hand if you're splinting a wrist or forearm).

A rule of thumb

If the part of a splinted or casted extremity is *painful, numb, or feels cold* after you've applied the splint, take the splint off or have it taken off to allow your limb to rest, and reapply it a bit looser. Never leave on a splint or cast or even an Ace bandage if pain, numbness or coldness appear below the boundary of the splint.

What to do with sprains

A sprain can be more serious than most people are willing to give it credit for. The most common is an ankle sprain, and it's usually the result of severely and forcefully twisting your foot inward. The ligaments and vessels on the outside of your ankle are commonly involved with this sprain. The inside of your ankle can also be involved by a severe outward twist of your foot. Knee sprains are tricky. If you've sprained your knee (using the definition I've given) you can almost bet that you've done damage to internal ligaments—the ones supporting the outside of your knee joint—and possibly to your knee cartilage as well. This is a common football injury and can be caused by any sudden severe wrenching of your knee where your foot is planted firmly in the ground while your upper body and thigh make a sudden movement in the opposite direction. This kind of movement produces a shearing force on your knee, and damage invariably results.

Another rule of thumb

All sprains should be X-rayed to make certain that the bones involved are not fractured as well.

I can't count the number of ankles and knees I've seen where trouble has started because of failure to follow instructions from medical advisors regarding weight bearing and splinting.

Dan A. learns the hard way

The case of Dan A. is typical of dozens I've seen, usually in energetic young men who view ankle or knee injuries as "kid's stuff" and end up paying for their skepticism. Dan had severely turned his left ankle during a physical education class in high school. His doctor made certain it wasn't fractured by X-raying it, and put his injured ankle in a walking cast. This is a plaster cast from the toes up to about midway on the calf, equipped with a rubber heel appliance molded into the plaster sole, as in Figure 5-2. Dan got tired of his cast and his ankle felt fine after only a week, so he took it off by soaking it in water and using shears to cut it away.

The trouble with this was that Dan went right back to physical education classes and his injured ankle, although it did not hurt, quickly

How You Can Relieve Pain

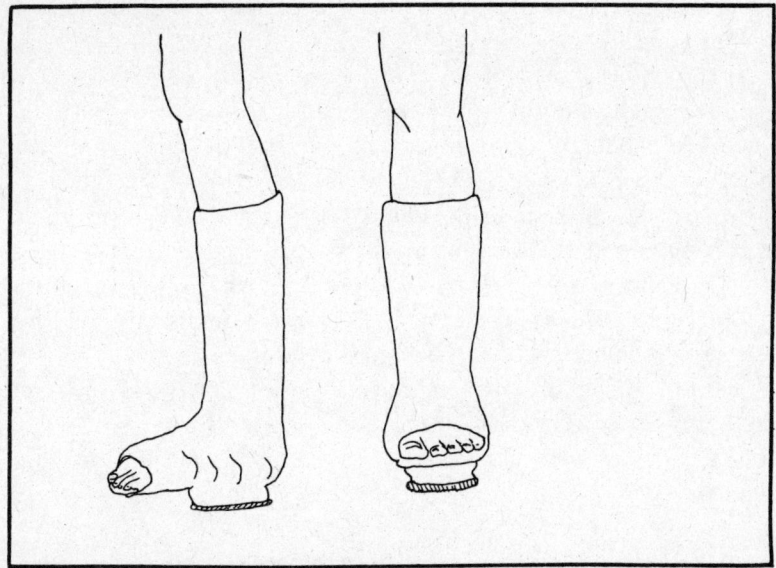

Figure 5-2

turned inward again because the supporting ligaments at the outside of his ankle joint hadn't healed (it takes at least six weeks to heal injured ligaments).

This time Dan wasn't so lucky (or unlucky). He fractured his ankle in three different places and the pieces had to be pulled together with metallic screws at surgery. Dan is sorry today that he was so headstrong and impatient—he has chronic arthritis in his left ankle. And all this could have been avoided had he listened to good advice!

How to deal with fractures: One more rule of thumb

If you suspect a fractured bone, try to immobilize (put at rest completely) the joint immediately above, and the joint or joints immediately below the area of the suspected fracture.

The reason for this is that the muscles that move the limb or other fractured part usually originate above the injured bone and they insert into the bone below the part that's fractured. If the upper and lower joints aren't put at rest, the muscles that arise and insert above and below may move the fractured bone and cause further damage.

There are many times, of course, when this isn't possible because of the unique location of the broken bone. Take the case of Lorrie P., for example. Lorrie was only 14 years old when she fell off a playground slide on extended arms and felt a sharp pain over the area of her left collar bone. By the time I saw her, a lump about the size of a hen's egg had developed over her collar bone about 2 inches from her shoulder joint. She'd fractured her collar bone.

Although this is a painful fracture, it generally isn't serious. What is needed with such an injury is a so-called butterfly strap. This can be made with an Ace bandage, a strip of any durable material cut about 3 inches wide and about 8 to 10 feet long, or with plaster over foam rubber (your medical advisor will need to use this latter method because it's tricky to apply). A square of sponge rubber may be placed over the fracture site. Figure 5-3 shows how this splint looks when applied correctly. The dressing should be an Ace bandage or strip of cloth applied with the shoulders forced backward so the strap will hold them in this position. In four to six weeks, this fracture will heal in a younger person. For the first two to three weeks, it also helps to place the arm on the side of such a fracture in a sling for most of the day as well. The technique for such a sling will be found in Chapter 6.

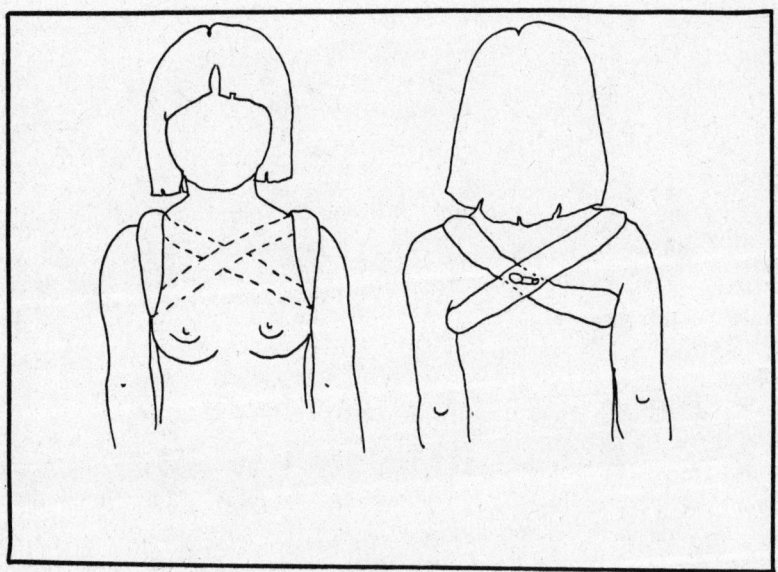

Figure 5-3

OSTEOPOROSIS

This sometimes distressing condition is most common in women between about 50 and 70 years old, although men may have it as well. The term osteoporosis has come to be applied to several rather unusual diseases of which osteoporosis (loss of bone tissue) is a part. By far the most common is the type that occurs without other disease, and try as medical scientists have, no good answer has been found as to what starts it off.

What happens is that the bones simply begin to lose their covering. The crystal lattice laid down onto the protein framework begins gradually and over long stretches of time to thin out. The process does not seem to be strictly a nutritional defect or to be caused by any other underlying trouble that we know.

Mildred fights osteoporosis

The case of Mildred J. is a good example of how osteoporosis starts, what it presents in the way of symptoms, and demonstrates, in my opinion, what is needed in the way of an attack on this vexing problem.

Mildred was a typical mother of three children who worked hard most of her life, who was a good and kind person to both her husband and her youngsters, and who, when her family was grown and mostly out of the house, gradually slipped into a much less hectic and slower life style than she'd had for the previous 25 years. Her family were patients of mine and fortunately none ever had serious trouble with their health. But the last time I saw Mildred for a yearly check-up, I noticed that she'd gained about 35 pounds over her previous weight, which was a bit high to begin with.

I had a long talk with her about this (as I'm sure you guessed by now), and put her on a diet and an exercise routine since she hadn't been getting nearly the amount of physical activity that she had even a year previously when her family was still in the home.

But I'm afraid Mildred didn't pay too much heed to this advice. She was socially active enough—took part in her Eastern Star work, was a member of a local bridge club, and enjoyed needlepoint and embroidery as hobbies—but all this, good as it was for Mildred's well-being, didn't get her up and moving as it should.

At any rate, about three years passed and though I had occasion to see her husband a couple of times in the office, I didn't see Mildred. Her husband always said his wife was doing well and was busily engaged in all of her "activities," none of which were physical kinds of activity. When Mildred turned 52, I had occasion to see her again. This time she had noticed some peculiar (for her) signs and symptoms. First of all, she noticed a sharp pain in her mid-back one night while turning over in bed. She thought it was a strained muscle, but the pain persisted—not severe enough to cause concern, just constant and aggravating. Some time later, she told me, she had some deep pelvic pain—distress over her pubis bone (the bone in front of the pelvis just behind the hair line of the pubis) and deep inside to this area. The pain was worse when she squatted down or walked for any length of time. Resting didn't seem to relieve it much.

There didn't seem to be any external signs of trouble, and Mildred was otherwise in the pink of condition—except for her weight, which she hadn't whittled down at all. X-rays of Mildred's back revealed that a vertebra midway down her spine was "wedged," that is, viewed from the side, the X-ray showed that instead of being the usual more or less square block of bone, the front part of the block was definitely narrowed down, making it look like a wedge instead of a square. Figure 5-4 shows the side view of a normal and an osteoporotic "wedge" vertebra.

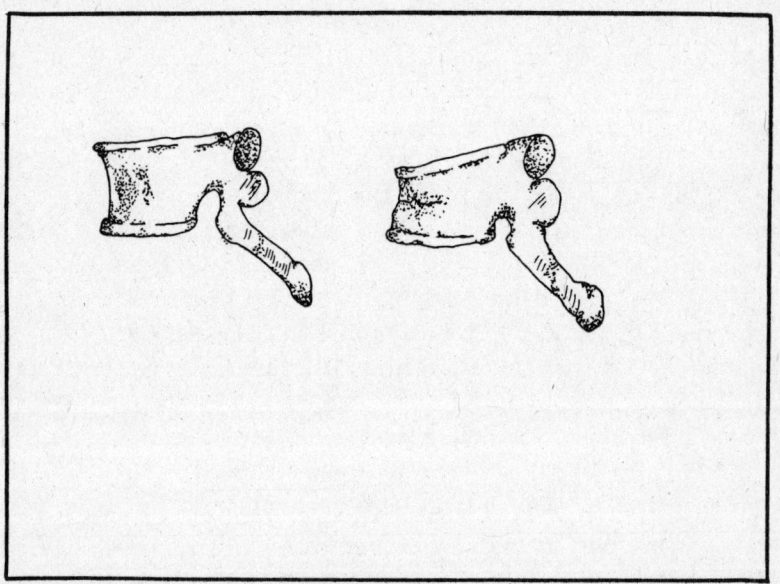

Figure 5-4

This wasn't serious, although it is a type of fracture called a "compression fracture," but it told the story. X-rays of her pelvic bones didn't show any fracture, but did show rather decided thinning out of the usual dense outer layer of all these bones.

What did all this add up to? A rather typical case of osteoporosis.

How Mildred managed her problems

As I said before, there seems to be no one specific cause for osteoporosis. Its main determinants seem to be as follows:

How You Can Relieve Pain

1. Comes on following menopause.
2. Comes on after a change from active to sedentary life style.
3. Is seen following anything that lowers nutritional status.
4. Is seen more often in people who let themselves get out of shape.

Mildred had let herself get into the rut of all four of the above danger areas. Let's take them one at a time.

Menopause

This quite natural state that women go through when they are done with childbearing is much maligned and much overrated as a cause of problems. This is not to say that it's easy—it's not. Some women have very uncomfortable hot flashes. Others go through an aggravating time with irritation and inflammation of the surface lining of their vaginas. Most have a siege with emotional instability—they're easily upset, nervous, and irritable.

The first two of these distressing symptoms, hot flashes and vaginal irritation, can easily be controlled with the addition of estrogen medication, and as a matter of fact, are the only two indications for using estrogen, in my opinion, during menopause. As they come under control, the estrogen dose should be gradually diminished until it's stopped altogether. The estrogen should be given orally—not by shots.

There are some who would recommend starting estrogen medicines for Mildred's problem, but I didn't and wouldn't now. Why? Because in my experience the possible dangers of side effects outweigh the very slight effect estrogens have been shown to have on osteoporosis.

Change in life style

It is tempting to slip into a "life of leisure" when the activities of raising a family are over (at least as far as the physical aspects are concerned). This commonly occurs at or near the time of menopause in women, but even if it doesn't, you readers who are women should take a vow today not to let it happen to you.

Take up at least one sport when your family of youngsters begins to grow up. It can be golf, tennis, hiking, fishing, skiing, camping or any number of others. Just pick one and stick with it.

Take a look at yourself in the mirror. Is the flab hanging loosely from double chin to thighs? Is there a jelly roll developing around your middle? Do those tissues sag and roll when you extend your arms? If so, there are diet and exercise routines to think about. Not only to think about—to start *today!*

Nutrition

It's true, of course, that the crystalline lattice—the outside layer of your bones—is primarily calcium. But since there is no evidence that ordinary osteoporosis is caused by a calcium shortage as such, there is no good reason to start gobbling down bunches of food containing calcium.

It does pay, however, to ensure that you do take in what is considered usual amounts of calcium. If you have anything like a well-balanced diet, it's difficult *not* to have adequate calcium since it is abundant in milk and dairy products, nuts and nut oils, green leafy vegetables, and fish. The amount found in most vitamin/mineral supplements should assure you of adequate calcium if you take one pill, tablet or capsule daily.

The same is true to a lesser extent of vitamin D, which is necessary for adequate calcium metabolism. Sunlight, with the production of a suntan, will add vitamin D as will pasteurized milk and fish liver oils. A single capsule of a vitamin/mineral supplement will provide adequate amounts of this vitamin as well.

It is also important that adequate *protein* be ingested. The reason for this is that the calcium crystals are laid down on a protein matrix in bone and this matrix (base layer) must be present before bone can be formed.

For details of a nutritionally balanced diet, see Chapter 14 in this book, as well as my earlier book, *The Biofeedback Diet: A Doctor's Revolutionary Approach*.

Conditioning

Yes, conditioning is quite important to the control of osteoporosis. A better term would be *pre*conditioning because, for example, if Mildred had paid some attention to this *before* she reached menopause, she would be having far less of a problem with her osteoporosis today ... and so will you if you'll start your conditioning program now!

Continued good muscle tone, as I've mentioned before, stimulates metabolic activity in the bones from which muscle tendons arise and into which they insert. The more of this activity you generate, the stronger your bones will stay. So the key to the control of osteoporosis is *to begin before it starts by keeping your entire body in reasonable physical tone through some kind of daily exercise routine*.

Figure 5-5 summarizes your best management and control of osteoporosis.

How You Can Relieve Pain 95

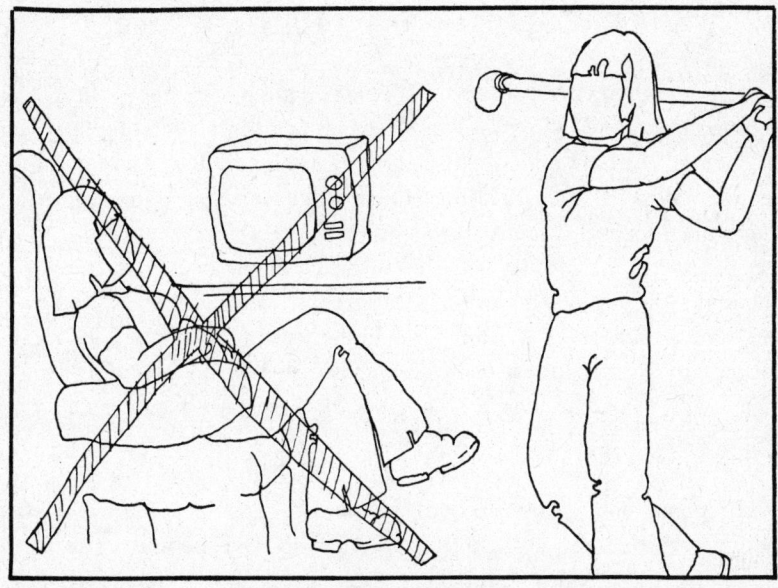

Figure 5-5

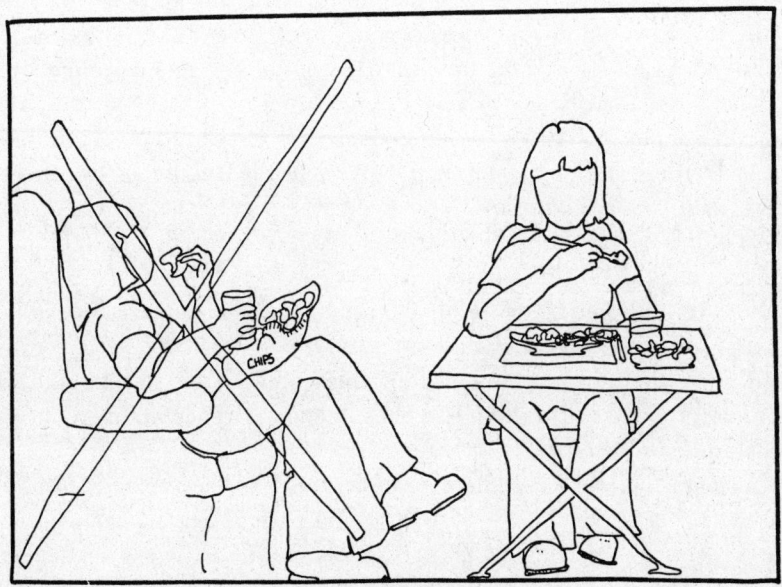

Figure 5-5 (continued)

THE PROBLEM OF THE PHANTOM LIMB

Problems that revolve around the so-called "phantom limb" are numerous and varied. The problem arises among those unfortunate enough to have something happen to them that requires amputation of part of a limb, sometimes most of it, in order to prevent serious, sometimes fatal consequences for your whole organism.

Serious trauma (injury) is the most common cause for having to amputate (sever) part or all of a limb. Such injuries usually occur as a result of vehicular or industrial accidents in which there is widespread destruction of tissues, muscles, nerves, bones, and arteries in an extremity—much more damage than can possibly be repaired even with modern surgical techniques.

Yet another cause for amputation of a limb is the aging process. As we grow older, we sometimes outlive our body's capacity to prevent some degenerative processes from taking place. This is especially true of the inside linings of arteries and veins, the vital blood vessels that course through your body and into your arms, hands, legs, and feet.

If the piling up of fatty tissue and the deposition of mineral salts in them reaches a certain point, a major vessel (for example, the one to your lower leg) might suddenly become unable to bring enough blood with its life-sustaining oxygen to your lower leg and foot. A condition called "dry" gangrene could set in, and the limb may have to be severed above the area that is not being supplied with enough blood.

Such surgery nowadays is safe enough and solves the problem quite well. And with modern artificial limb manufacturing techniques by experts in their field, you have an excellent chance of being able to get around and do most of the things you used to be able to do even though almost all of a leg or arm may have to be sacrificed.

However, in some people who undergo this kind of surgery, a peculiar and aggravating situation may develop some time after surgery—generally delayed until well after the wound from the amputation is healed and the stump is sound and well again. The phenomenon of "phantom limb" takes various routes.

In some, there is a definite sensation that the removed leg or arm (or hand or foot) is still present—as though the severed part appears like a ghost (hence the term "phantom") and feels as though it has reattached itself. Most amputees have a certain amount of this after their surgery but the process gradually and steadily fades away with the passage of time.

With others, however, there is more than just the "phantom." There is pain in the ghost foot or hand as well, or there may be a burning sensation, a

How You Can Relieve Pain

feeling of icy coldness, a feeling of needle pricking as though the phantom part has "gone to sleep."

I've seen patients in whom the pain in the phantom part disappeared only to lodge on the true stump that remained and then finally disappear. I've seen others in whom the phantom was still hanging around for as long as two years after the surgery.

Al McK. exorcises phantom

A young man I know named Al McK. had a heavy iron ingot dropped accidentally onto his lower leg and foot at the foundry where he worked. The injury crushed his left ankle and foot quite badly and surgeons did everything they possibly could to save his foot, including a delicate bridging of one of the main arteries from his lower leg to his foot that was destroyed in the accident.

The operation worked well for a few days; then, without warning, the new vessel formed a clot and the blood supply was severely compromised to Al's left foot. The surgeons amputated at a point above his ankle where the blood supply was still adequate to meet demands. Al came through the surgery well and his stump healed without incident. But his "phantom" began to visit him and it was quite painful.

His stump was examined carefully and no problems were seen. The bone ends were well rounded and the muscles carefully brought around the

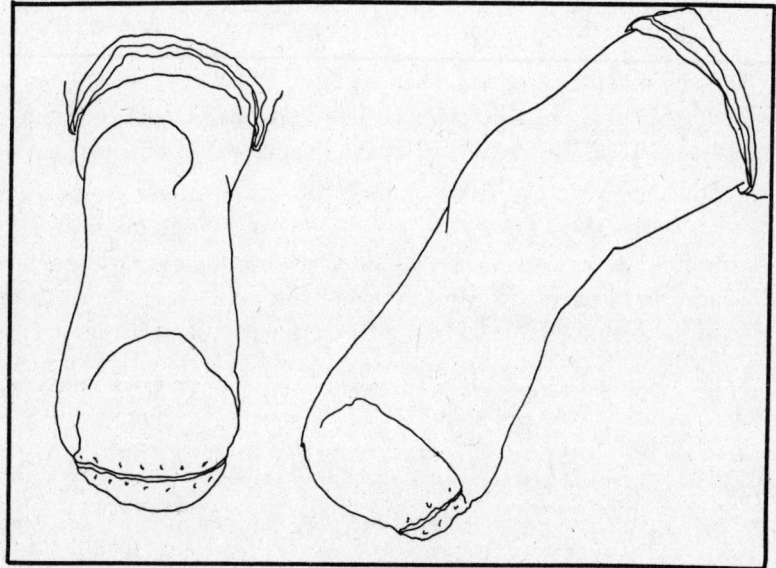

Figure 5-6

end of the stump where they formed an adequate cushion. There was no sign of neuroma—blobs of overgrown nerve tissue that sometimes occur at the ends of severed nerves—and the blood supply to Al's stump was very good. Figure 5-6 shows a well healed amputation stump like Al's.

His doctors tried local injections of anesthetics and cortisone to reduce any possibility of inflammatory reaction. This worked for a time, but then the phantom pain returned. Vigorous physical therapy was begun—massage of the stump, exercise of the lower leg muscles, local moist heat packs and the like—all to no avail.

Then one of the doctors called in a colleague who had been using biofeedback techniques with good results in other conditions to see if this might possibly help reduce Al's distressing phantom pain. The following technique was used to teach Al a biofeedback method he could use himself:

1. With the lights dimmed in his hospital room and with no visitors to distract him, Al was taught to concentrate on his missing foot and ankle, now amputated. He formed a picture of it in his mind's eye and allowed no other thoughts to enter. He concentrated on the pain that the "phantom" was causing.

2. He next allowed the picture of the severed foot and ankle to slowly disappear in his mind's eye. He concentrated on the thought: "My foot and ankle are gone. If my foot and ankle are gone, they can produce no pain or discomfort." He repeated this thought over and over in his mind as the "picture" of the amputated foot and ankle gradually disappeared.

3. For reinforcement, Al was then taught to concentrate on this thought: "There will be complete and total numbness from my stump down." He repeated this over and over in his mind as well.

4. Following step 3, Al was tutored by the therapist to completely erase the picture from his mind and concentrate on anything he wanted (except for his foot, ankle, or anything connected with his accident or surgery), usually something pleasant such as camping in the mountains, a favorite pastime for Al before his injury.

At first nothing happened. Al was discouraged and not at all convinced that such "nonsense" would work anyway. However, his therapist saw him every day for two weeks and convinced him that it was at least worth a try. Soon Al was doing his biofeedback routine three times a day: on waking up in the morning, during the middle of the day, and just before dozing off to sleep at night.

Within two more weeks, Al admitted that his painful phantom was much better. In six weeks he had no pain at all! His therapist instructed Al

How You Can Relieve Pain

to continue his routine at least once a day even though he was rid of his pain, preferably just before going to bed.

In another two weeks, Al was fitted with a prosthetic device (artificial lower leg and foot), and in another month, with diligent practice and the help of the Physical Medicine Department at the hospital, his gait was so smooth that no one could tell he wore an artificial limb.

In my opinion, this technique, or one similar to it, has great potential for all kinds of problems concerning chronic pain and distress. I've used it many times on patients with a variety of ailments of bone, muscle and joint with success at least equal to all the other techniques and therapies I've seen employed.

It can't and shouldn't be classified as a miracle cure or as a panacea for all ills. And it doesn't work for everyone who tries it. Sometimes this is because individuals who try it aren't convinced it *can* work. This is a must if success is to be forthcoming. At other times, it fails because the person directing its use isn't too convinced himself! And such lack of confidence rubs off on his patient.

But if you don't expect miracles right away, and if you're willing to open your mind to new things even though they may sound "weird," you may be pleasantly surprised at how various biofeedback techniques can help.

We'll be talking further along in this book about how others have applied this technique to their problems with success; not always total success, but success nevertheless.

CAUSALGIA PAIN

The term "causalgia" was coined many years ago to describe the kind of pain and discomfort often felt in a limb—hand, foot or leg—following the passage of some time after an injury.

Causalgia can follow a healed fracture, for instance. Or it can be seen with a severe wrenching injury, such as in your neck following a sprain after a rear-end collision in a car. The pain and distress (causalgia can also take the form of "burning" and just plain irritability of the skin over a certain area) can be near the original injury or it can be quite a distance away from the injury. In a sprained neck, for example, the distress may be felt in your shoulder, upper arm, or even in your forearm and hand.

It isn't always clear why causalgia plagues some people following injury, and fortunately it's not common. But when it occurs, it does raise Cain in the limb involved.

Most medical people feel that causalgia has something to do with injury or trauma to the special nerve endings located in the walls of surrounding blood vessels in the extremity that has sustained an injury.

These special nerves are known as autonomic nerves and they control the size (the inside diameter) of arteries and veins. They also control such functions as sweating, the sensations of heat and cold, and the supply of blood to tiny hair follicles. It isn't uncommon in causalgia to notice that skin hairs surrounding the area involved fall out, creating a bald spot on an arm or leg. Nor is it unusual to notice the absence of sweating in an area of an arm or leg.

In any event, it's possible that in a fracture (even though it heals perfectly well) or in a severe sprain, the roots of large nerves (their beginnings higher up in an extremity or close to the shoulder joint, for example) may be bruised or traumatized. This indirect injury to the nerve endings in blood vessels may be the cause of causalgia.

Rose R. duels with causalgia

A patient I recall named Rose R. fractured both bones of her lower right leg while skiing one winter. This type of "skier's fracture" is quite common on the slopes of winter resorts where skiing is popular. Figure 5-7 shows this rather common fracture. Rose's fracture wasn't especially bad nor was it complicated. It healed nicely following reduction under local anesthesia, the application of a plaster cast from her toes to mid-thigh for four weeks, and a shorter plaster cast from toes to just below her knee for another four weeks. Physical therapy and an exercise routine following removal of the second cast seemed to restore normal strength and stability to Rose's knee, calf, ankle, and foot muscles that were weakened by the prolonged inactivity of being in two casts.

About nine months later, her leg having returned to an apparently normal state, Rose began to notice very uncomfortable "shooting" pains beginning above, directly over, and downward from the old fracture site just below the middle of her lower leg. At first they were mild and often accompanied by a burning sensation, and there were changes in the sensation of her skin around the old injury site.

Examination failed to turn up a reason for these distressing symptoms, which over the course of two months seemed to be worsening rather than getting better. Rose didn't notice any difference in the function of her foot, ankle or leg. The muscles worked fine and there was no evidence of shrinking of any of her leg or foot muscles that would indicate damage to the muscle nerves. Rose had entered into a siege with causalgia.

Over the next six months Rose's orthopedic surgeon tried local anesthetic injections around the area of the larger nerves that convey

How You Can Relieve Pain 101

sensation from the foot and lower leg. This failed to alleviate the pain. Next, he tried physical therapy: contrast baths in a whirlpool machine (both hot and cold water), massage of Rose's lower leg muscles, and diathermy (heat generated by radio waves). Rose noticed some relief but not anything that sustained itself for more than a couple of days.

Finally, a neurosurgeon was consulted and he performed a test with a drug injected into Rose's major leg artery. This drug mimics the effect, for a time, of blocking the autonomic nerves.

The relief was both instantaneous and gratifying for Rose, and it proved to the neurosurgeon that a permanent interruption of the autonomic nerve pathway near the lower spine might be what was needed in the way of permanent relief.

Rose was glad to try this procedure because of the miserable time her causalgia had given her. The surgical interruption was done and today Rose has an occasional twinge of pain in her lower leg, but by and large she is free of causalgia.

Unfortunately, such surgery isn't always successful, though it is worth a try when all else has failed. Biofeedback techniques are just now beginning to be used for this condition, but it's too early to say if they will be helpful.

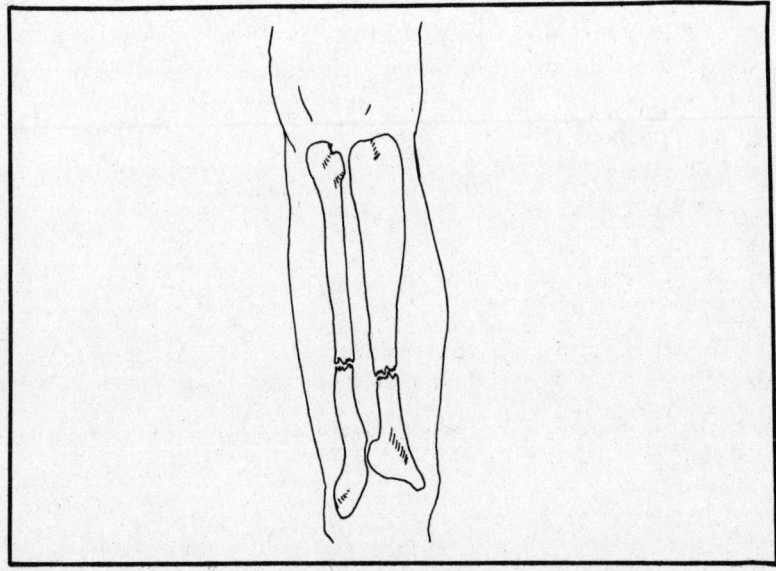

Figure 5-7

SUMMARY

1. Mild pulls and twists (strains) and more severe wrenches and tearing (sprains) involving ligaments, tendons and muscles can be handled, at least at the outset, at home. Sprains around joints should generally be X-rayed to make certain that a fracture hasn't also occurred.

2. Ice initially, followed by heat after the passage of three or four days will help most strains and sprains. To splint these injuries, including suspected bone fractures, the joints above and below the injured bone should be put at rest where possible.

3. Osteoporosis is a thinning of bone and is best treated by prevention of it in the first place through keeping your body in reasonable physical tone before it has a chance to start. This is especially true for women, in whom osteoporosis is quite common following menopause.

4. The use of biofeedback techniques can control the distressing pain of injuries, amputations and bruising of extremities. Its mastery takes time and patience, and often guidance from a medical advisor, but biofeedback may pay huge dividends in time.

5. Causalgia in limbs usually follows an injury, and may be delayed for some time after the original injury is healed. It may take an expert to help you with this problem, and surgery may eventually help if other methods fail.

6

How You Can Use Helping Devices for Ailing Joint and Muscle Problems

Many times, you'll find it necessary to use splints and special bandages for various arthritis, muscle and bone disorders. When these occasions arise, it will be of help to know how to devise them on your own and what to use to make them work. We'll talk in this chapter about various ways of splinting and bandaging.

Occasionally, the use of canes and crutches may be necessary to help you through certain injuries and afflictions of your skeletal system. The use of these aids is usually temporary, although some conditions may require their use more or less permanently. We'll have a look at many of the processes that make canes and crutches a necessity.

Sometimes paralyzed or partially useless limbs present special problems in getting around. You'll find the discussion of walkers and canes especially helpful. In addition, you'll gain some firsthand knowledge of how you can make your household safer and more easily navigated, and a look will be had at what you can do to make the chores of everyday living much easier.

USING SPLINTS TO ADVANTAGE

When you need to take one or more joints or muscles out of commission for a time, splinting is an effective way to do so. As long as splinting is done correctly, and the whole function of the involved limb is taken into consideration, you'll have little trouble in mastering the techniques.

Figure 6-1 represents the fingers, hand and wrist in the so-called "position of function." It's very important to learn this position since any time one or more fingers, the hand itself, and the wrist need to be put at rest for any reason, this position should be maintained at all times. The reason for this is that whenever you immobilize the fingers, hand or wrist, a certain amount of stiffness—even in the joints and muscles that aren't involved with the injury or disease—will set in. When it does, you'll want to retain the best function of your hand and wrist when you take the splint off. If you've used the position of function, your hand will at least be "stiff" in the position in which it works most efficiently.

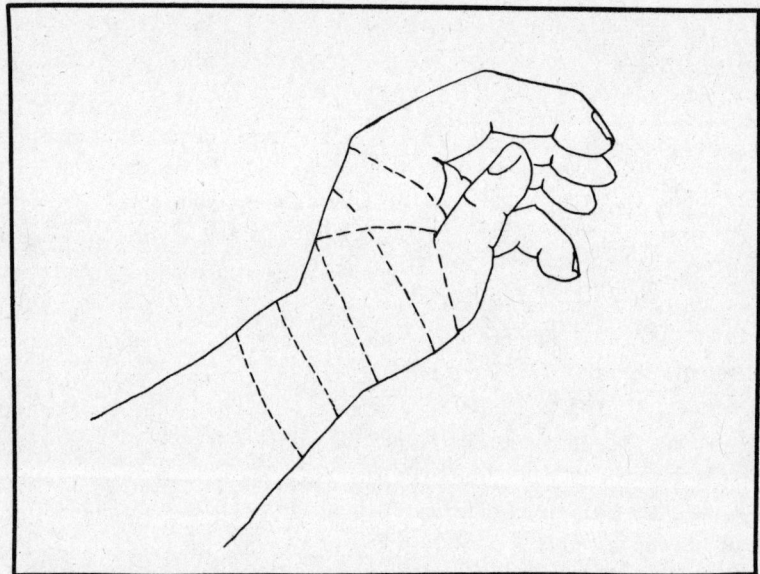

Figure 6-1

One man's solution

Ted G., a man with an old wrist injury, had recurrent trouble with traumatic arthritis involving his left wrist. When his wrist would be quite sore and stiff and his fingers and thumb difficult to use because of the pain in his wrist when he used them, he found a very simple way to tide himself through these periods, which lasted only two or three weeks. He fashioned a splint utilizing stiff cardboard for the forearm portion. He first wrapped the cardboard carefully with several layers of plain gauze so the edges wouldn't chafe his skin. He made the splint long enough to extend from mid forearm up into the palm of his hand, but not beyond the last palm crease. Then he laid a ball of knitting yarn about 3 inches in diameter over the cardboard in

How You Can Use Helping Devices 105

the palm. He secured the yarn ball and the splint with an elastic bandage as shown in Figure 6-2.

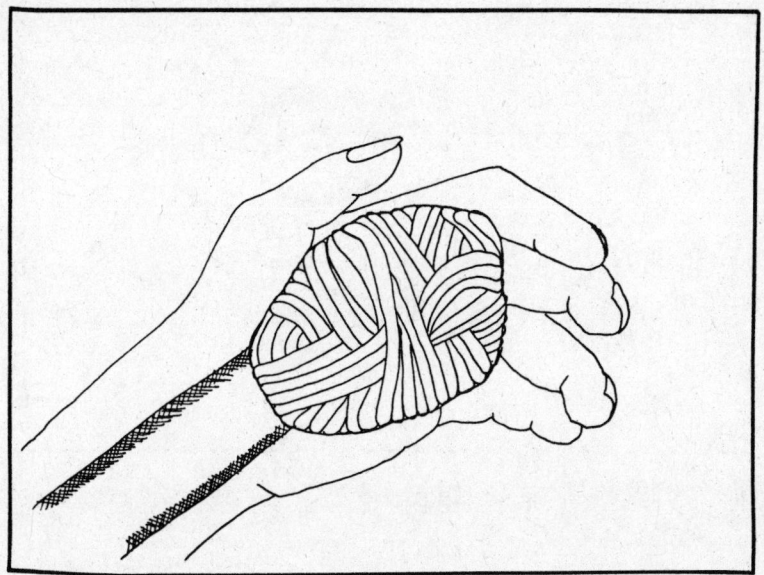

Figure 6-2

Such a splint will work nicely for any condition, including an injury where more than one finger, including the thumb, or the hand itself, or the wrist needs to be put at rest *for a short period of time*. Ted simply placed the splint in position and kept it in place by winding a rolled elastic bandage around the splint including the yarn ball to keep it snugly in place. You can use a rubber elastic bandage or a cotton elastic bandage, or even plain cloth cut in a strip about 2 or 3 inches wide and about 5 or 6 feet in length, rolled up for easy use. Notice how Ted left enough of his fingers and thumb out of the wrapping so he could still move them easily.

Other splinting solutions

Instead of a yarn or string ball, a rolled-up elastic bandage can be used in the palm of your hand to curl your fingers around, as shown in Figure 6-3. A second bandage is then used to secure it in place. Rolled gauze can be used rather than elastic bandage, made snug with adhesive tape. Instead of a rolled bandage, simply packing the palm and fingers with clean layers of any smooth material may suffice—just as long as the position of fingers, hand and wrist ends up looking like the one in Figure 6-1.

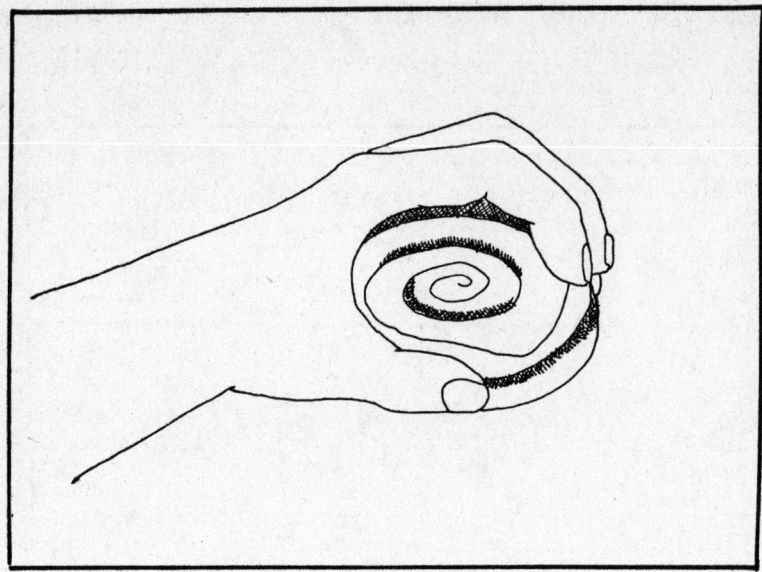

Figure 6-3

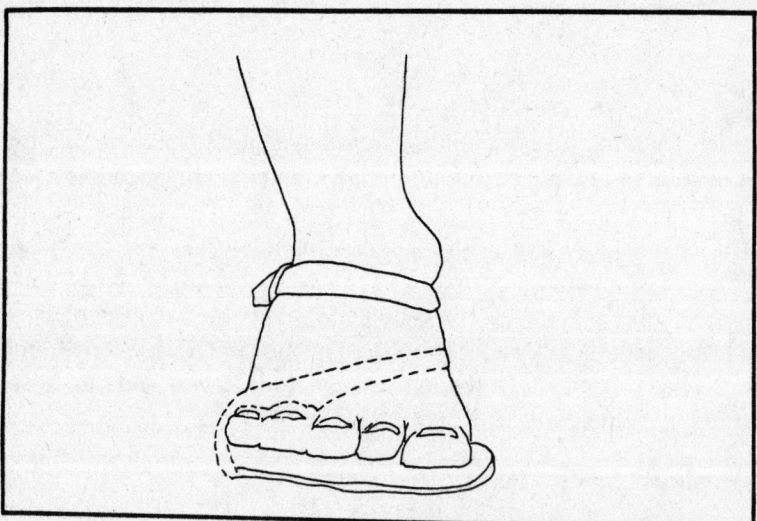

Figure 6-4

Either the thumb or index finger can be splinted by itself fairly comfortably. You can use a smaller rolled bandage to curl the thumb or finger around and simply fix them with adhesive tape after painting the skin with tincture of benzoin first. Benzoin helps protect your skin against

How You Can Use Helping Devices   107

irritation from adhesive tape and should always be used where tape is to contact your skin. Paint the skin thoroughly and let it dry before applying the tape.

The best splint for painful toes is simply a stiff-soled shoe or sandal. Nora W. found, for example, when she broke two of her toes, that stiff-soled sandals with the two toes fixed with transparent tape from the top of her foot around and to the bottom of her sandal permitted her to walk in comfort for most of the day. Figure 6-4 shows how she did this.

In general, if weight bearing on an ailing foot or ankle is uncomfortably painful, don't do it.

Major upper joint splints

Both elbow joints and shoulder joints are best splinted with the use of slings. There are any number of ways to make slings, one of which will suit your problem best.

Vince E., for example, had a propensity for getting tennis elbow—a usually short-lived, but exquisitely tender condition reflecting overstretching of the muscle tendons of the forearm at the elbow. When he came to my office the first time with this painful condition, he had fashioned a sling as shown in Figure 6-5. Other variants of arm slings for either elbow or shoulder disabilities are shown in Figures 6-6 and 6-7.

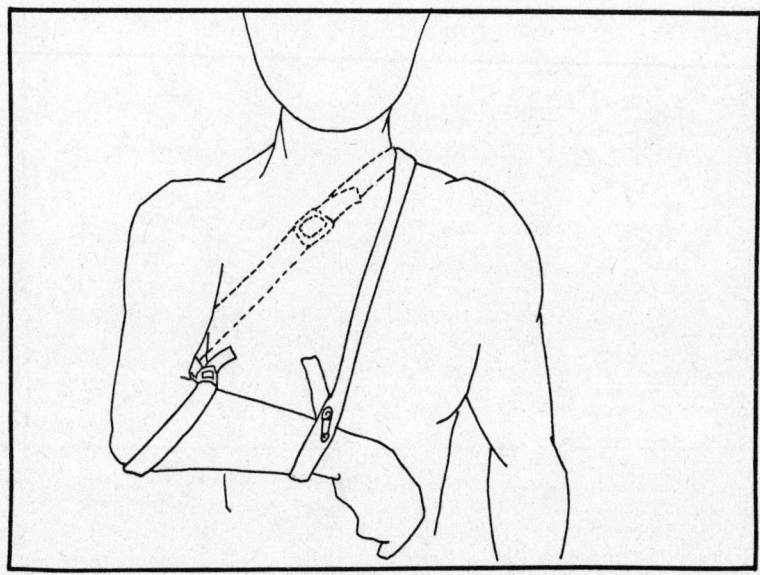

Figure 6-5

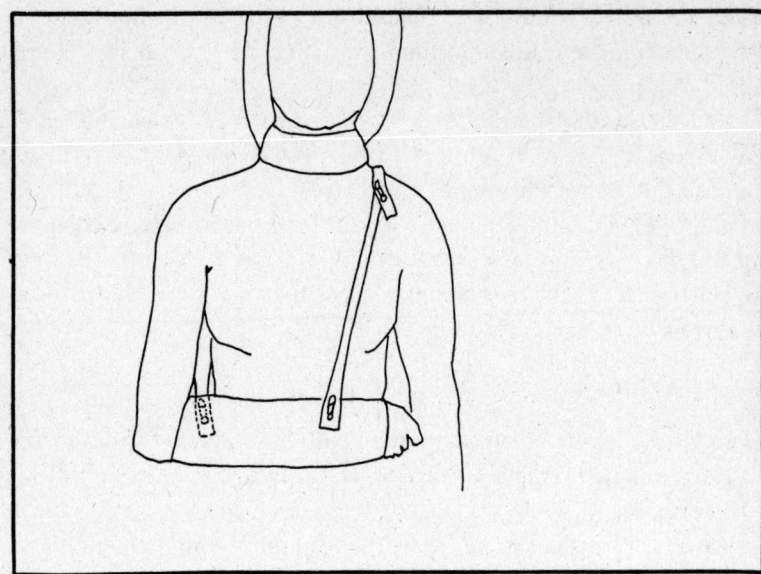

Figure 6-6

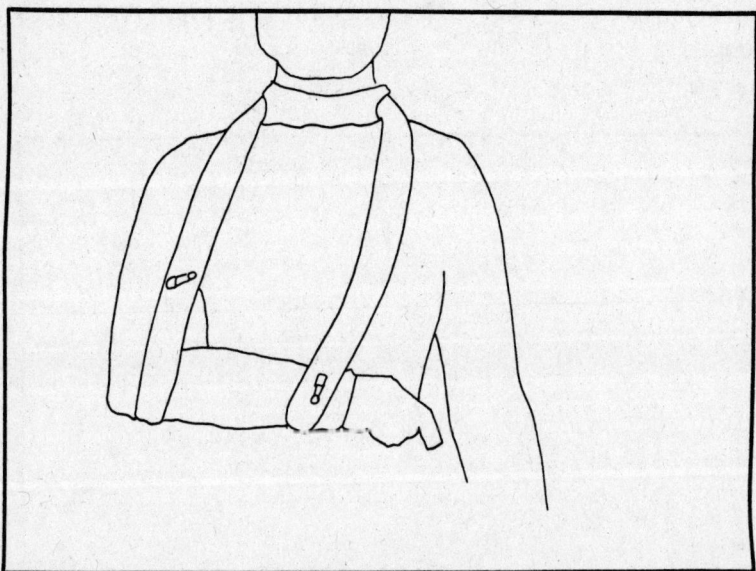

Figure 6-7

How to splint lower joints

Your hip joint is the largest major joint in your body and is also the most difficult to "do without" if you consider your ability to walk around one

How You Can Use Helping Devices

of the most important things you do every day. The only practical way to splint your hip joint, yet retain your ability to walk, is to use two crutches and not bear any weight at all on the involved leg. We'll take up the use of crutches later on in this chapter.

Anything you can do to your knee joint that keeps it from bending while walking around will often effectively splint this joint. Two firm pieces of cardboard from 3 to 6 inches wide and stretching from your midthigh to just above your ankle will do this nicely. Since your thigh is bigger than your lower leg, you should take measurements with a measuring tape at your midthigh, at the middle of your knee joint, and at the lowest point of the splint on your lower leg. When you cut the cardboard, it will appear tapered—widest at the top, narrowest at the bottom. This type of splint will cause you to walk "straight-legged," so that you'll have to swing the splinted leg outward and around while walking. One or two 6-inch wide elastic bandages, starting the wrap at the lower end of the two pieces of cardboard and working up, will effectively hold the splint in place. Adhesive tape will help to hold the two pieces together while you wrap them.

Mona finds relief from ankle pain

Mona Y., a middle-aged lady I know, injured her left ankle some years ago and it left her with traumatic arthritis in this joint—that is, left her with injured ligaments on the outer side of her ankle that flared up about three or four times a year. She finds relief for this distress by using a strapping splint

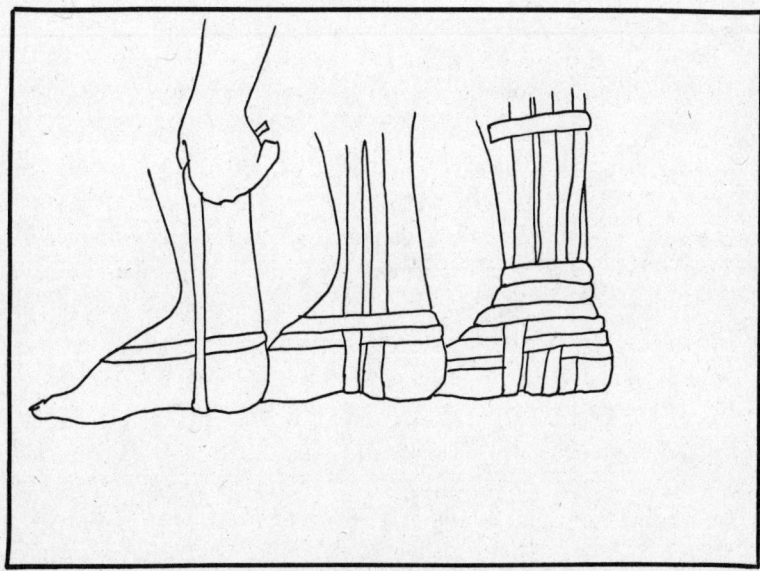

Figure 6-8

that she applies herself. Mona Y.'s strapping technique is demonstrated in Figure 6-8. She thoroughly paints all of the skin involved with tincture of benzoin first and lets it dry. Then she tears the tape in the lengths she needs and applies them as shown. A 2-inch square felt or gauze pad over the painful area can be used for added protection as can a strip of gauze or felt over the heel cord. She is relieved of pain and retains her ability to walk around for normal activities of the day by keeping this splint in place for five to ten days. After this time, the flare-up is past and she can remove it. The splint also works well for sprains on either side of your ankle.

Things to keep in mind with splints

1. Splints are *temporary* measures to limit motion at one or more joints, thereby putting joints at rest so they will heal.
2. If the part of an arm or leg involved in any splint *becomes painful or feels cold*, or both, immediately remove the splint completely and reapply it when the pain and coldness have disappeared, *being careful to wrap it more loosely than before.*
3. Any firm object you use in a splint (cardboard, metal, wood, and the like) *should first be padded or wrapped generously with enough gauze bandage or smooth material layers* to prevent your skin from being irritated or pressured.
4. When you've finished with the day's activity, you may remove the splint for the night and replace it the next day.
5. When splinting for a recent injury remember that if there is doubt as to the seriousness of the damage, the splint is only a *temporary measure* until you can have your medical advisor examine the injury.
6. Before applying a splint of any kind for any reason, it's always best to try and reduce any swelling that may have occurred around the area involved. *This is best done with ice packs applied intermittently for 20 or 30 minutes at a time* for as long as it takes to bring the swelling down. Heat will only increase swelling, and should be delayed.

MORE IMMOBILIZATION METHODS

Rib injuries and chest wall injuries may sometimes pose a problem with pain. Sometimes just taking in a breath of air makes the injury hurt so

How You Can Use Helping Devices   111

much that you may cut your breath short rather than inhale completely. Here's how to help relieve such a problem.

With the person sitting on a stool (and, if a man, his chest hair gently shaved off with a safety razor), measure up from the sore area on the chest about 7 inches, and down from it about the same, paint the area in between—front, side and back—with tincture of benzoin, and let it dry. Be certain to cross the middle of the chest in the front and cross the spine in the back with benzoin painting, in both cases about 3 or 4 inches.

Then, with the air in the chest exhaled, apply a 2-inch strip of adhesive tape from front to back, crossing the midline in front and in back about 3 or 4 inches. Let the patient breathe normally, and then have him breathe out all the air once again. Apply the second strip in the same fashion, overlapping the first strip by about ½ inch. Repeat this for the 5 or 6 inches above and below the sore area. When you're through you'll have immobilized the chest on one side as well as can be done, much to the relief of the patient. See Figure 6-9 for the technique.

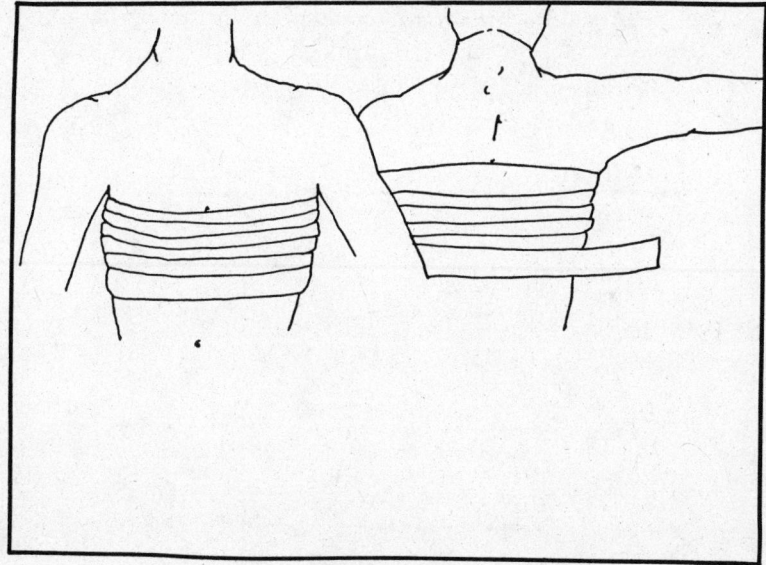

Figure 6-9

If the patient is female, her breast on the sore side may be padded with cotton and incorporated into the adhesive tape strapping, the nipple and center of her breast being left free of tape; or the breast may be held upward and left free of tape altogether, whichever feels more comfortable.

Phyllis gets in shape for brace

Phylis J., a woman in her 60's who had a stroke, was recuperating at home in the small town where she lived. She was getting better, but noticed that her left leg seemed to bow backward at her knee joint when she'd try to exercise or bear weight on her affected left side, and that her left foot tended to drag, a common weakness following stroke. To help overcome these tendencies the following helping device was applied. (See Figure 6-10 for the application technique.)

1. Using an elastic bandage 6 inches wide, her husband applied it as though starting an ankle splint. After the second turn around her ankle, her husband brought the bandage up to Phyllis's knee along the *outside* of her lower leg.

2. He then wrapped a turn around her knee joint, over the part of the elastic bandage he held in his other hand, and stretched up from her foot.

3. With each turn around her knee, he stretched up the vertical part a bit more and turned the wrap around the portion held taut. When this was done, he pinned all bandage junctions with safety pins.

4. Applied properly, the "lift" had the effect of pulling her weak left ankle outward and upward and also braced her knee joint.

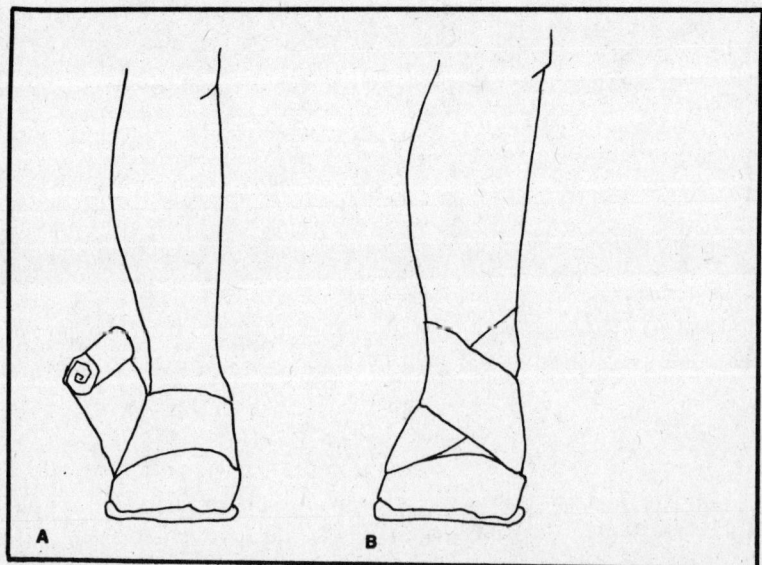

Figure 6-10

How You Can Use Helping Devices 113

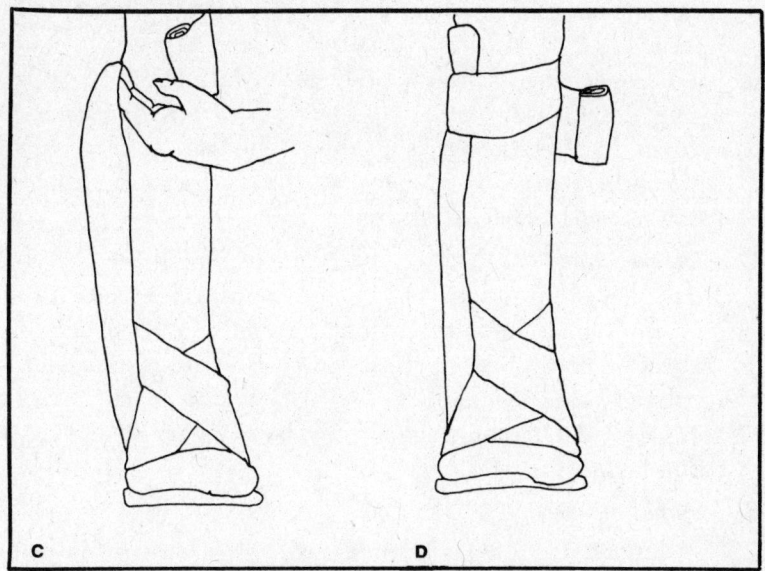

Figure 6-10 (continued)

5. Later, when Phyllis became "steady" with this splint, she knew she was ready for a permanent brace to help keep her walking.

WHEN LIMBS ARE PARALYZED

One or more limbs can sometimes be completely or partially paralyzed from such things as injuries to the nerve that makes a particular muscle group work, diseases like polio (thank God we don't see many new cases of this anymore, but there are plenty of older cases still handicapped by it), and strokes—the blood vessel accidents that occur in the brain and affect the nerve cells responsible for our "willful movements."

With any of these ailments that cause paralysis, it's useful for you to consider them as progressing from one state to another just like a story or a movie.

1. *Acute stage*

   This is the period immediately following an accidental injury to a nerve, for instance, in your wrist that affected the movements and sensation in part of your hand or in your fingers. Remember that the farther toward the end of a limb so affected, the fewer muscles are involved, and the closer to your body the injury may be, the more muscles and nerve endings will be involved.

In a disease such as polio, the acute stage would begin with high fever and severe pains in the muscles involved. It would end with the disappearance of these signs and with the leftover paralysis. In a stroke, the acute stage would start with the usual headache and dizziness, and perhaps with numbness and tingling in the right or left half of your body. It ends when these signs are gone and paralysis and numbness remain.

2. *Recovery stage*

This is the stage during which your body tries to restore things to normal. Wounds heal, strength and stamina slowly return to the uninvolved nerves and muscles, and muscles at first thought to be paralyzed begin to move again. This is usual for stroke, where appearances at first are generally much more severe than they turn out to be later.

3. *Rehabilitative stage*

This is *your* stage! This is the time to bear down on all the things that affect your organism so that you may recover to the fullest. Your psychological outlook, your mood, your will to do the things you know must be done, and your common sense—all these and more must now be brought into play. You can do it!

Herb forgets

Herb T., a patient I dealt with following a severe fracture of his upper arm about 3 inches below his shoulder joint, had an injured radial nerve from this fracture. This is the nerve in the arm that supplies the muscles that extend (straighten out) the upper and lower arm (wrist) and fingers. He'd been away from home when the accident occurred and the treating physician had put Herb in a "hanging cast," which means that it began at his upper arm near the armpit down to just above the wrist, and was suspended from a neck sling so the weight of the cast kept the broken upper arm bones together and stabilized. Herb was aware of the trouble in straightening out his wrist and fingers, but had done nothing about it—he'd given up!

I pointed out that the nerve that caused his wrist and fingers to curl up (flex) wasn't injured, yet he wasn't doing anything about moving or exercising either the wrist or fingers. I started him in on squeezing a rubber ball and on the passive straightening out of his wrist and fingers, using his good hand to move them. In addition, I had him do abduction/adduction exercises, moving the fingers sideways away from his hand and then toward his hand.

How You Can Use Helping Devices

In four weeks, when the fracture had formed a good callus (bridge of new bone), I started him moving his shoulder, which likewise wasn't involved in the nerve injury. I made Herb do these workouts six times a day, and by the time he was ready to come out of the cast, at least all of the joints not involved with the nerve injury were fully able to be used, a condition that wouldn't have existed had he not taken the time to *move all of the joints* not involved in his cast.

His bruised nerve finally came back and with further physical therapy mostly at home, he got back 90 percent of the function of extension at his fingers, wrist and arm.

In Herb's case, his main helping device was *his good hand*!

HOW TO USE WALKING DEVICES

Walkers

Sometimes the condition of lower limbs requires the use of a walker. This device is a four-legged metal frame designed so that weight bearing can be done entirely or almost entirely with your hands, arms and shoulders. Walkers may be the only device that will allow ambulation around the house for you folks who also have difficulty with balance, who need to support more than half of your body weight to move around, who may have serious trouble with a hip or leg such as fracture with surgery, who suffer from a general disease with involvement of both hips or legs (as with arthritis or multiple sclerosis), or who may be elderly and somewhat weak. Walkers have the disadvantage that they can't be used to navigate stairs or on uneven ground. As you stand straight beside a walker, its top should be about at hip level. A high stool without foot rests and a smooth grab bar rather than a solid seat are about all that is needed.

Standing up at a walker

If you have one good leg, keep this foot firmly planted near your chair, rise up with your good leg and arms grabbing the chair arms, swing your good leg forward with your good-side arm now grabbing the walker bar, move your bad-side arm to the walker and swing your bad leg forward, keeping this foot off the floor if you're not supposed to bear weight on this side.

Moving with a walker

Using your arms, swing the walker forward about 8 or 10 inches, your weight on the good leg. Shift your weight to your arms, and swing your good leg forward, then your bad leg forward.

Sitting with a walker

Being certain that your good leg is against the chair before trying to sit, bend your good leg and then transfer your bad-side arm to the chair arm.

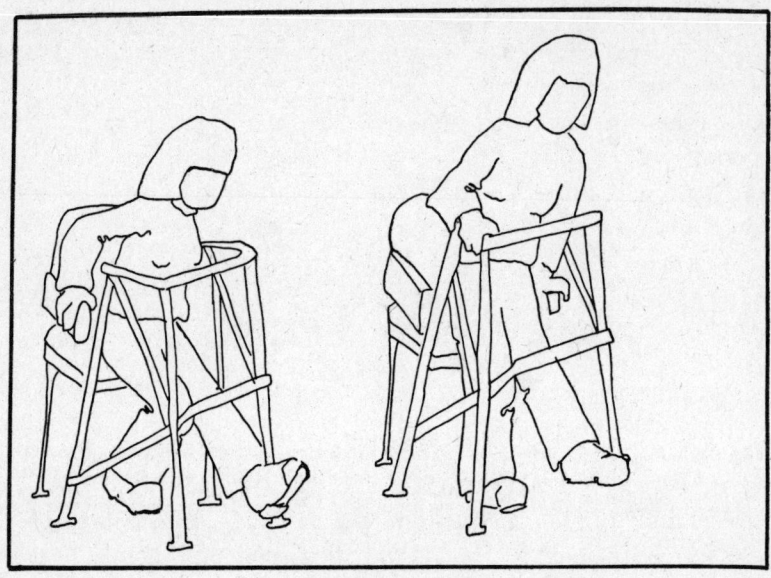

Figure 6-11

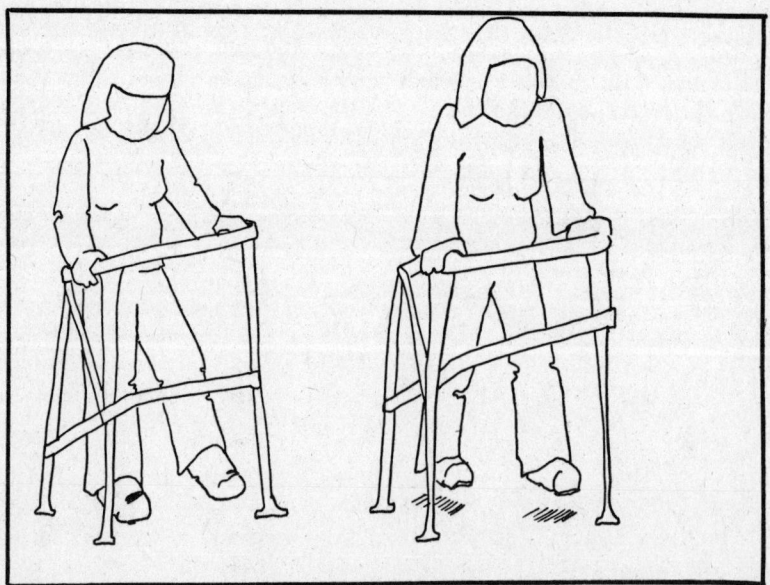

Figure 6-11 (continued)

How You Can Use Helping Devices

Begin to sit down with your good-side arm on the chair arm and lower yourself into the chair.

Figure 6-11 shows this procedure.

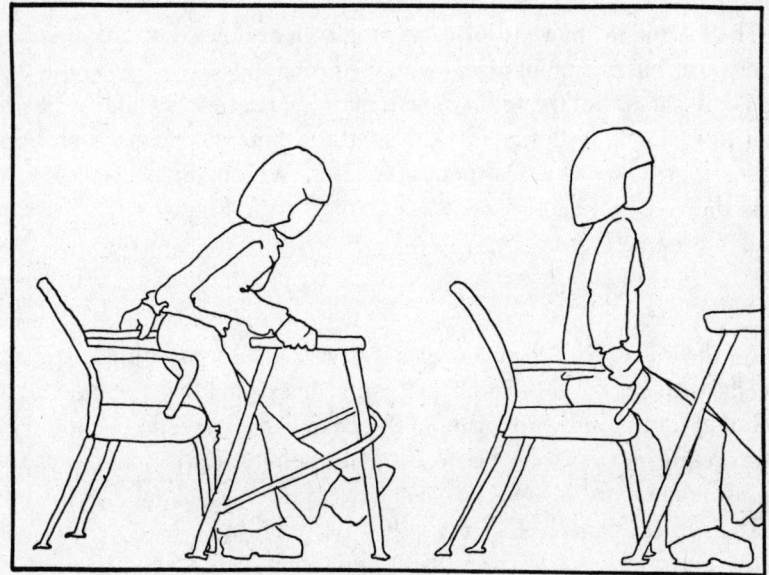

Figure 6-11 (continued)

Crutches

Basically, there are two kinds of crutches—the axillary (armpit) crutch and the forearm crutch. Either can be used as a single or double crutch; that is, on one or both sides. If you use the standard axillary crutch, you should be certain that the part that fits into your armpit is well padded, preferably with foam rubber. The tips of either kind of crutch should, of course, be fitted with rubber caps for safety's sake. It will be easier on your hands if the axillary crutches are also fitted with foam rubber grip pads. The forearm crutch has the advantage of being easier on your armpit since it is used by contact only with your forearm and your hand, and is more stable than a cane.

Moving with crutches

The common method of moving with crutches involves moving both crutches forward, then swinging the good leg forward slightly ahead of the crutch tips. You can either bear some weight or no weight at all on the ailing leg and foot.

In the "four point" move, the left crutch is placed forward, then the right foot forward followed by the right crutch forward and the left foot forward. This may be useful when speed is not important and your balance may not be too good.

In the "two point" move, the right crutch and left foot are moved forward together, then the left crutch and the right foot are moved forward together.

The "swing to" move involves moving both crutches forward, then both legs forward, but to a point just *behind* the crutch tips. The "swing through" move is the same, but the legs are both moved forward to a point *beyond* the crutch tips. Each is designed to meet the different strength and agility qualities that those who use them may have. Whichever move serves you best is the one you should become familiar with. Figure 6-12 shows the various moves with crutches.

Canes

As the rehabilitative phase of an injury, disease or surgical process proceeds with regard to a lower extremity or extremities, a cane may be substituted for the walker or crutch. The cane is designed for use when just a little weight needs to be borne with the helping device, or when your sense of balance or "sureness of foot" isn't quite normal yet.

The typical cane has a curved handle; there are also three- or four-legged types of canes, which furnish a somewhat more stable base and are

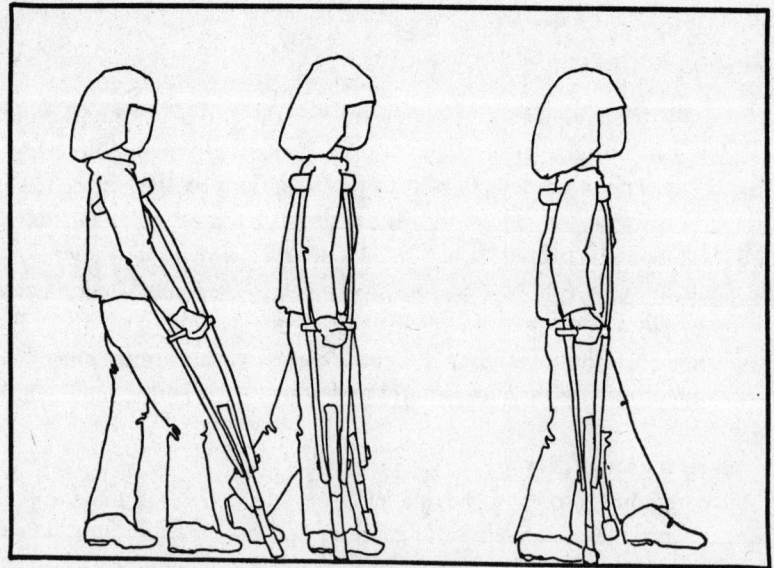

Figure 6-12

Three point gait.

How You Can Use Helping Devices

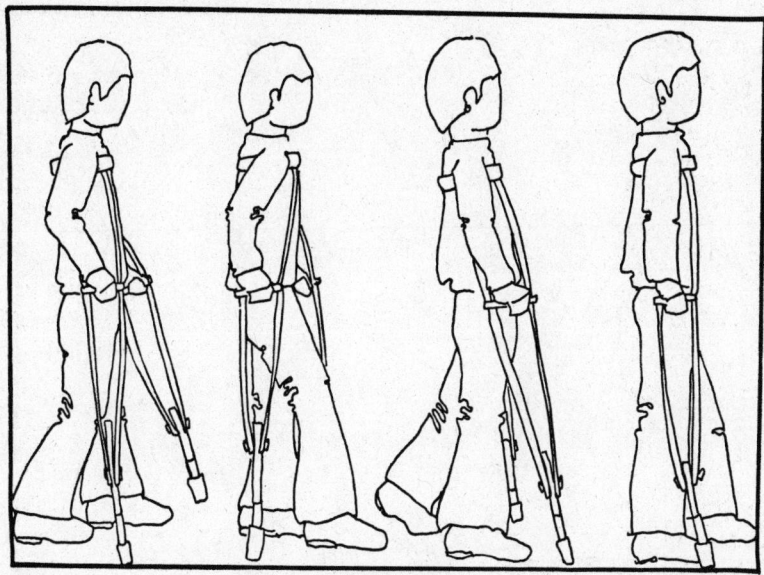

Figure 6-12
Four point gait.

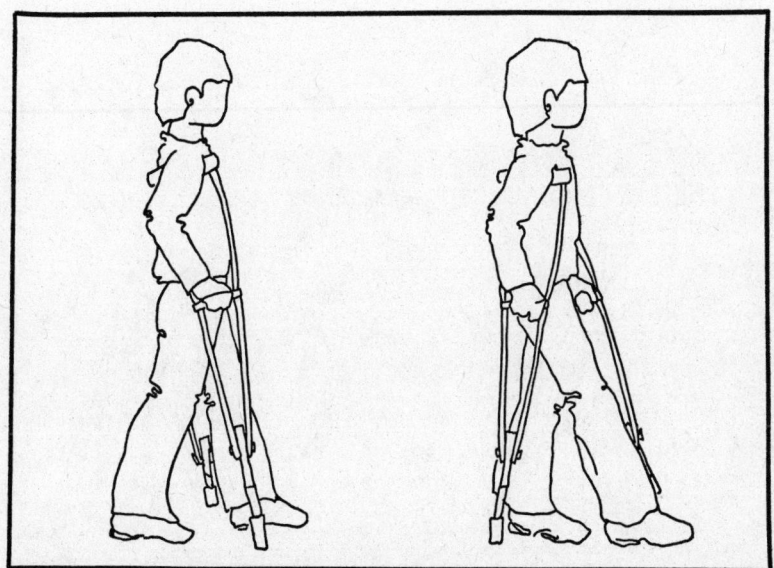

Figure 6-12
Two point gait.

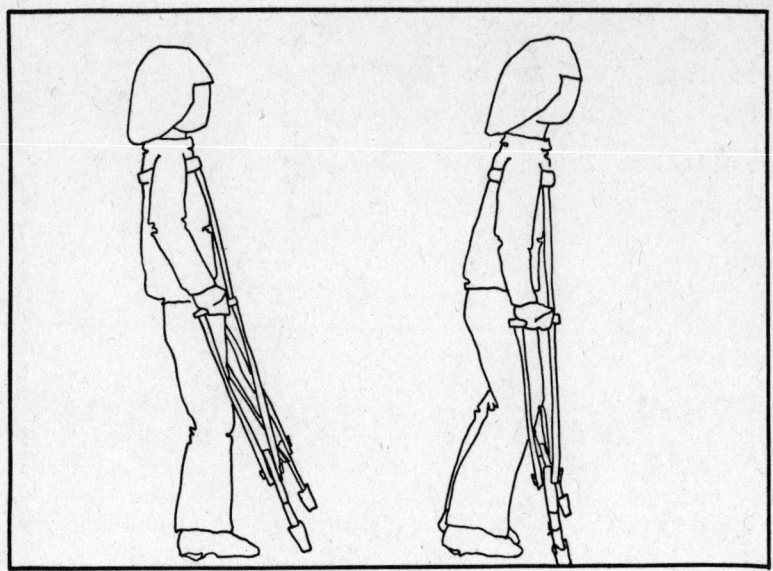

Figure 6-12
Swing to gait.

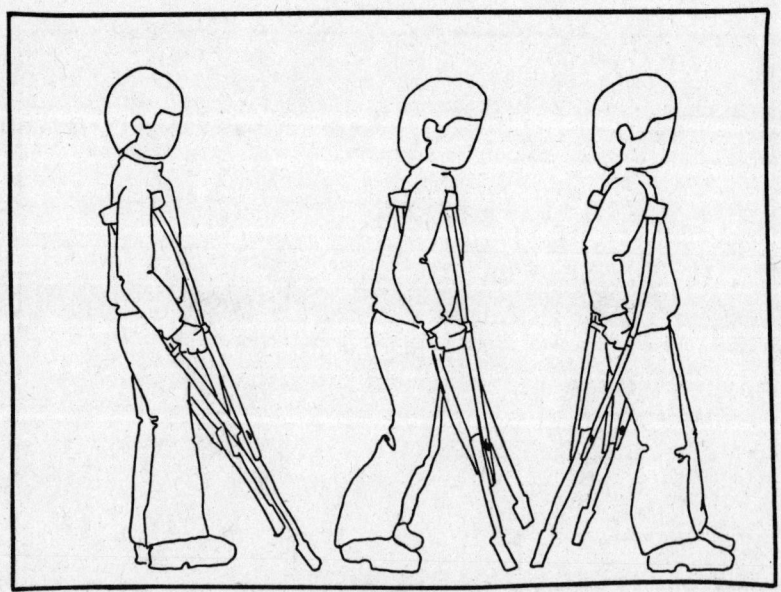

Figure 6-12
Swing through gait.

How You Can Use Helping Devices

free-standing if you have to let go to do something else with the arm or hand that's holding the cane.

Moving with a cane

A cane should be held with the strong-side arm. The cane and the ailing leg and foot are moved forward at the same time; then the good leg is brought forward. This may seem clumsy at first, but doing it this way will help balance and give a smoother walking pattern without lurch.

Note: For navigating stairs with regular crutches, canes or forearm crutches this rule applies for optimum safety and comfort: up with the good leg, down with the bad. Move the crutch or cane *with* your bad leg.

Figure 6-13 demonstrates stair navigation with crutches or cane.

HOUSEHOLD AIDS AND HINTS

There are many things you can do around your house to make it a more comfortable and efficient place to work and relax when you need to use assistive devices to get around. It may not be possible for you to do some of these things for yourself, so you may have to ask your spouse, a friend, or a relative to come around from time to time to help you get things in order. Don't be shy about asking for such help—people who don't have to worry

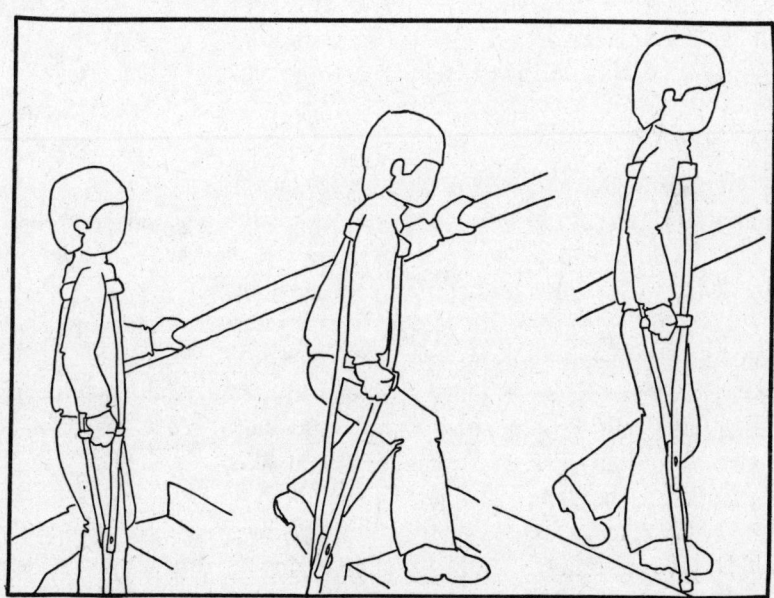

Figure 6-13
Upstairs

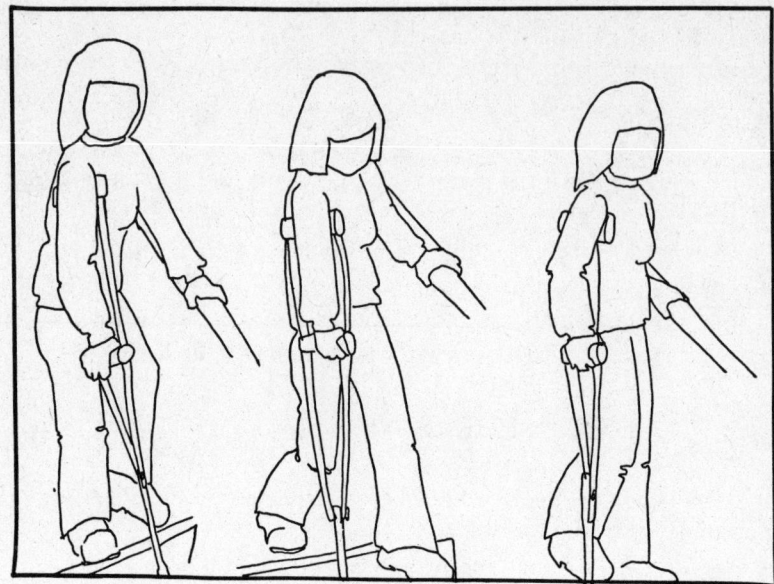

Figure 6-13
Downstairs

about such things themselves are lucky and most of them realize it. They will be only too glad to help out, and many will come up with new or unusual ideas that will really help you with your particular problems.

The house generally

If you use a walker, cane or crutches, it's a good idea to completely remove all throw rugs, children's toys, books, and magazines from the floor. And if you have linoleum or wood floors showing, or have no carpets on the floors, don't let anyone talk you into waxing them.

If you have one good arm and hand, and you use walking devices, it's a good idea to install rails at your front porch, if you have one, and all stairways up and down in your house as well as the back stoop. Consider getting hand rails for both sides of steps and stairs. When navigating steps and stairs you can shift both crutches to the weaker side and use your strong arm and hand to support yourself on the climb up or down.

Rails are also good to have in at least two positions in the bathroom: at the bathtub and toilet to further support your use of these two facilities as you climb into the tub and out, and onto the toilet seat and off. The rails, of course, should be positioned where you can grab them easily with your strong arm and hand, and the walking devices should be near enough to both tub and toilet so you don't have to stretch too far to get hold of them.

How You Can Use Helping Devices

Dressing

When one or more legs are weak or paralyzed, or when you have only one good arm or hand, the usually simple act of dressing can be a chore. For shoes or appliances that slip when you're trying to put them on, a heel stop can help—a small quarter- to half-inch piece of wood, a little longer than the width of your shoe heel nailed into the floor near where you dress will prevent slippage when the heel is shoved up against it when you're putting your shoe on. Zippers or hooks and laces for shoes will help when it's hard to master tying a one-handed shoe-string.

The use of a button hook or switching to Velcro fasteners for shirts, blouses, dresses, and pants will greatly simplify dressing yourself. The Velcro holder is a thin strip of material sewn onto either side of a buttoned garment in place of buttons. One side of Velcro has tiny hook-like projections, the other has tiny eyelets. When one side is pressed against the other, they stick together automatically until pulled apart.

In the kitchen

When you have arthritis, bone or muscle conditions that make you a "one-armed" person or make both arms weak, there are some things you can do to help in cooking and preparing meals.

For example, to hold pots in place while stirring the contents with one hand, rubber suction cups with two upright metal or wooden prongs placed close together can hold the pot handle while you stir.

Two nails can be driven through the back of one of your bread boards to impale potatoes, carrots, and most vegetables that must be pared—this will hold the vegetable while you're cutting or slicing or paring with one hand. On this same board, two short pieces of quarter-inch wood strips can be glued to one corner at right angles to each other. This will hold bread slices while you're buttering or making sandwiches with one hand.

Brushes of all kinds can be made or purchased that stick by suction to the bottom or sides of your sink. They can be used to wash dishes and silverware with one hand. By hanging towels through drawer or oven handles at convenient places in your kitchen, you can use them as one-handed dryers for your good hand.

SUMMARY

1. Splints and special bandages help to immobilize sore and injured or weakened and diseased parts. They can be made by you to suit your particular needs, or they can be purchased. They are temporary tools to help you manage through painful times. They can often be

removed at night and reapplied the next day if necessary. They should be permanently removed when rehabilitation of joints and muscles begins.
2. The best helping device is your hand, arm, leg, or foot that is the strongest or least affected of the two.
3. A variety of crutches and canes enable you to support a little or most of your weight while you get around. You should always adhere to the rules of safety for using these items. Rails help with these devices, especially with stairs; grab bars in specific locations also help.
4. Simple devices that hold a hundred things in place when you can use only one hand or arm at a time are most helpful around the house. Special devices such as one-handed can openers and rolling pins may also help.

7

Keeping Your Mind As Flexible As Your Muscles and Joints

In this chapter I want to talk about how you can keep your mind in good running order at the same time as you're keeping your muscles and joints limber. We'll also talk about how you can use biofeedback techniques to confront the hang-ups that are apt to rear their ugly heads when you're laid up for one reason or another.

We'll look, too, at ways to maintain motion and flexibility in spite of rather severe ailments such as multiple sclerosis—how to keep those parts of your body that are not affected by the ailment in good tone so that they will remain limber and usable.

We'll discuss methods and techniques to keep you out of the "tea and sympathy" rut as well. You'll learn how you can prevent yourself from getting into that dismal state of mind where you begin to believe that others owe you for something they had nothing at all to do with in the first place. And we'll talk about how you can turn what seems at first glance to be a tragedy into active and productive energy.

ACTIVITY AT REST

When you're laid up for whatever reason, your mind usually goes through three stages: the stage of depression and shock from the ordeal you've been through, the stage of remorse and self-pity for your sorry plight, and the stage of rehabilitation.

Depression and shock

It really matters very little what may happen: a broken leg, an arthritic hip, a strained neck. Anything that lays you up for a while raises havoc with your emotional apparatus. Why is this? Can't you protect yourself against it? Of course you can! Depression, remember, is usually caused by feelings of anger or guilt about something, and when this is turned inside—aimed at yourself instead of something outside yourself—you get blue and depressed. So the first thing to do is, if illness, infirmity, disease, or injury gets you down for a time, turn *out* your anger and guilt—let it all out right from the beginning. Even if you have to ask your spouse or others to leave the room for a while, do it. When they've gone, scream! Yell! Beat on an overstuffed chair back or pillow with your fists! Let your anger out. It will help your recovery and you'll start to feel better right away even if that casted leg or that inflamed hip or that stiff sore neck still hurts. At least you won't be making it worse or asking for chronic trouble to set in if you get the gall out of your system right from the start.

Make a pact with yourself from this point as well: Decide right here and now that this temporary infirmity and what caused it isn't punishing you for something and isn't something you need to go over and over in your mind, thinking how narrowly you missed "meeting your Savior" or how terrible a blow from fate you got. You're lucky! You can at least think about what happened—many people can't. And you have a beautiful opportunity to start doing something positive about what you know will happen if you don't start in now to head it off.

Remorse and self-pity

Human nature, with every one of us, makes us want to be taken care of—like a baby—when we're laid up for almost any reason. It seems natural that we regress—go backward in time to a stage in our lives when we were truly entirely dependent on someone else for our care and attention. We may well remain rational and mature in almost every other way, but we're taught from youth that it's bad to cry or get out of control in any emotional way when we're older. We've got to be sensible about everything and bottle up what we really feel.

This works out fairly well in most situations except when we're laid up. Then it makes children of us once again. And that's one reason for what I said a minute ago: Let it all out at the beginning. Admit to yourself and everybody else in the household that, yes, you're hurt and mad as heck, and even shed some tears if this helps to relieve the feelings building up inside. Then you're ready to start taking care of yourself.

When you get to the stage where you start feeling very sorry for yourself—when you begin to indulge in self-pity, the "poor me and all my troubles" type of thing—that's real trouble! All it gains you is a *worsening* of whatever may be wrong physically, the distinct possibility that whatever is wrong now won't get very much better, even when the physical causes have been healed. And it gains you the one thing you don't want in those around you: loathing. Why? Because the people who have to put up with such a sad pitiful thing day in and day out begin to react against you if all they hear is complaints and woe from you.

Rehabilitation

Once you've gotten over the first two humps, you're ready for rehabilitation. What does rehabilitation mean? It means overcoming whatever is wrong—even though part of your ailment may be permanent—and coming back to the best possible state of function that you are capable of.

There are many kinds of rehabilitation. Physical, mental and even vocational rehabilitation each brings its particular problems and solutions, but *you* have to supply the spark, *you* have to say "I will," and *you* have to keep up the drive and determination to bring about your rehabilitation.

I can't recount the number of people I've seen after a stroke, after a severe injury, or after learning that they've contracted a chronic disease of one kind or another who just seemed to have given up completely. And often these folks are aided and actually encouraged by well-meaning friends and relatives! The easy way out—the child's way out—is to lie back and be waited on hand and foot. Soon this gets to be a habit; a little later, a way of life; and finally, the way you want to live. If you're getting something—a little more attention, a little more sympathy, even a little more money every month in the form of a compensation check following an injury on the job—this "something" becomes the end point in your life. It becomes the ultimate and final goal.

What else is there if you're being paid to sit and do nothing but vegetate, and being lavished with kindness and sympathy as well? Or does being ill appeal, somehow, fill some kind of need inside that you didn't quite have enough of up to now? Well, don't feel badly; a lot of people become chronic porch-sitters for this very reason. And the funny thing—or I should say, the tragic thing—about these people who get to thinking someone else owes them a living is that it's quite plain as you talk to them that they're very unhappy, miserable people. They just don't care for anyone or anything. They become self-centered cranks, expecting others to do and to care and to love, but they've lost the capacity to be fully human.

If this is what you really want to be like as a person, then please don't waste time reading the rest of this chapter. This chapter is for people who enjoy life, who enjoy feeling for others, who enjoy loving and being loved in return. And it's for people who feel pride in accomplishment even if the accomplished feat is simply learning how to fend for themselves around the house even though they're paralyzed from the waist down.

Tom V. struggles and wins

I knew a young man named Tom V. who fell about 65 feet from the scaffolding beside a building on which he was standing to use a sand blasting machine. He fractured his right ankle, his right hip, his left ankle, his pelvis, and injured his back in the fall. To further complicate matters, Tom developed bladder problems from his pelvic injuries and had to wear a catheter—a tube placed inside his bladder to drain off urine. He got into trouble with infection from his catheter and the organisms rapidly became resistant to antibiotics so that newer, rather toxic medicines had to be used to control the infection. Tom developed a severe allergy to the new antibiotics and went into shock from the allergic reaction. The shock state damaged part of his brain before it was brought under control. All in all, Tom almost died, but when he did recover from the critical condition, you may imagine the state he was in, what with two legs and both feet encased in plaster, weakness and wasting of the muscles of his left side from brain damage, difficulty in talking and swallowing, trouble with his vision, and so on.

Not too many years ago, such a patient as Tom would have been relegated to a back ward of some institution if he'd recovered from all the physical and mental insults that he endured over the 16 months after his fall. Because of a highly dedicated team of specialists, Tom managed to learn to fend for himself. He learned to get from wheel chair to bed and on and off the toilet, to feed himself, to manage his bladder and rectal functions, and finally, to speak and be understood again.

But the really amazing thing that Tom did during his agonizing recovery was that he managed to keep his wits and his brain busy, with a cheery, optimistic outlook that amazed his many therapists. Tom knew without having to be told, for example, that he would never do sand blasting or any form of physical labor again. When he had regained his speech and was well on his way to getting out of his wheel chair with braces and crutches, he began a correspondence course in accounting, having always had a certain flair for working with figures. It took Tom eight months to finish what people going to regular college courses would finish in three months. Before he would finish the courses required to obtain a degree in business administration with a major in accounting, Tom would spend eight years!

Before two years had passed, Tom had begun to look for work. He ran ads in the newspapers, he wrote letters to businesses, and he had people put in a word for him whenever they could.

The result was that Tom landed a federal job with a local armed services accounting center. Within six months of getting his job, Tom was up and out of his wheel chair for most of the day with the help of a long leg brace and a forearm crutch (see Chapter 6). Sure, his walking was slow and laborious, but *he could walk*. Certainly, his mind hadn't entirely cleared from the damage, but *he could think and work*. And yes, his visual problems did persist, but he could see well enough from one eye—the eye that wasn't damaged—*to do a job*.

How long did it take Tom to reach this point? Three years and four months! Was he always bubbling over with optimism and a zest for life? Of course not, but he learned by observing those around him in his long visits to hospitals and rehabilitation centers that when you give in to *depression and anger*, you might as well throw in the towel ... and Tom enjoyed himself too much for that.

Today Tom visits such rehabilitation centers as an instructor during his spare time. His government employers are only too happy to give him extra time away from his regular job as section head of the accounting office where he works. When he visits the places where sufferers of the really complicated and severe results of bone, muscle and joint ailments have gathered to attempt to salvage themselves, Tom won't let his "patients" rest for a minute. For those who are so depressed that they can't or won't help themselves, Tom uses their inner anger to make them so mad that they've been let down that they're only too eager to pull themselves up when he gets through with them. Rough? Unsympathetic? Even mean at times? Yes, all of these. But that's sometimes what it takes to start yourself fighting back!

BIOFEEDBACK AGAIN

I've mentioned biofeedback before and demonstrated what some people were able to accomplish for themselves by using this technique. Now I want you to take a careful look at this thing called biofeedback and see if you may be able to use it to your advantage for whatever ails your frame and its levers, pulleys and hinges.

Biofeedback is based on logic, and on something doctors have known for decades—probably for hundreds of years—but have never reduced to what it really is so that you and I could understand it.

First and foremost, biofeedback is based on common sense and observation. Obviously, you can't make yourself fly over rooftops or perform other feats like Superman, nor can you cause yourself to become invisible at will. This is fantasy and fiction, which entertains us all when we need to escape the real world for a while, but what we're dealing with here is the reality of life as we must face it.

Secondly, biofeedback is based on human physiology and anatomy. For many years doctors were taught that there were certain functions of the human body that couldn't be altered by will, that such functions as breathing, heart beat, the size of blood vessels, digestion, and the like were taken care of automatically by certain brain centers not responsive to willful volition.

Then certain practitioners of "ancient mystical arts" began to appear on the American scene who were capable, apparently, of remarkable control over many of these very functions. Some people had control over them to such an extent that they could alter them almost any time they wanted. At first these people were labeled as frauds and little attention was paid to them. Slowly, however, a few others began to look a little closer and found that they weren't frauds at all, but people who had developed their control by practice and design.

Experiments started. Observations were recorded. Modern gadgetry was employed to actually show that various functions of the body could indeed be altered with a bit of practice.

Thirdly, biofeedback is based on the technique and experience of the individual who wishes to use it. What may work for one person in approaching biofeedback therapy, may not work at all for the next. This is another fact of life we all face every day. It's a fact faced by your medical advisor every day of his life as well. No two people are constructed in quite the same way, have thoughts and feelings of quite the same intensity, or view life in quite the same way. What your medical advisor does in practicing his art for you and your family is to manipulate odds. He knows *most* of his patients will respond a certain way to a certain method of treatment appropriate to what may ail them. He's counting on you being one of the majority.

This isn't always true, as most of you know. There is just enough variation among the few hundred patients that your medical advisor sees over a period of time that what may seem like just another example of a disease or ailment or injury he's seen dozens of times before and that has responded well to a certain approach of therapy, will seemingly blow up in his face and will not work at all for that particular patient.

Biofeedback is no different in this respect. You must first understand the basics, then determine the best method of approach for *you*. You must

Keeping Your Mind As Flexible As Your Muscles and Joints

steel yourself against apparent failure. What doesn't work the first time around can be discarded and another approach used. Maybe this won't work either, but you can try a third, a fourth, or whatever it takes to discover methods that do help.

Laura experiments

Laura F. is a young woman who illustrates what I mean. Laura was only 22 when she began to notice what she at first took to be just irritation to the "crazy bone" nerve in her left elbow, causing numbness and tingling in her forearm, hand and fingers. She'd experienced this kind of sensation before when, like most of us, she noticed such irritation in her fourth and little finger when she leaned too long on her elbows. And that's what it would have been—just pressure on the nerve as it passes close to the surface of the elbow—had it not been for the next set of symptoms: a progressive problem with speech and vision over the next six or eight months.

Laura had multiple sclerosis. Fortunately, her symptoms went away fairly rapidly when she began treatment with high doses of steroids (cortisone-like drugs) gradually tapering the dose over four to six weeks.

Laura and I had a long chat about her disease. There is no known cure for it, but it can usually be controlled during its "bad times." Between flare-ups, I told Laura, there would be periods of relative freedom from problems, but with time the problems that were left when the flare-up subsided would gradually worsen. There was no way to predict what these problems might be or how rapidly they might make their appearance.

But I stressed to Laura that no matter what course the disease might take, the better physical and mental condition she kept herself in when she felt reasonably well, the easier it would be for her in the long run. She started a toning routine. It was a bit tough since the first go-around with the disease had left her left hand and her right thigh muscles somewhat weaker than they had been. The muscles in these two areas still worked in most of the movements she wanted them to make, but they felt weak.

Shortly following her second flare-up, about a year later, Laura noticed more weakness in her right leg and left arm. And she definitely had more trouble pronouncing some words. It was then that I broached the subject of biofeedback with Laura, not as a way of trying to control the inevitable progress of her multiple sclerosis, but to help her to keep up her exercises—she really had lost interest in doing them following her second attack.

Her right thigh was beginning to wither a little—some of the main muscles were wasting from involvement of nerves that made them work. The same thing happened with her left hand muscles—she noticed that her grasping power was diminished.

I encouraged Laura to experiment with ways to help her just before her twice daily toning routines. She told me later which things helped her the most:

1. Simply concentrating on "wanting to exercise" didn't work. She just didn't have any response to this though she tried for about six weeks to make it work.

2. She found that if she concentrated on the nerves to her leg and arm—the ones that were weakened—some improvement was noted. That is, before her exercise routine, Laura concentrated in her mind on a picture of her spinal cord flowing down from her brain, carrying nerve fibers originating in her brain outward in large nerves through her pelvis and into her leg.

3. The large muscle in front of her thigh—the main muscle that straightens the lower leg when it contracts—was weakened, so she concentrated on another muscle, a smaller muscle that curves around the thigh and crosses the knee. She concentrated on this muscle working harder, helping her to move her lower leg.

4. She also concentrated on a similar picture of the nerves that flow from the spinal cord at the neck, coursing down through the underarm area into the arm and hand. The muscles that moved part of her wrist and fingers were weakened, but those that moved the part of her wrist and hand on her thumb side were all right. She concentrated on these muscles responding more vigorously and with increased power.

By sticking with this method before exercising, Laura was able to make the muscles that were not affected by the disease work harder during exercising. The ball squeezing with her left hand and fingers, and wrist flexion exercises done while holding a small weight in her hand—a kitchen skillet in this case—became easier and more vigorous with practice.

Of course, Laura didn't alter the natural course of her disease with this technique, but she discovered a way to stimulate the muscles that were still functioning to work even harder and get even stronger.

In observing Laura's disease for over seven years, I'm pleased to say that when the time came for her to spend part of her life in a wheel chair or using crutches to get around with, Laura was not only well conditioned and took to both with ease and dexterity, but she was also able to maintain complete self-sufficiency in her job and her home in spite of these restrictions.

Keeping Your Mind As Flexible As Your Muscles and Joints 133

Laura confided to me later that mastering biofeedback helped her with the depression and periods of panic that often go along with chronic afflictions such as multiple sclerosis.

TOO MUCH ATTENTION

One of the most common causes of disability among younger men who are used to a vigorous physical style in their work and play is a back injury. In fact, back injuries are almost, if not completely, an exclusively American phenomenon whose victims often demand and receive more attention, more settlements from employers following injury, and more sympathy from those close to them than any other I can think of.

Why is this? There are many reasons, and after observing back injuries for over 27 years, my opinion is that the main cause for lingering problems with relatively minor back ailments, especially among younger men, is the *attention* they get at home and elsewhere.

Wrapped up with all this attention is fear that somehow a back injury necessarily means that there will be sexual loss and masculine deprivation, and therefore is a sign of weakness and shame. There is also the fear that somehow a back injury means crippling for life.

In addition, the employers are very sensitive to the "bad back" employee, and not only do employers want claims settled at whatever the cost, they don't really want to see or hear from the person with the back injury again—at least as far as their particular place of business is concerned.

And so we have the makings of a very large problem. It is an industrial problem, a problem of our society, and a problem for the person who has a "bad back."

I'll deal with this special problem in more detail in Chapter 12, but I raise it here to show you how the mind gets into the act in back injuries and how you can use your mind to help you over the hump of a "bad back."

Brett T. responds

Brett T., a young man who was in his late 20's when I first met him, worked at a rubber manufacturing plant. His job was a heavy one—he trundled around 200- and 300-pound drums of rubber hose on a wheeled carrier, among other duties at the plant where he'd worked for six years before his injury. One day, one of the drums tipped over on the cart and Brett tried to steady it. He hurt his back.

Although no one would say that Brett's back didn't hurt plenty for a day or so, he really didn't injure it severely—there were strained muscles and ligaments and they hurt. But Brett's employers immediately sent him to a doctor whom he didn't know for a special examination to determine the extent of the injury. This doctor told Brett that he should stay away from heavy work for a while. The one thing his doctor failed to do was to reassure Brett that he really didn't have a serious back injury.

The next thing Brett knew, his case was turned over to the Workmen's Compensation people for "handling." These are the folks who administer state compensation insurance for injury laws in every state. Brett soon found himself in yet another doctor's office, and he had more examinations and tests and X-rays. Later this doctor told Brett that his injury would prevent him from returning to his job at the rubber plant.

Meanwhile, Brett became the focus of attention at home: His wife waited on him hand and foot, his kids insisted on doing all the household chores that Brett used to do as a matter of routine. Brett soon became convinced that his injury was more serious than he'd been told and further convinced himself that he'd never do laboring jobs again. Unfortunately, no one he had consulted up to this time endeavored to indicate differently.

The days grew long and Brett became a "mental invalid." His back pains actually got worse! And there was a matter now of settlement with the company regarding his injury, which Brett by now had come to think of as their fault. He developed an attitude altogether too common nowadays that "someone was gong to pay dearly for my hurt."

By the time Brett's wife convinced him to come to my office to see if there was something I could do for Brett's nagging pain (by now it went from his back into his buttocks and thigh), Brett was fixed in an attitude of defensiveness and stubborness.

I examined Brett and detected nothing seriously wrong. There was pain all over his back and anywhere I touched hurt him. He moved like a man over 50 and was the classic example of a depressed person.

I asked Brett point blank: "What would you be willing to give up if you could get rid of your back trouble?" He finally asked what I meant. So I told him. I said would you give up lying around the house all day like a retired stud horse? Give up all the attention you once had from your family, now turned into something like disgust because of your attitude? Give up your fantasy of being taken care of like a baby for the rest of your life?

Brett didn't like to hear this, of course, but after much hemming and hawing around he admitted that he would like to get back to normal, but his back just wouldn't let him. To this I said "Nonsense"! and I taught him the simple relaxation techniques of biofeedback. Within four weeks he was able to make his tense lower back muscles relax and control about 50 percent of the pain. In eight weeks, he was out looking for a job. In three months, his family life was back to normal and he was working. Brett does have an occasional back twinge, or a night's backache after a hard day's work, but so does practically everyone else.

Most importantly, Brett dug himself out of a worthless, useless life style by facing up to his supposed disability.

USING WHAT'S LEFT

Sometimes just switching from what you once had to what you now have is all it takes to keep your mind active and your emotions in a healthful state.

You've seen many people, I'm certain, who have lost the use of legs, hands, arms, and the like, and yet seemed to have that spark ignited at some point to snap them out of the sea of despair that such people usually find themselves in. Not that this state is at all unusual—anyone gets into this rut after an accident or disease takes away a part of what used to be a whole you. Again, what counts is how you *respond* to the misfortune

Nancy L. is unlucky in auto

Nancy L., a young lady of 20, was an "in-betweener." She was finished with school and, like many young people her age, hadn't the slightest idea what she intended to do with her life at this stage of the game. She did know one thing, however. She knew she was going to spend as long as she could having a whale of a good time before making any long range commitments. And this she did with great gusto. She liked all sports and was good at several. She liked traveling and did plenty of it with several young men who liked to do the same. She enjoyed parties and went to three or four every week.

But all this ended abruptly one day when an auto in which she was a passenger went off the road after trying to take a curve much too fast. She fractured her spine at about waist level.

Now began the healing process, the rehabilitation, and the depths of despair as Nancy realized she would never walk again on her numb, lifeless legs. Her fracture healed without mishap. The problems with lack of bowel and bladder control were overcome. And she even made the adjustment to the idea that the young men in her life, and many others to follow, would be unable to carry on much of a relationship with her again. But there Nancy was, with no educational background beyond high school (she didn't do too well there because she was busy having a good time), no interests she could pursue now that her legs wouldn't work, and no goals in mind.

Depression hit with a bang. One day when Nancy's mother brought her to my office in her wheel chair so that I could look into a minor problem with the skin on one hip, I decided to see what was on Nancy's mind. She seemed more sullen and morose than previously.

Nancy began to talk and she began to cry. She moaned and lamented about how cruel the fates had been to her by taking away her legs. She went on like this for a time as I dressed her skin wound, bandaged it and helped her to a sitting position on the examining table. I said, "Well, the fates didn't take away your shoulders, arms, or hands, did they?" and helped her mother move her to her wheel chair. Nancy didn't reply, but later her mother told me that she had suddenly announced she would learn typing and shorthand. She did, and later got a job as a secretary at which she's done quite well and is still working.

Sometimes a person has to be jolted into action!

Vern H. makes sacrifice

Take the case of Vern H., a young man who had the misfortune to pitch over in his motorcycle in a complete circle off a hill, fracturing the middle of his seven neck vertebrae.

The accident left him with only slight motion in his right shoulder and very weak ability to lift his left wrist. His was, of course, confined to a power wheel chair which he operated with his chin. He needed almost complete care for eating, getting into and out of bed, reading, transportation, and other such functions.

Vern's mood, too, was at low ebb when he reached the end of his rehabilitation. His decision was unique: He heard someone at the rehabilitation hospital, where he went at intervals to have his kidneys and bladder checked, mention some research that was going on in a city distant from his own home town. The next day he sent a letter off to the doctor who was in charge of the research. I never did learn what was in the letter, but it convinced the research doctors. He became a full-time employee at the center, which was researching problems concerned with reestablishing nerve function in paralyzed victims with spinal cord injuries!

Today Vern has the feeling of accomplishment in doing something useful with his life. It is this sense of *doing something useful* that is important for you at this point, both in helping yourself and in helping others who are similarly involved.

SUMMARY

1. In keeping your mind on an even keel to cope with muscle, bone and joint disabilities, depression, remorse and self-pity must be

Keeping Your Mind As Flexible As Your Muscles and Joints

continually battled. Once started on this path, your rehabilitation falls naturally into place.

2. Biofeedback techniques are an important ally against the emotional roadblocks to getting back to production and activity. Biofeedback can help you see what you're doing and then correct it.

3. The specific biofeedback technique you use may vary from what helps others, and from what helps you one time, yet fails the next. By exploring the nature of your muscle, bone or joint disorder, you can learn what works best and use biofeedback regularly to help you over the humps.

4. Biofeedback techniques are not miracles or panaceas for all ills, nor are they capable of doing everything you might wish. They can, however, aid you immeasurably once you understand the details of your particular trouble and apply the techniques wisely.

5. Often, minor handicaps can be magnified and made to become disabilities simply by giving them too much of the wrong kind of attention. When this situation develops, you must face up to the question: "What will I give up to get better?"

6. Often, the simplest is the best. With your particular ailment, ask: "What do I have left to work with, and how can I train them to full capacity?"

8

How to Reverse the Weak Stiff Limb Syndrome

This chapter presents a prime consideration in keeping bones, muscles and joints limber and useful—useful, I mean, in the sense of keeping them *able to be used*.

We'll have a look, for example, at what arthritis does to joints, tendons and cartilage and how to counteract the process so that you can have useful limbs and avoid letting them get stiff and weak, hence, useless for the things you want to do and should do.

We'll have a look at what stroke does and does not do to nerves and muscles. For example, a stroke doesn't necessarily "knock out" all muscles on the side it may involve. I want you to learn methods of reconstituting useful limb motion by utilizing those muscles that aren't affected so that your arms, legs and face may remain functional.

We'll also have a closer look at amputations and injury—how they generally affect limbs and what you can do to help restore them to usefulness.

Finally, we'll look at some extreme problems to see what can be done if you decide you will make the great effort to do something.

ARTHRITIS: THE STIFFENER

Like most other ailments, arthritis can and does span a broad scale from just "a touch" in a single joint on the one hand to severe involvement of multiple joints on the other, and just about every shade of gray possible between the two extremes.

In considering the anatomy of arthritis, it's obvious that any ailment that inflames cartilage and joint lining (often called the synovium) as does

How to Reverse the Weak Stiff Limb Syndrome

arthritis is apt also to involve tendons, because tendons frequently originate from or insert into their muscles across a joint. The arthritic process may also involve bone surfaces that make up the joint, and may involve muscles themselves, especially those that span a joint or originate and insert near a joint.

At any rate, your arthritic joints get stiff because of a series of events usually starting with pain. Pain causes you to "baby" the affected area. This is good to a point, but then the babying must stop. Why? Because if carried on too long, the muscles that work your babied joints will begin to show signs of weakness because of disuse. The diagram in Figure 8-1 illustrates what happens in this process.

You may see from this series of events that it is essential to size up your particular problem from several points of view. You may need help from an expert—your medical advisor—to do this, but the effort will pay dividends.

Pain

Some pain accompanying the arthritic process may, as we've seen, be fairly constantly present. But the real go-around with arthritic pain—the excruciating, incapacitating type—is generally on a cycle of some kind. The cycle may be short, every two or three weeks, or it may be once or twice a year or longer. Pain cycles may or may not be connected with seasonal changes such as the first big storm of winter or the April and May rainy season. Flare-ups may also be triggered by emotional upheavals, by physical strain or minor injury, or by sitting or standing for prolonged periods.

Whatever causes it, it is essential to get the pain under control rapidly so that you may do what is necessary to avoid the consequences depicted in Figure 8-1.

Recall the previous discussion on pain:

1. Aspirin or one of the non-aspirin counterparts (containing acetaminophen) used in adequate doses (up to six or eight a day at evenly spaced intervals over two- to six-week periods without interruption) and buffered with any of several antacids to protect your stomach from irritation (containing magnesium trisilicate, magnesium carbonate and/or calcium carbonate or perhaps all three) is your first line of defense.

2. Rest is important. If it's your knee joint that has flared up, a dressing such as we've discussed to keep your knee from bending (walking stiff-legged) may suffice. If not—if bearing weight on your knee causes moderate or greater pain—then you may need one or

two crutches temporarily to take your weight completely off the involved knee.

3. If your elbow or wrist is involved, a simple sling may put the part at rest adequately. But remember: This phase of resting treatment should not last longer than it takes to get any pain and swelling under control. When both have been *controlled* (not stopped completely), start using the joint!

4 Hot and cold contrast packs or baths will help to control pain and alleviate stiffness. Use them to your advantage with each go-around of the pain cycle. Remember, if redness and swelling are also present around a joint, *delay heat* until both are diminished. Ice packs or cold water, however, may be used immediately. Spend 30 or 45 minutes with ice and/or heat. Repeat three to six times a day. You may find that a hot water bottle wrapped with a towel is better than soaking in water—or you may find the reverse to be true. The electric heating pad may help you more than the hot packs. Whatever method does *you* the most good is what you should use. Use one or another of them and spend some time at it!

Now you're ready to limber up those joints.

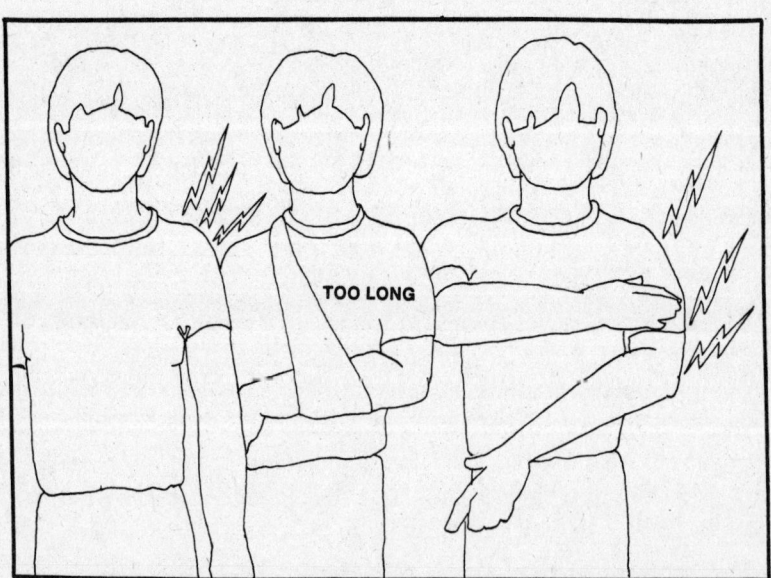

Figure 8-1

How to Reverse the Weak Stiff Limb Syndrome

May T.'s method could help you

May T.'s problem, typical of rheumatoid arthritis, was located in her right ankle, her left knee and both hips. May was 47 when I first met her and she had had her problem for about five years. She rolled into the office one day in a wheel chair with the complaint that once again her ankle, knee and hip were "flared up."

When I examined May, I found the usual signs of the disorder: swelling, redness, pain, and more. I found muscles in her foot, her lower leg and both thighs that were atrophied (shrunken down in size). This bothered me. I asked May how long she'd been in a wheel chair and she replied that it had been for about a year, ever since her last attack—"Just couldn't get around afterward," she said. I thought May might get mad enough to go elsewhere when I really began to scold her for having let her muscles get into such lousy shape.

"Why, Doctor," she said, "how could anyone do otherwise after what you see in those joints?" May had tears in her eyes, partly from pain and partly from my harsh-sounding words. I'd been purposely harsh to impress May first of all that she needed to focus her attention on a problem that was within her power to control.

Then we began to get down to brass tacks. The following regime is the one I put May on for reversing her problem:

1. *Her swollen left ankle.* May's ankle had become involved only recently and was not deformed except from the swelling of this particular episode. When the swelling was down (in her case, she took acetaminophen, eight tablets taken two at a time every six hours around the clock and buffered with two antacid tablets with each dose), I started her on passive and then active ankle joint motion to be done by her husband three times each day as shown in Figure 8-2.

   In this therapy, the joint is moved first by another person and then followed with motion by you, using your own muscles to imitate the motion carried out by whomever is helping. In the case of May's ankle, the first motion was pointing the sole of her foot toward her opposite leg, then it was pointed outward to her left. The third and final motion was a circular motion involving the first two and, of course, all positions in between.

2. *Her right knee.* May's right knee was larger, she explained to me, than her left even between flare-ups. Some deformity had set in as

may be expected after a lapse of time with rheumatoid arthritis. So I had her husband take it much easier on May's knee joint, but put it through the motions just as with the ankle. In the case of a knee joint there is only one motion involved: straightening the lower leg

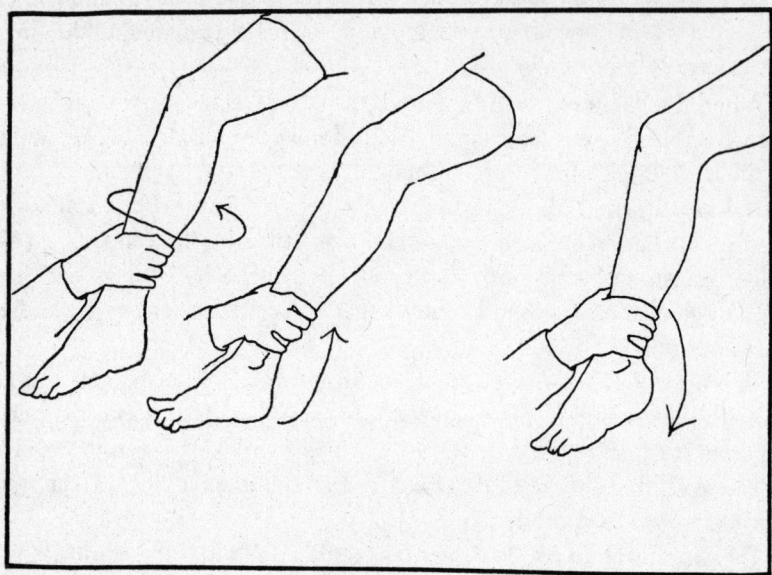

Figure 8-2

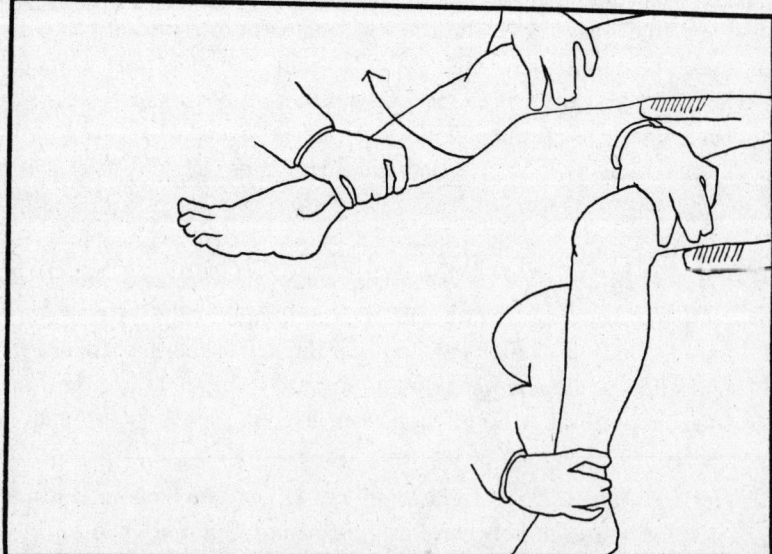

Figure 8-3

How to Reverse the Weak Stiff Limb Syndrome 143

up, horizontal with the floor, then back down again and back up. Of course, May's knee joint wouldn't go through a normal full range of this type of motion because of the deformity that had already started and the discomfort of her recent flare-up. So her husband was carefully instructed *not to force* this joint beyond the point where it felt tight when he moved it, but nevertheless to move it through the up and down motion three times a day for at least ten minutes. May's knee motions are depicted in Figure 8-3.

3. *May's hips*. Hips have movement in three directions: flexing (bending) your thigh upward toward your abdomen and downward; moving your thigh out to the side and back across the midline of your body toward the opposite side; and a circular motion with your whole leg or thigh (the motion is harder with your lower leg straight out than with it bent down). May's wheel chair, of course, would inhibit movement at her hips, so I instructed her husband to help her out of the wheel chair and onto a stool or armless chair for hip motion therapy. Furthermore, I encouraged May to remain out of the chair as much as possible, to use the stool, her bed, a straight-backed chair without arms, at least during motion therapy. May's hip motion is illustrated in Figure 8-4.

I instructed May and her husband to continue this regimen for five days, and then switch to weights. May's husband purchased a bag of sand at

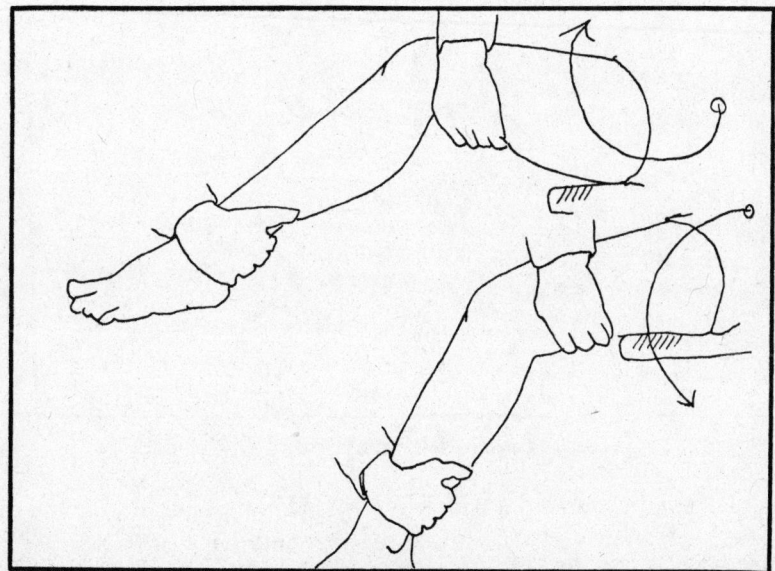

Figure 8-4

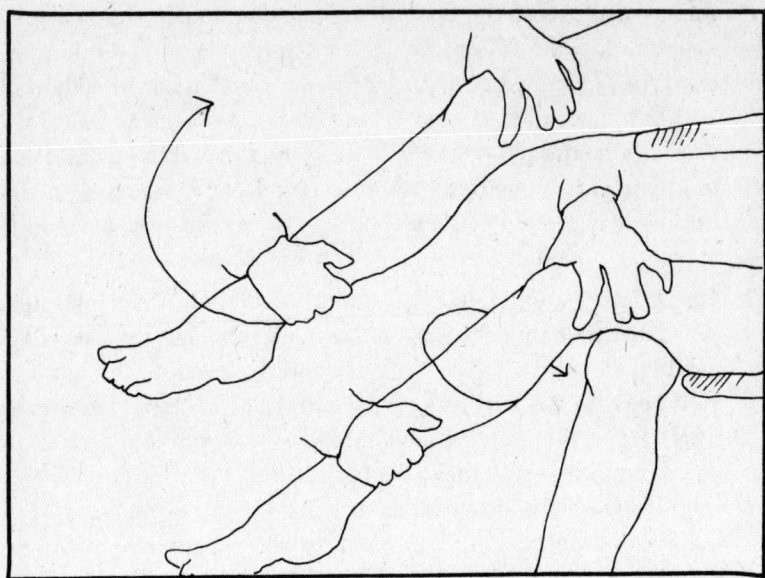

Figure 8-4 (continued)

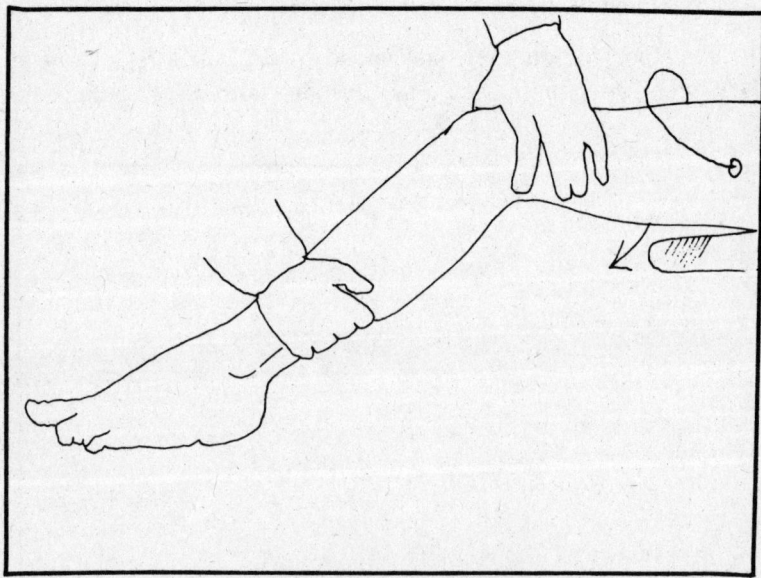

Figure 8-4 (continued)

a local hardware store and a couple of yards of canvas material at the dry goods store. May sewed the canvas together into bags (with heavy duty thread) that generally fit the sole of her left foot; they were of such size as to hold one pound, three pounds, and five pounds of the sand. After five days,

How to Reverse the Weak Stiff Limb Syndrome

the motions for each joint I've described were done with a one-pound bag of sand strapped to her left foot (to exercise her ankle and hip) and to her right foot (to exercise her right knee and hip). These exercises were to be done using only May's muscle power with no assist from her husband.

When she could do them easily and well with one-pound bags of sand, she was to progress to three pounds and then to five pounds, each time putting each of her involved joints through the same motions as in the illustrations, only with the added sand weights.

At no time was May to decrease her acetaminophen and antacids, and if there were signs of increased pain after the motion therapy during the day, she was to use warm soaks in the bathtub provided the redness hadn't returned. If it had, May was instructed to use ice packs and no heat.

Within six weeks, May was walking! She wasn't walking far, but enough to do all her household work and cooking, and with enough reserve energy left over to take a daily stroll using short strides and moving slowly but steadily.

Gary O's dilemma

When you don't pay attention to your medical advisor, you sometimes get yourself into trouble. This happened to a young man named Gary who sustained a fractured midthigh bone after a fall from a horse.

The method for treating a broken midthigh bone used to be, and sometimes still is, to encase the person in a plaster "spica"—a sort of jacket made of plaster of paris extending from the waist down over the back and groin to encircle the injured leg down to the lower leg such that both hip and knee are immobilized while healing progresses. Nowadays, this method has largely been replaced by traction—fractured bones pulled together by weights on a rope attached to wires through the lower thigh bone, followed by steel plates screwed across the fracture, or a metal rod driven down through the entire length of the thigh bone.

Gary was advised of the method of treatment (traction/screw plates) and that he would be in plaster for only a short time, followed by crutches for some time to allow for a healing callus of bone to form firmly around his fracture site.

His advisor also took pains to warn him that during this crutch session (for taking the weight off the injured leg) his leg would grow weak and his knee joint stiff, and that as a result he would have to make up his mind that when the plaster came off and when he was able to bear some weight again, much time would necessarily have to be spent getting the leg muscles back into shape—not from the standpoint of the injury itself, but from the standpoint of the weakness we've discussed resulting from non-use of the healing limb.

When Gary's plaster cast came off, he began his limbering up exercises well enough, but he figured that since he still had to use crutches for another eight weeks, he could put off doing them as instructed (three times a day for 30 minutes) until he could bear full weight on his leg.

His thigh healed without difficulty and finally his crutches could be stored away in the closet. But he'd neglected his advisor's instructions. When I saw him four months later, Gary was still limping and had no stamina at all in his left leg. He complained bitterly that something was wrong and his orthopedic surgeon was keeping it from him. A quick examination revealed Gary's problem. It wasn't "something wrong" or any complication at all from the surgery or the accident. His entire leg musculature was atrophied from disuse!

It took Gary about three months to regain strength and stamina in his left gluteus (buttock), hamstrings, thigh and lower leg muscles, and even today his left knee doesn't bend quite as far as his right knee—living proof that if you neglect your toning following any appreciable rest phase you may regret it! It cost Gary at least a half year to remedy his folly.

STROKE: THE STIFFENER

It is a grim blow, to say the least, when a stroke strikes and you suddenly find an entire side weak or paralyzed. In addition, stroke often, though not always, leaves you with speech problems, thinking problems, and sometimes with hearing and vision problems as well. The fortunate thing, perhaps, about a stroke is that it generally involves only half of your body's muscles and limbs. Still, it's a depressing reality when you have to look at your good right hand and leg, for example, and note that not only won't they move when you "will" them to, but they also have little or no feeling in them. You find yourself shifting your limp right arm with your still functioning left hand, or you find yourself moving your "lifeless" right leg around with your still functioning left foot.

In so doing, you've actually discovered one secret of the return of any function that may remain in your right arm and leg—*the idea of moving all non-functioning limbs through their entire range of motion even though they may appear useless for some time*! And if there's no one else around to do this, your good left side is as good a "physiotherapist" as you'll find.

Why is moving around so important? Because in so doing, you maintain a certain level of muscle tone in the large muscle groups affected by the stroke, and you keep those joints limber! Just moving a joint routinely day in and day out may mean the difference in an elbow, for instance, that is stiff and sore and refuses to work anything like it once did and an elbow that does what you want it to do even though the muscles that

How to Reverse the Weak Stiff Limb Syndrome

work it may never be quite as strong as they once were. In order to learn to maneuver a paralyzed side around to your fullest advantage, you may want to recall the following discussions we've had:

1. After a stroke, the muscle groups that at first appear to be paralyzed may only be *partially* unable to work. Other groups of muscles that ordinarily might not take a major part in moving, say, your shoulder, may be brought into an important role by virtue of having strength still left in them.
2. A weakened muscle group, such as the biceps muscle that brings your lower arm and hand upward toward your shoulder may not work if it has to work against gravity. The muscle may not be able to pull up your forearm and hand if your arm is hanging by your side, but it may be able to pull your arm upward if your whole arm is *supported* in a sling or *resting* beside you on the bed, or floating in water by your side.
3. The use of a simple pulley or pulleys operated by your good side will increase the efficiency of your affected side several fold.
4. Parts of limbs that are weak or paralyzed and which bear the brunt of pressure, even on bed sheets, or the arms or seat of a chair you may be sitting in, need special protection to prevent "pressure sores," especially during limbering routines.
5. You must also take special precautions in the application of heat or cold to partially or fully paralyzed limbs: If the ability to distinguish heat and cold has been diminished or is absent (as it often is at first, sometimes even after muscle power may partially return), you may burn or frost an area of an extremity, being unable to tell when the limits of heat and cold have been reached or exceeded in the limb being treated.

Sharon F. pulls through

A lady I knew named Sharon F. typified the five areas of concern in stroke that I've just listed.

Sharon was in her mid-60's and was a widow when she had a right-side stroke. She was alone in the house and her children were scattered to the four corners of the country. She lived in the old family house at the edge of a small town, and though she had many friends, they were unable to be with her all the time. With the most welcome help of two of Sharon's neighbor friends, we were able to start physiotherapy almost immediately after her stroke, which was moderate, partially paralyzing the muscles in her left arm and leg and leaving the right side of her face weak.

As in many strokes, there was at first a stage of limpness in the affected muscles, then a certain amount of spasm (rigidity) of the muscles set in. During the flaccid (limp) stage (about three weeks in this case) each and every one of Sharon's joints were routinely put through their entire range of motion three times a day, being careful to gently massage the skin of upper and lower limbs and back, buttocks, and face with a facial cream or lotion following this activity.

I taught Sharon's friends the following principles of physiotherapy:

1. *Face.* Sharon's forehead muscles were kneaded gently upward and downward on the weakened right side. Her cheeks were gently massaged in a circular motion, both clockwise and counterclockwise. Her drooping mouth on the right side was pulled up and down and her jaw opened and closed. Figure 8-5 shows how this was done.

2. *Shoulder/arm.* Sharon's shoulder was drawn upward and then depressed downward and her upper arm was rotated, flexed, extended, and carried to the side and across her body. Her forearm was rotated at the elbow. Her wrist was flexed, extended and rotated. Her fingers were flexed and extended at the end, middle and knuckle joints and spread, then bunched at the knuckle joints. Her thumb and little finger were repeatedly opposed (touched). Figure 8-6 shows how Sharon's motions were accomplished. Note

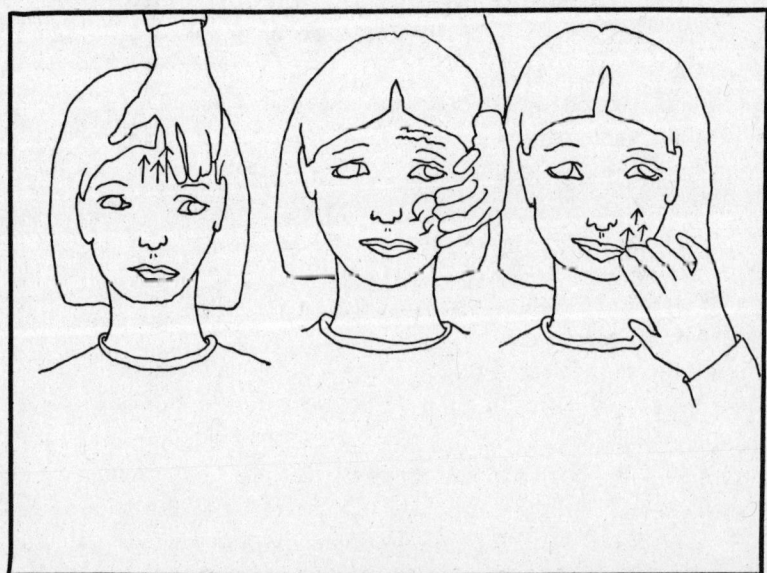

Figure 8-5

How to Reverse the Weak Stiff Limb Syndrome 149

that motions at the shoulder and elbow and at the wrist are done *both with the arm rotated outward and rotated inward at the shoulder joint.* This aids in the recovery from spasm that often sets in with muscles affected by stroke.

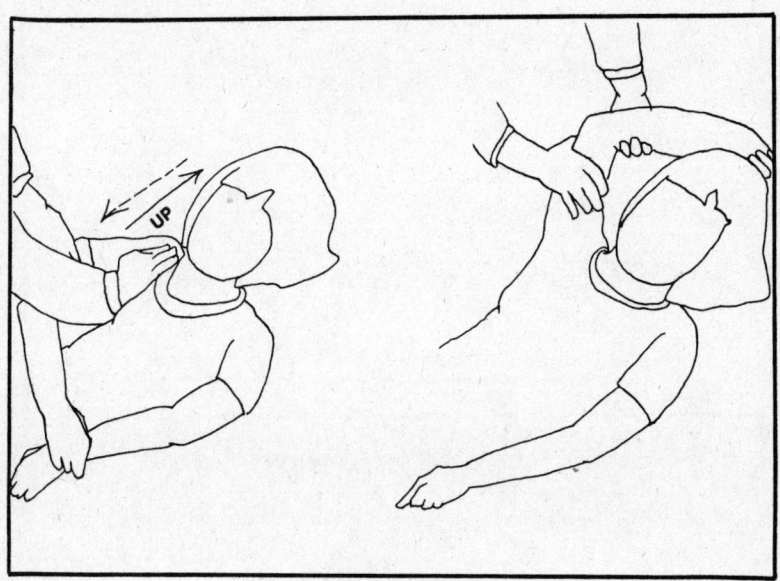

Figure 8-6

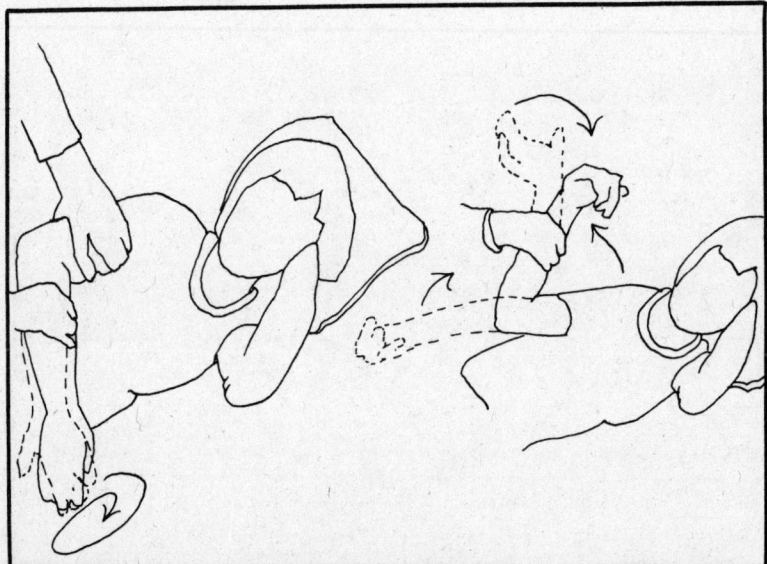

Figure 8-6 (continued)

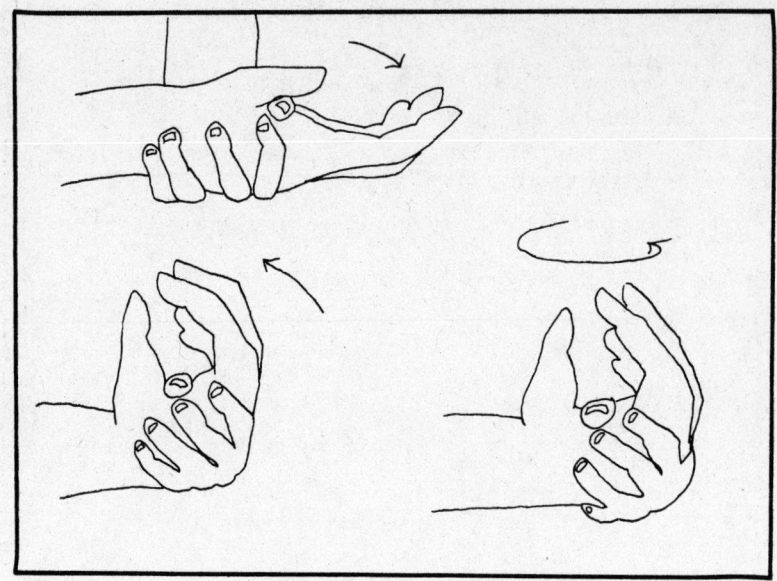

Figure 8-6 (continued)

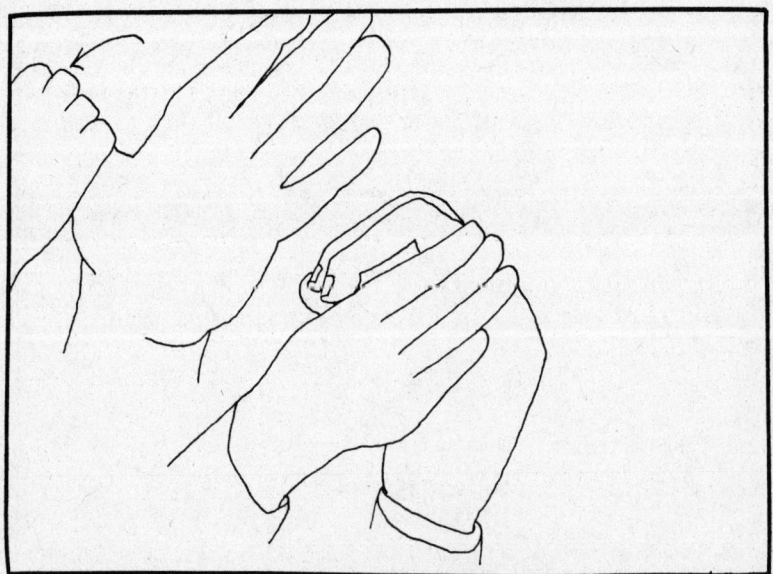

Figure 8-6 (continued)

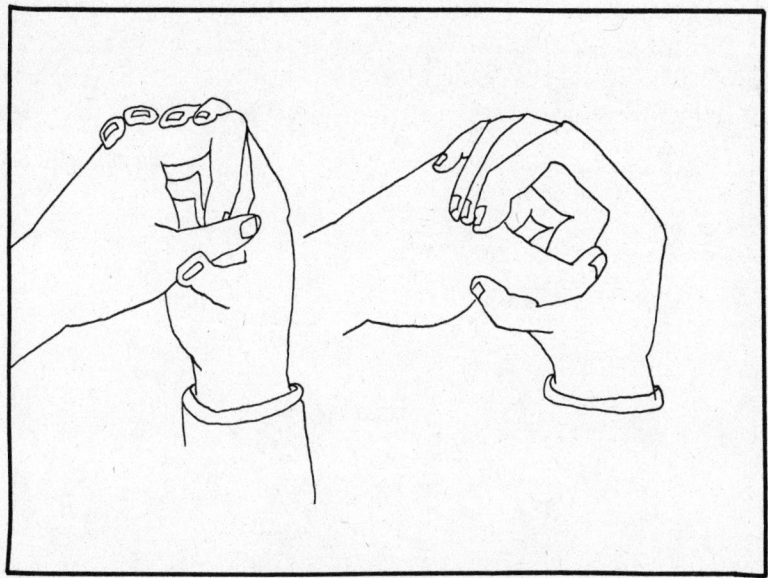

Figure 8-6 (continued)

3. *Leg/foot*. Sharon's leg was flexed and extended at the hip and moved in a circular direction. Her knee was flexed and extended. Her ankle was flexed, extended and rotated. Her toes were both curled up toward the sole of her foot and extended upward. Figure 8-7 shows these movements. Note that in the cases of both arm and leg, some of the motions were accomplished with Sharon lying on her good side, others while she was lying on her back, and still others while she was supported in a sitting position.

Although Sharon didn't have too much loss of sensation, there were patches of numbness. This numbness can be much worse or it may be practically absent after a couple of weeks. In any event, generally the more numbness, the slower the recovery of the muscles, so don't be discouraged at all if limb function seems to be quite slow or even at times does not appear to be progressing at all.

Sharon's persistence, and that of her friends, paid off. She began to feel some of her muscles returning very slight at first, then more and more as each week passed. By the sixth week following her stroke, Sharon was able to start *active* exercises consisting essentially of the *passive* movements described above, but now against the resistance of the therapist's own hands and arms. Soon Sharon progressed to a single tripod crutch and in two months she was walking around the house and doing some of her usual work. Her rehabilitation was begun with joint and muscle toning even though they didn't work at all in the beginning—the joints and muscles were ready for the effort of learning to use them all over again! If they hadn't

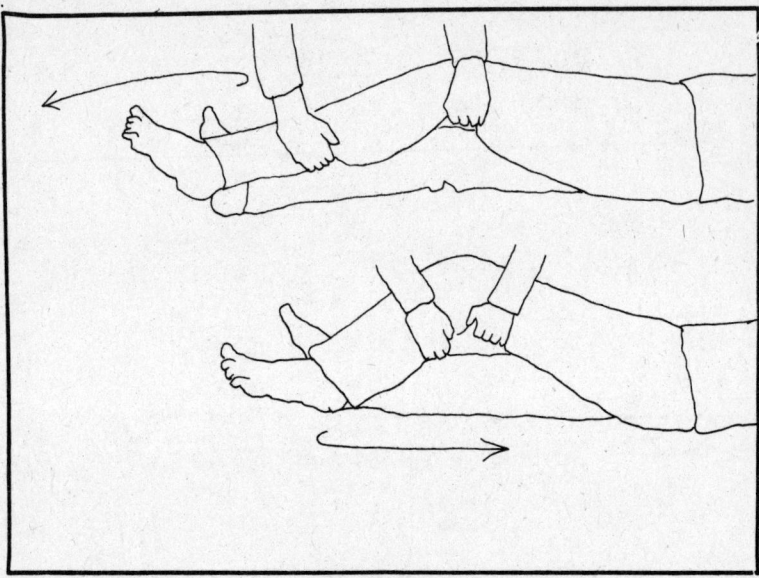

Figure 8-7

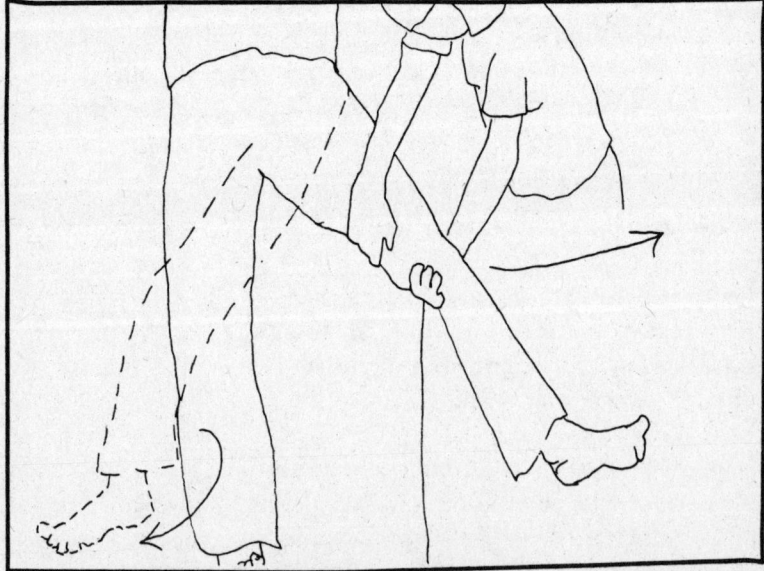

Figure 8-7 (continued)

How to Reverse the Weak Stiff Limb Syndrome 153

been, Sharon's left side would certainly have withered away to nothing, and when her recovery did take place, there would be no limber joints or toned muscles to encourage and develop useful activity again.

Today Sharon has lingering muscle weakness in her left arm and leg,

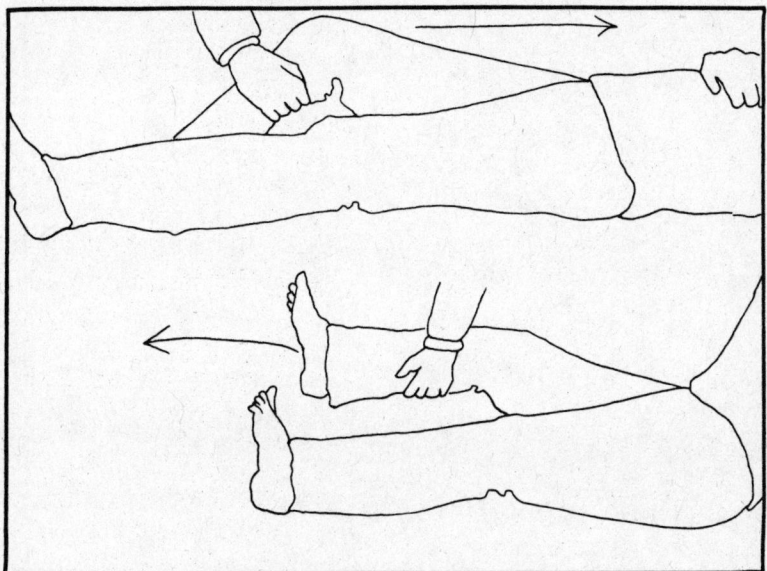

Figure 8-7 (continued)

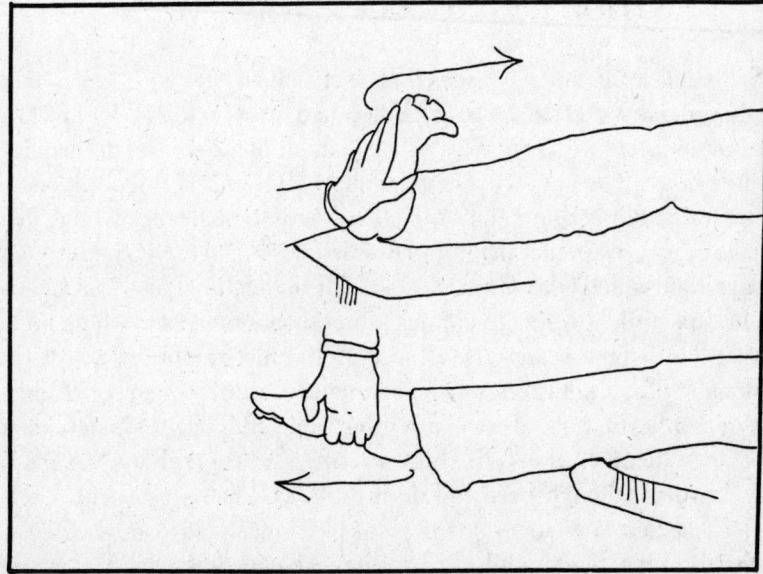

Figure 8-7 (continued)

but a casual glance wouldn't detect it. She walks almost normally without a crutch and uses a cane only when she is fatigued. Her left hand is useful to grip and hold objects, though her fingers are somewhat stiffened. A far cry from useless, lifeless limbs just dangling from their sockets!

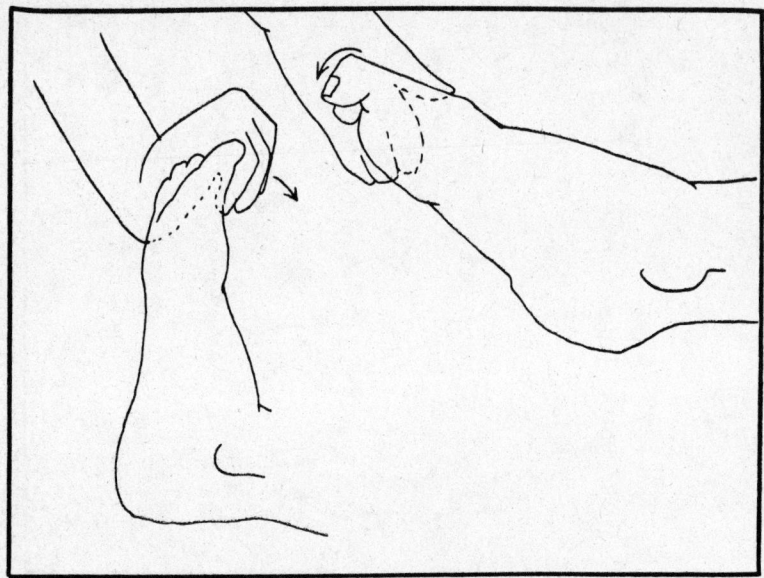

Figure 8-7 (continued)

DOUBLE TROUBLE FOR MEL W.

Sometimes, the fates just seem to be set against a person. A man in his early 40's named Mel W., for example, had heart surgery for a slowly increasing problem with two heart valves that all but kept Mel an invalid at home in a chair. The surgery was quite successful and Mel was like a new man, returning to work and almost the usual activity that most of us enjoy at that stage of life. Two years later, however, he developed high blood pressure and had a right-sided CVA (stroke) as a result, much like Lois B. in Chapter 2. He lost his ability to speak and was rather disoriented as to where he was and what day it was at any given time. Mel's chief trouble was stiff right shoulder and elbow joints after about six weeks of partial recovery of speech ability and only slight recovery of a sense of time and place. He understood what was said to him quite well. He had a difficult time replying through the use of his voice, though he could do it quite well by writing with his left hand—a feat that took some practice, but Mel mastered it thoroughly.

For his stiff shoulder and elbow, a simple device was rigged up at home that Mel was able to use by himself. Figure 8-8 shows how the device

How to Reverse the Weak Stiff Limb Syndrome   155

worked. Mel used the pulley arrangement with his good left hand and arm pulling the rope and moving his shoulder and elbow through the various planes of their motion.

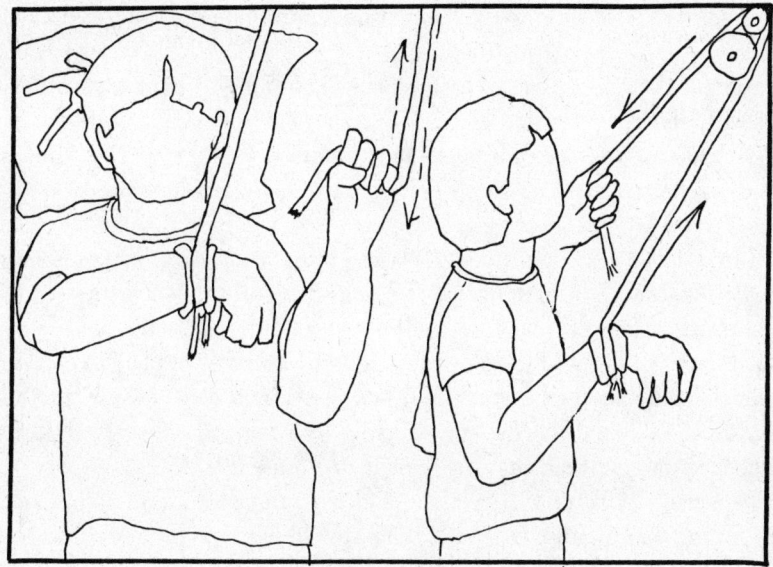

Figure 8-8

He started by using the device while lying flat on his back in bed to reduce the pull of gravity (as it would act were he standing). When Mel became stronger, he was able to use the device standing up. All this kept his two stiff joints from "freezing" and when he began to have some return of muscle power in his shoulder and elbow, he achieved fairly good use of both joints, though not as good as they had been prior to his stroke. The point is, *some function returned.* Had Mel allowed his shoulder and elbow to dangle uselessly during his recovery phase, even that partial return of function would have been to no avail: Mel wouldn't have been able to move those two stubborn joints which would have "frozen" permanently.

SAND: STILL VERSATILE

I suspect many of you will recall someone you know (perhaps yourself) who had an elbow injury as a youth. Whether it had been dislocated or fractured, when the cast came off after some weeks of carrying your injured arm around in a sling encased in rigid plaster, you observed how stiff and unyielding that elbow was even though healing was almost complete. You may also recall how withered some of the muscles in the upper arm and forearm were. This is evidence of what I've said before: Even though muscles and joints not involved directly with the injury are put at forced rest (as in a cast), they get lazy and weak and undergo atrophy—shrinkage of mass. It takes a real effort to overcome this unfortunate, but necessary state of affairs.

You may have had or seen others carrying around "a bucket of sand" to help straighten out stiffened elbows. This remedy is crude, perhaps, but effective nonetheless. Probably the most common mistake was the amount of sand used in the large three-gallon bucket usually procured for this purpose.

A little sand weighs quite a lot. When you start using a bucket (a large coffee can with a carrying strap—such as a dog collar pushed through two slots at either side near the top—will do as well) for that stiff weak elbow and arm, limit the weight to one or two pounds at first. Get used to carrying this around the house with you when you move from one place to another. When you've adjusted to this, start curling with the container of sand, that is, repeated motions like those depicted in Figure 8-9.

With time—one or two weeks—add a pound and then another until you're up to five pounds. The trick is to add enough weight and effort with curling such that some discomfort occurs right at first—not severe pain, just uncomfortable pull. Within six weeks of such effort on your part, that stiff

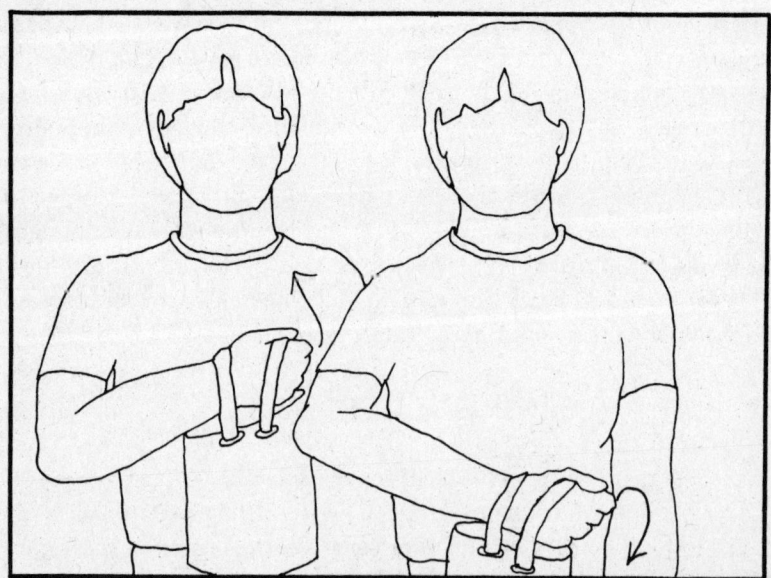

Figure 8-9

How to Reverse the Weak Stiff Limb Syndrome

elbow will allow full straightening out (extension), and the curling exercises will help with full flexion.

Even with amputation

I helped a young man named Chuck M. to regain upper arm and thigh strength by using sand following an accident in which his right arm and left leg had to be amputated surgically just below the elbow and knee respectively.

When using heavy weights of any kind in this way, you should be cautious in *protecting all the pressure points.* In Chuck's case, he used an ordinary piece of 1-inch thick foam rubber to rest his elbow on while exercising his arm, and a piece of the same foam rubber across the stump (well healed by now) where the strap fit. The same applied to his leg stump.

Chuck was able to get fitted for his prostheses (artificial arm and leg) in record time with the strength and vitality he restored to his arm and leg by utilizing this method. And he mastered the use of both of these artificial limbs much sooner as a result of the added strength in the muscles above his two stumps.

THE BENEFITS OF WATER

I suspect that there are many sports as strenuous, or even more so, but none quite so beneficial or versatile as swimming for those who may have certain problems with stiff, weak limbs caused by nerve diseases, such as multiple sclerosis. With such diseases, the trouble is generally spotty—that is, you're apt to have an area of numbness, say, in one hand and a left lower leg that is weak. Or you may have some difficulty with focusing your eyes or moving your tongue the way you'd like and an area of numbness on your abdomen or in the rectal or vaginal areas. Moreover, the areas involved may change from time to time with actual improvement in the numbness and weakness that first appeared. Severe weaknesses, even bladder and rectal disfunction, may improve following the natural flare-ups which may be severe, but often recover, especially following treatment with newer drugs. Unfortunately, such medicines don't cure the process; they do, however, control it, often to a surprising degree.

The time to start involving both the weakened muscle groups and those that remain untouched is right now! And swimming is one of the best ways I've found to do just that. You may even need help at first, but accept it. All that's needed is a pool and someone to aid you at first. Even if you only swim 15 feet, or even 6 feet at one time, you're doing your body a tremendous favor. The reason for this is that with swimming, there are very few muscles that aren't used. And more importantly, you're taking advantage of the natural buoyancy of water. Haven't you noticed how much easier it is to lift someone up in the air when both of you are standing in a pool? How much easier your own body is to handle when you allow the water to support your weight? This is because you actually weigh less in water—the water relieves your muscles of having to move against a good percentage of gravity, freeing them to push, pull, lift, bend, and flex your body weight with much more efficiency.

In fact, you can do a lot at home with a bathtub that is a half to two thirds full of water in the way of limbering stiff joints and exercising flabby muscles weakened by disuse and disease. Simply climb into the water and do your exercising with the limb buoyed up by the water! You can't swim, of course, but you can exercise both legs and arms in your own bathtub. And by regulation of the temperature, you can have the double advantage of heat to go along with the antigravity effects.

I knew a lady, Florence R., whose flare-ups with MS forced her into a wheel chair and to need help even with eating. Nevertheless, Florence had discovered the benefits of the pool long before and would insist on being wheeled right over to the pool twice a day where she was helped to slide from chair to pool and, while being supported on her back in the water, she was able to kick and exercise her buttock and thigh muscles. With support on her stomach in the water, she was able to exercise both shoulders and arms.

I can't say what Florence might be like today without her zeal and willingness to fight the odds with the pool conditioning, but I do know that when Florence's MS goes into remission (a lessening of symptoms following a flare-up), she is able to bounce right out of that wheel chair and carry on a fairly normal life with vastly improved muscle tone.

SUMMARY

1. Not using your joints because of the pain of arthritis may cause stiffening. When the pain is controlled, you can help your joints and the tendons that span them by seeing to it that they're put through exercises and toning at an early stage.
2. Following injury, as with acute attacks of arthritis, you can make it a point, and a daily routine—even though it may cause distress and *some* pain—to put the involved joint or joints, together with the muscles that move them, through their full ranges of motion lest they stiffen and permanently weaken.
3. Strokes are serious business, but recovery of at least partial function of involved limbs depends absolutely on your ability to

stick with toning and use of these limbs even though you may feel clumsy and awkward at first, and even if what you end up with is not as efficient as what you started with. After all, any useful function of a limb, no matter how insignificant you may think it is, is far better than no function at all.

4. There is much you can do at home to help with stiff, painful joints by utilizing heat, cold, simple pain medicines, pulleys and rope, sand and water.

5. Remember that no matter how you may feel following injury, disease, or stroke—no matter how discouraged you get at first—keeping up with toning and the use of those joints and muscles may mean the difference between wheel chair and walking, or between the ability to care for yourself and needing others to do it for you.

9

Keeping the Rest of Your Body in Top Shape

I want to point out in this chapter how you can keep the rest of your body—the parts not involved with muscle, bone or arthritic problems—in shape. I'll talk about common things that come up while you're recuperating from various ailments of the skeleton, things that bring on hemorrhoids and constipation, for example, and some of the problems associated with paralysis below the waist—the bladder and rectum that don't work normally and other disorders.

We'll also go over toning your "good limbs," and talk about specific things you can do to keep the non-involved muscles, bones and joints working in even better order so that they can bear an extra burden as your involved extremities recover and heal.

We'll also discuss certain heart and lung problems that recurrently plague persons with special disorders such as curvature of the spine. We'll take a look at what you can do to prevent, as well as deal with such problems.

YOUR DIGESTIVE TRACT: ITS CARE AND FEEDING

One of the most common areas of your body that consistently causes trouble along with ailments of bones, muscles and joints, is your digestive system—the part of your anatomy from mouth to rectum. This lengthy tube is called the gastrointestinal tract, often abbreviated as the G. I. tract.

Since your G. I. tract begins with your mouth, let's look for a minute at this organ and see what happens to it.

Teeth

Teeth are probably the most neglected part of your G. I. and skeletal systems. I use the word "skeletal" here because your teeth are formed and

Keeping the Rest of Your Body in Top Shape

anchored in your upper and lower jaw bones. Teeth are lost by Americans at far too early an age, generally because of neglect. They're made to last a lifetime, but they seldom reach the golden stage of maturity.

This seems especially true in people with arthritis and other bone and muscle disorders—particularly those that keep you confined for periods of time, or those that cause one side of your body, usually the "dominant side," to be temporarily out of commission, as in a stroke. So it's important to remember your teeth—even more than ever—during a bout of trouble.

The following rules will guide you during problems with your limbs and back, as well as serve as a guide for when you're well:

1. Brush your teeth thoroughly with salt and baking soda, mixed in equal parts, once daily followed if you wish by your favorite tooth paste. Brush with a fairly rigid tooth brush. During the tooth paste brushing, you should make it a point to brush mostly your gums, the inside of your cheeks, and your tongue. This should be done in the morning after breakfast or before bedtime at night.

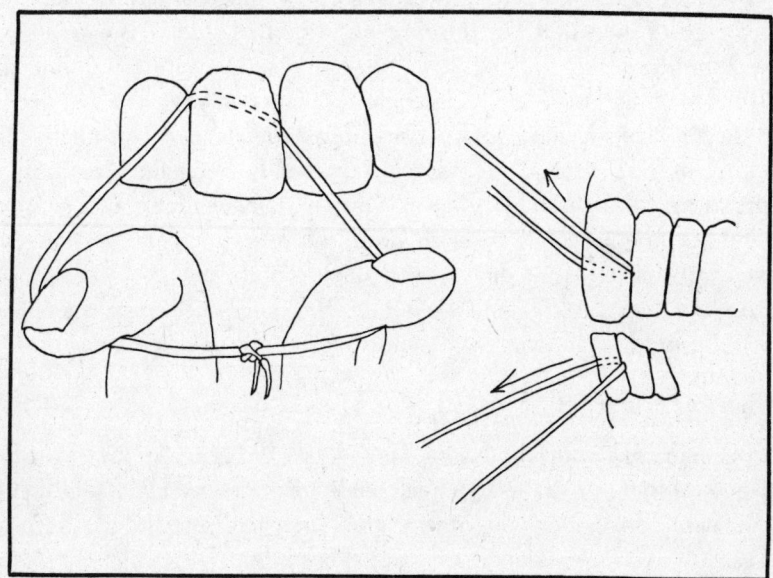

Figure 9-1

2. Floss your teeth thoroughly and daily with unwaxed dental floss. If you brush in the morning, floss at night after supper. If you brush in the evening, floss in the morning after breakfast. Flossing means to take a piece of dental floss (purchased at most drug or grocery

stores) about 12 inches long out of the tube and tie a double knot in the two free ends. The loop thus formed is easily controlled and is stretched so that the floss is wedged into every one of the spaces between your teeth and pulled, first against the side of one of the two teeth, then the other, back and forth to dislodge food particles that collect there and to remove plaque—the film containing bacteria and acids that start cavities. This maneuver *will save your gums* from disease and will toughen them to resist atrophy (shrinkage) *which is the most common cause of tooth loss.* Figure 9-1 shows the flossing technique.

3. Visit your dentist at least twice a year for check-ups. You will be rewarded by teeth that last long and wear well.
4. If one arm or hand is not working well, concentrate on using the other hand to perform tooth hygiene. It can be done, including flossing, with one hand using the loop method I've described.

Mouth

In stroke and certain other nerve disorders, one side of the mouth may lose its feeling as well as the chewing power on that side. The caution here is to eat and chew carefully at mealtime—you can bite into your numb side with your teeth and not feel it. This doesn't mean that you shouldn't use the numb side if your jaw muscles will work, but it means to do so with caution. Following meals, inspect the side of your mouth that's numb or partially paralyzed to make certain you haven't bitten your tongue, cheek or lip. If you find that you have, use a cotton swab with hydrogen peroxide to keep it cleaned out, and healing should take place rapidly.

As an alternative to using the numb side, chew only on your good side for a while until some sensation comes back to the affected side.

Swallowing apparatus

Occasionally, your swallowing apparatus will be involved with various arthritic and other problems. This is usually temporary, but some difficulty may persist. During the phase of your problem when swallowing is difficult, stick mostly with liquids and very soft foods such as jello, junkets, smooth cooked cereal, and ice cream. Usually these foods will pass down when others won't.

By using protein supplements (milk shakes with eggs mixed in them, yogurt preparations) you can achieve a balanced diet for an indefinite time if you have to. (See the section in Chapter 14 on diet, or see my recent book, *The Biofeedback Diet: A Doctor's Revolutionary Approach*, for details.)

Keeping the Rest of Your Body in Top Shape

Recall, too, that when your swallowing apparatus is involved with any disorder, it is well to eat and drink *slowly*. This allows the slowed down action of your gullet (esophagus) to carry nutrition down to your stomach for initial digestion.

Stomach

During periods of altered activity—such as when you're temporarily confined to a bed or chair for a short time—your stomach continues to produce acid and digestive juices as it did before your affliction. This will sometimes bring on an acid stomach condition because you don't put as much bulk food into it for the juices to work on. If you have problems with acid stomach or heartburn, as it's sometimes called, remember that there are many antacids—medicines that neutralize acid—that can be purchased at your drug store or grocery store. These preparations usually contain aluminum or magnesium carbonate, or both, and the labels on antacid containers can be read to see if these ingredients are in them.

In case such preparations can't be found, you can use milk of magnesia to help acid stomach. But be certain to read the label on the milk of magnesia bottle (liquid form) or box (tablet form). It will give you directions for the *antacid dose* and the dose to use for *constipation*. If you happen to have both an acid stomach and constipation, this is an ideal medicine to use, following the constipation doses given on the label.

When your stomach is upset or acid-feeling, it's better to eat or drink your liquid and soft diet more often—every hour or so, for example—rather than to let long lapses of time pass by between feedings. This puts something into your stomach for the digestive juices to work on so they won't irritate your stomach lining. It is better *not* to use baking soda to help an acid stomach.

Bowels

Periods of bed rest and inactivity generally bring on sluggish bowels. This condition is usually caused by two problems: not enough physical exercise and not enough liquids in addition to your regular diet.

The following hints will help to see you through constipation:

1. Train your bowel to move at regular intervals as close to the same time of day as you can. Your bowel is much like a dog in this respect: It can be trained to empty at intervals, to give you a "feeling" that you have to move your bowels at certain times.

2. Get as much physical exercise as your particular ailment will allow. Even if you're confined to a bed or a chair, you can utilize certain

Keeping the Rest of Your Body in Top Shape

isometrics for your abdominal muscles that will materially help you to move your bowels, as we'll see later in this chapter. If you can walk at all, even with crutches, do so as often and for as long as you possibly can each day.

3. Keep your bowels softened. This is done naturally by drinking plenty of liquids each day—the hotter the weather and the more exercise you can get, the more liquids you need. Water is readily available and should be taken in generous amounts, including with meals, frequently between meals, last thing before bedtime, and first thing on arising from bed. Remember that milk and dairy products, as nutritional as they are, tend to bind your bowels Strive for proper balance with dairy products when you're constipated.

4. If stool hardness is still a problem, reduce the fiber content of your diet until softening occurs. The fiber content is high in meats, vegetables, and cereals and lower in other foods.

5. There are medicines, perfectly safe to use, that physically soften your stool without any other effect, and they are not absorbed from your bowel. These medicines act by attracting water into the stool itself. Consult your medical advisor about the best one for you. You can feel safe in taking such medicines over a prolonged period of time if you need to and since they are not laxatives, they won't cause a "laxative habit."

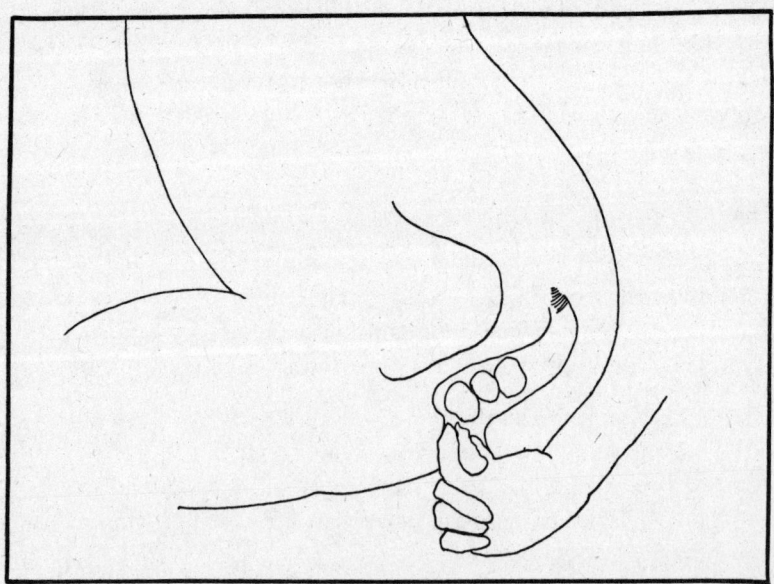

Figure 9-2

6. If you occasionally do need a laxative, just plain milk of magnesia taken as directed on the bottle or on the package should be sufficient.

Sometimes a hard knot of stool will collect in your rectal canal just up inside the anal opening—the outlet controlled by the circular bands of your sphincter muscles. If this happens, simply put on a rubber glove or finger cot (a single rubber covering for one finger), lubricate the finger well with plain Vaseline or mineral oil, and gently insert your finger up inside the rectal canal. When you've located the hard knot of stool, try to break it up with your finger into smaller chunks, and then gently pry them out, piece by piece, until the hard knot is eliminated. Figure 9-2 shows this movement.

Hemorrhoids

These pesky protrusions are perfectly normal vein structures that become congested just up inside your rectal canal and then bulge out. Sometimes they protrude outside your anal opening. They're called hemorrhoids because they are the normal hemorrhoidal veins that belong in your rectal canal. They can be quite an aggravation at times, especially when you're debilitated for any reason. The following will help in the care of hemorrhoids.

1. Keep your bowels soft and move them regularly. Straining to move hard stools makes hemorrhoids worse.
2. Don't prolong the session on the toilet at bowel movement time. Just sitting there too long can make hemorrhoids protrude. Perform the job rapidly and then get off the toilet.
3. If you have protruding hemorrhoids following a bowel movement, take a clean piece of toilet paper after cleansing your anus and place a generous portion of Vaseline or facial cream on it. Place the paper with the emollient on your hemorrhoids and gently with your fingers through the toilet paper, push them toward your anal opening and keep firm sustained pressure on them. They can often be made to return back up inside the rectal canal. At the same time as you're doing this maneuver, concentrate on your anal sphincter muscles to *relax*. This allows the hemorrhoidal veins an easier passage back into the rectum.
4. Suppositories can help after hemorrhoids are pushed back inside the rectal canal. The suppository should be gently inserted *after* you've pushed the hemorrhoids back in place, and can be used at

bedtime again if desired. The best suppositories contain medicines designed to sooth the irritation hemorrhoids usually bring on and in addition are designed to cause the veins to contract, thus shrinking down the size of the hemorrhoids. Your medical advisor or druggist can instruct you on the best kind of suppositories to use.

5. A little bleeding is not at all unusual with hemorrhoids. Sometimes the veins break and bleeding occurs. This is seldom a cause for alarm. It usually isn't a lot of bleeding and generally stops in a short time. If troublesome hemorrhoids continue to plague you in spite of continued care as outlined here, you may want to consider having them removed surgically, a simple procedure that when properly done will obliterate the troublesome veins.

Stella J. fights back

Stella J. was only 26 when she was involved in a serious car accident. She fractured her lower back and was paralyzed from the lower abdomen down, including both legs and pelvis.

In the process of rehabilitation for her injury, Stella was confined to a wheel chair; her willful control of both bowel and bladder was gone. When this became a reality, Stella panicked. "How will I eliminate my wastes?" she wondered. How can anyone cope with such a problem? Well, they can and do, all the time and every day.

Each day at a prescribed time, Stella was taught to manually empty her lower bowel using exactly the same technique I've described for dealing with hard knots of stool. Stella placed a finger cot over the first finger of her right hand (it could be either hand), lubricated it with mineral oil and gently emptied out her rectal canal. And she's done this every day for five years! Stella was horrified at first by "the mess," but she soon learned, as you will if you must use the technique only now and again, that "mess" is only in the mind of the beholder—you do what must be done. And when you've accustomed yourself to it, it's no longer a mess, but the normal way you do it for your particular problem.

Stella developed hemorrhoids shortly after returning home from the hospital. She wasn't able to feel the area around her anal canal well enough to control them as efficiently as I've described because the nerves that convey sensation in this area were numb along with the rest of the nerves from her waist down. But her sphincter muscles had some tone left in them since they're also controlled by a second set of nerves that work automatically.

Keeping the Rest of Your Body in Top Shape

I had Stella climb into a tub of piping hot water twice daily for a while when her hemorrhoids developed, and instructed her to keep the water as hot as she could. She tested the temperature with her fingers and elbow since, of course, this sensation, too, was lost to her below her waist. This technique (sometimes called Sitz baths) plus local care brought Stella's hemorrhoids under control. Figure 9-3 shows positioning for a Sitz bath.

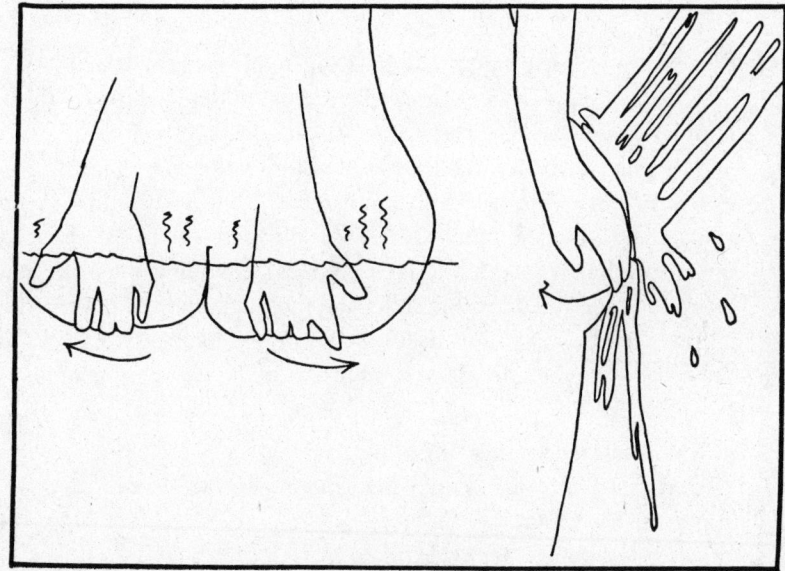

Figure 9-3

THE URINARY TRACT

The urinary apparatus needs attention as well during periods of prolonged bed rest and debilitation.

For example, in Stella's case, she lost the ability to willfully empty her bladder. The use of a catheter was necessary. Stella was trained to empty her bladder at regular intervals each day by means of a hollow glass rod carefully and gently inserted into her bladder via her urethra—the outside opening of the tube leading from the bladder outside. This type of catheter is one of several types, but it is the safest for repeated use as in Stella's case. Of course, the glass rods needed special attention between uses to keep them clean and sterile.

In your case, assuming you haven't gone through what Stella did, you should remember that to keep a healthy urinary tract during periods of ailments when you don't get around as well as usual, you need to keep *drinking liquids in large quantities.* Make a habit of drinking two full glasses of water—large glasses—between each meal and during your meals. In hot weather, increase this to three glasses. Anything liquid will furnish the necessary water—coffee, tea, juices, malts, pop, egg nogs, milk, and other beverages.

The following list may help you keep your urinary tract in good running order:

1. Sometimes following a spinal cord injury or disease, your bladder may empty "on its own accord" and rather suddenly at times. If this happens, wear an absorbent material like a baby diaper or Kotex pad in your perineal (crotch) area. Following the emptying, be sure that your perineum is dried thoroughly—urine is irritating to the skin, and will cause much distress if left there. The best agent for this procedure is a bland (no perfumes) emollient such as skin cream or Vaseline on cotton following thorough blotting of the urine on the skin by absorbent tissue paper. You should leave a little of the emollient cream in place on your perineum between treatments.

2. For washing your perineum area, use plain soap and water—a soap to which no deodorants or perfumed substances have been added. They're hard on your skin. Rinse thoroughly with water, dry, and apply the emollient.

3. *Do not* attempt to place anything, including a catheter, into your bladder without first having been taught the technique by your medical advisor. Once you learn such techniques (and it's easily mastered) for your particular problem, you may then confidently and safely do it yourself at home.

4. If you notice that your bladder isn't working properly during any ailment that forces you to be at prolonged rest, and you can feel your bladder protruding as a grapefruit-sized bulge above your pubis bone, don't delay—consult expert medical help!

In Stella's case, after some problems with recurrent urinary tract infection, her medical advisor put her on some medicine designed to reduce the number of bacteria in her urinary tract and bladder. She continues to take the medicine even today and has only occasional problems with infection.

If you notice sudden irritation or frank pain during the act of urinating or just after urination, increased frequency of urination, chills and/or fever, a urinary infection may be the cause and your medical advisor needs to be consulted. Remember, too, that one of the most important rules in treating

Keeping the Rest of Your Body in Top Shape

urinary tract infections is *doubling your intake of fluids until the last traces of infection are gone.* This may take two or even three weeks. But don't let up, and continue to follow medical advice.

Urinary stone

Kidney (renal) stones and bladder stones are not uncommon problems, especially for those who are debilitated. It is best when they can be prevented, of course, but sometimes they will form in spite of the best preventive efforts. The first line of defense against urinary tract stones is our old standby: fluids, and plenty of them, in your diet and as much physical activity as you can muster.

Physical activity is the second line of defense against the formation of urinary stones, but sometimes because of your particular infirmity enough physical activity simply can't be gotten in each day. It has been shown time and time again that just getting out of a horizontal position and standing up, even if just for a short time several times a day, will help keep your urinary tract free of stones. This is one of several important reasons why I've emphasized the role of muscle toning and exercises while you are taking care of arthritis, bone and muscle ailments.

For people who are paralyzed for any reason, the most common place for urinary stones to form is in the bladder. Bladder stones, unlike the smaller urinary stones that form higher up in the urinary tract, aren't noted for their spontaneous passage out of the bladder. This is why people with both legs paralyzed, like Stella for example, need to visit their medical facility routinely at least twice a year so that such bladder stones can be looked for, and if found, crushed inside the bladder and flushed out, a relatively easy out-patient procedure.

Gus R. prevails

Urinary stones can be caused by things other than inactivity, however, as Gus R., a man in his early 50's who had a stroke, found out. During his stroke recovery, in which Gus's left side was paralyzed for a time, he began to pass urinary stones—formed near his kidney and passed through the tube from kidney to bladder and thence outside.

Gus became a stone former. Fortunately, the stones in Gus's case weren't large—in fact they were little more than ordinary fine "gravel"—but they felt to Gus like the Rock of Gibraltar when they were being passed! Gus's doctor had his stones analyzed, subjected to tests to learn what his stones were made of. Each stone has its own "fingerprint" or chemical salt of which it is mainly composed. It was found in Gus's case that a particular salt containing phosphate was the culprit. His doctor prescribed a medicine that removed phosphate compounds from his diet (Gus took the medicine with his meals) and his stone forming came to an end.

CARDIOPULMONARY TRACT

The term "cardiopulmonary" refers to your heart and lungs. That both need a little more attention during times of bone, muscle and arthritic ailments is attested to by the fact that in hospitals the most common complication following any surgery involves this system.

Consider what happens when you have to be at rest for any reason beyond what is usual for you. Your heart, a most efficient muscular pump, isn't required to work as hard when you're lying down in bed. It works harder when you're sitting up in a chair or on the side of your bed; and even harder when you're standing; it works harder still when you are standing and moving around. Now it's true that any muscle, including your heart, can be strained beyond what is good for it. On the other hand, when it is allowed to go flabby, any muscle, including your heart, suffers. What I'm trying to get across here is that you need not go to either extreme (too little or too much exercise), but you should strive to settle on a point somewhere in between.

Your heart must also pump blood through literally hundreds of miles of your blood vessel "pipes." When they are at prolonged rest, these vessels also get "flabby" and the blood inside them becomes "stagnant." The trouble may start at this point.

What you should try to do in periods of disability when you aren't getting your usual exercise by being up and moving around is to mimic being up and around. This helps to restore tone to your heart and blood vessels and it keeps your blood circulating through its vessels in a more efficient manner so that the blood isn't so apt to congeal.

The same applies to your lungs. Your heart pumps all of your body's blood through your lungs every few minutes. The reason for this is to allow your blood to pick up oxygen from the air you breathe in, and to give up carbon dioxide (the final product of your body metabolism) so that you can breathe it back out. It is difficult to talk about heart and blood vessel action without also considering your lungs, so we'll discuss them as a single system, working as a smoothly running pump to deliver oxygen to your tissues and to eliminate carbon dioxide from them.

At bed rest

When you're lying in bed, from a flare-up of arthritis in one or several joints, or from a stroke, or from any condition that puts you down for a

Keeping the Rest of Your Body in Top Shape 171

while, there are things you can do to help your pump system keep performing for you at higher efficiency. The following list describes what I mean:

1. All muscles not involved with your ailment need toning at least twice during the day. Even spending 30 minutes or longer at this three or four times a day isn't too much time to devote to it. You can use isometrics for this—that is, forcibly contracting a group of muscles against any resistance. An example of this is to scoot down in your bed far enough so that both legs must be flexed at your knee and so that the soles of your feet rest against the foot of your bed. Now simply force your legs to push against the foot of the bed and then relax. Repeat this activity several times, pushing harder each time, even using the afflicted leg if that's possible, as much as you can without causing severe pain. With such isometrics, you need to start at your toes, your feet, and your lower legs and work up systematically to thighs, abdomen, chest, shoulders, upper and lower arms, hands and fingers, and finally your neck and face. Put all the muscles you can through their paces in this manner. Jim D., a man in his mid-50's with a left-sided stroke, accomplished this by using his wife as "something to push against." Following her efforts three times a day at moving Jim's partially paralyzed limbs, his wife would move to Jim's good side (his right side) and he would exercise his muscle groups systematically from his toes to his neck by forcing them to push against her hands and arms. For example, with Jim's right arm extended out on the bed and flexed at his elbow, she would push against his lower arm while he forced out against her hands. She would then position her hands so that they pulled his forearm toward her, while Jim pulled in the opposite direction with his forearm.

2. It's a good idea to further stimulate the circulation in both legs by wearing a pair of well-fitted elastic stockings during the entire time that you're confined to bed or to a chair. The stockings, to work properly, should extend from the area where the toes join your feet upward to well past midthigh. They should fit snugly, being neither loose nor too tight. Your medical advisor, hospital, local drug store, or surgical supply house can see that you are supplied with such stockings. Furthermore, as you become more active—up and out of bed and chair—you should put the stockings back on at bed-time until you have become fully ambulatory again.

3. At least three times a day, following your toning exercises, use this routine for your lungs: Force in 12 deep breaths of air into your lungs, using your diaphragm muscle (the large muscle that sucks in air when you breathe in) to pull in as much air as possible (much more than a usual breath); then push all this air out of your lungs, again using your diaphragm muscle to push every last bit of the air out. At the end of this deep breathing session, give at least three good deep coughs ("come up from the bottom each time"). Figure 9-4 shows some of Jim's toning routine.

4. Another good idea, during your toning routines and while lying flat on your back in bed or sitting up on the side of your bed or chair, is to do several belly isometrics. Suck your entire abdominal muscle area inward until you can't pull in any farther; then force the muscles outward again as far as they'll go. Repeat this several times. At first your stomach muscles will feel sore following this exercise. But you will not only have toned your abdominal muscles (at least the unaffected side of your abdomen, if you have had a stroke), but you will have aided your intestinal tract to help you avoid constipation. Such abdominal muscle contraction also makes your intestine contract and squeeze its contents toward your lower bowel, a double bonus when you're incapacitated!

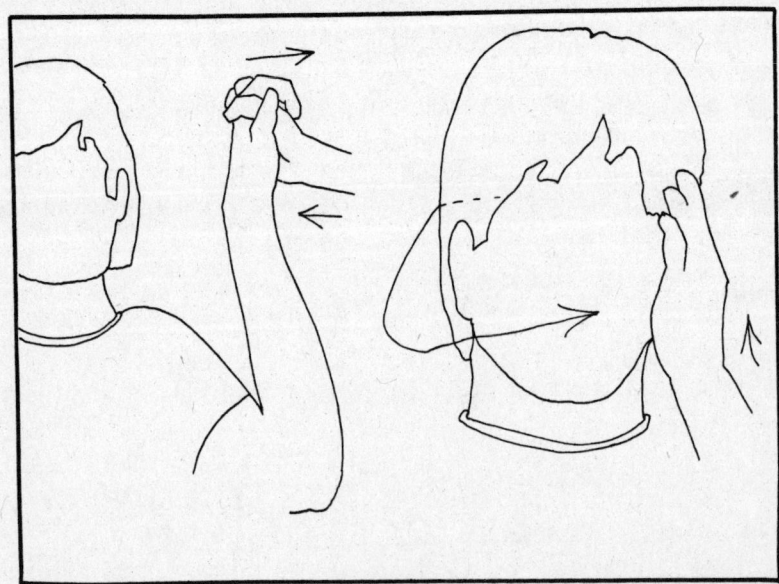

Figure 9-4

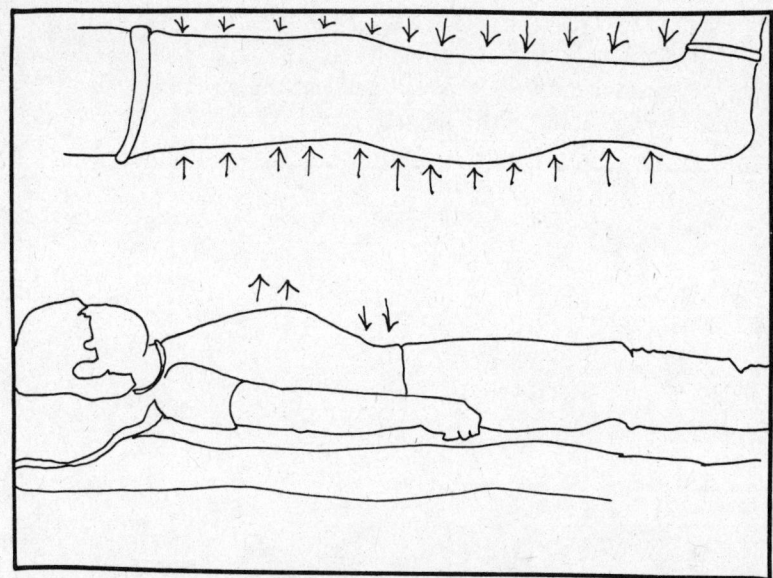

Figure 9-4 (continued)

5. When you're confined to bed for more than two weeks, you should seriously consider getting hold of an orthopedic bed. This is a special bed used on the orthopedic floors of hospitals where, for example, people must recover from injuries and surgery in which one or both legs are enclosed in plaster casts, or when the lower spine has been injured and neither lower limb is working properly. The main feature of such a bed (and it can usually be rented from your local hospital or surgical supply house) is that it has a metal rod extending from head to foot which is clamped to the bed frame. There is an adjustable "trapeze" bar hanging from the center rod that you can grab with one or both hands to pull yourself upright and do all sorts of toning exercises with. The trapeze bar also aids in getting yourself to a sitting position at the side of the bed as well as helping you to get out of bed and into a chair. I recall a patient of mine, Ed N., who had rather serious leg injuries and found himself depending a good deal on his wife and friends for help in changing positions or getting out of bed with both legs encased in plaster casts from thighs to toes. A friend of his was handy with tools and constructed such an apparatus for Ed's own bed by using rope strung between two 2x2 boards screwed into the head and foot of his bed. Then the friend fashioned two movable ropes to hang from the main trolley and tied them to an axe handle. It worked quite well, though it wasn't as fancy as the bed in the hospital where Ed had

been. But fancy doesn't matter; what does matter is function. Ed's trapeze functioned well enough to keep him in good muscular tone and to make him less dependent on others during his recovery. Figure 9-5 shows Ed's apparatus.

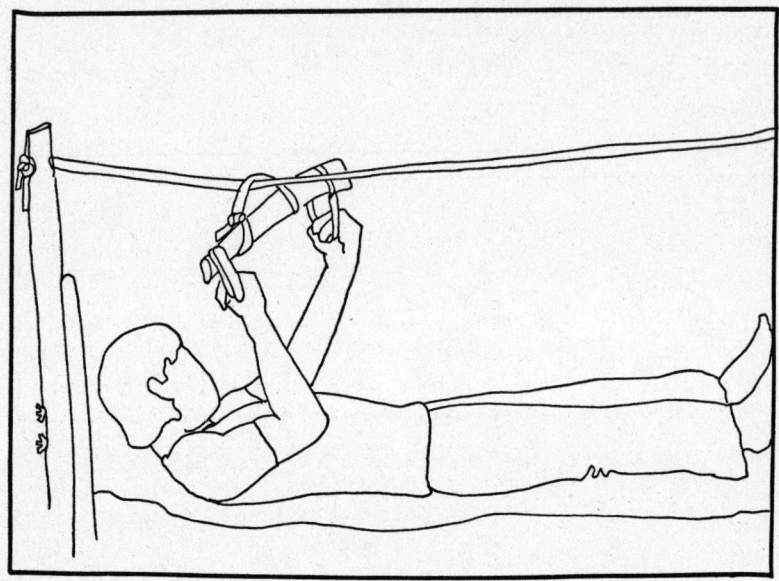

Figure 9-5

Sitting up

You can do many things more easily and efficiently when you are sitting than you can lying down as far as toning and moving around is concerned. Your abdominal isometrics (described previously for toning abdominal muscles and aiding to prevent constipation) are more easily done if you are sitting up. You can squeeze your belly muscles harder, and gravity pulls your abdominal contents downward when you're sitting, thereby making the toning more efficient.

You can twist at your waist when sitting, a difficult maneuver when you're flat in bed. And you can do isometrics by pitting your own muscles against one another more efficiently sitting than you can lying down.

It's also easier—much easier—on your helper, whose aid you may still need in sitting up if one side of your body is partially paralyzed or out of commission for any of several other reasons. He or she can do much more for you with you sitting up and doing more to help yourself than if you're

Keeping the Rest of Your Body in Top Shape 175

lying in bed. In addition, the movements you make while sitting up must work against gravity—something they didn't have to do since your bed supported your limbs lying down. This adds more effort on your part.

Eve W. gets in shape

The case of Eve W. illustrates what has to happen during recovery from the debilitation brought on by some types of problems corrected by surgery. And it shows how each step of a general plan with a goal in mind helps you to plan your days.

Eve was only 24 when she had a newer type of surgery done to correct a condition called scoliosis of the spine. This means that Eve had a double curvature of her backbone that started when she was an early teenager. No one knows exactly why. She began to notice a hump in her back near her right shoulder that got slowly but progressively worse with each passing year. At the same time, she noticed increasing upper and lower back discomfort and stress. The process that was curving her upper spine to the right side was causing a compensatory curve of her lower spine in the opposite direction. Braces and casts seemed not to do too much good and surgery was done that involved "remolding" the spine and holding it securely in place by means of metal rods fastened to her spine.

When Eve was in her third day of recuperation after surgery (she came through it with no problems), her doctors started her on leg exercises while Eve sat on the side of her hospital bed—the kind I've described in previous sections—where increasing weights were added to her shoes and she raised each leg from a hanging position to straight out, then back down again. Why this particular toning? Because Eve's legs would have to be extra strong for the next phase of her therapy which turned out to be riding a stationary bicycle—a machine with wheels, seat and pedals like an ordinary bike, but with the wheels elevated off the floor. This was because the curvature of Eve's spine had begun to compromise her lung breathing capacity, as is common with this deformity. And if Eve were ever going to regain her lost lung power, she would have to get herself into a position of doing pulmonary demand exercises (sometimes called aerobic conditioning). This means particular exercises that cause your body to move through space—jogging, swimming, bicycle riding, rowing a boat and similar activities. Such exercise eventually would help restore Eve's lost "wind." And it did. Today Eve has normal lung power, thanks to early planning and insistence (often against Eve's wishes) on proper rehabilitation procedures. Eve will live longer and be healthier for having gone through it.

SUMMARY

1. When you're recuperating from a variety of ailments involving bones, muscles and joints, your digestive tract must be cared for to aid in recovery and prevent complications.

2. Taking care of your digestive apparatus starts with your teeth and ends with your rectum and involves your stomach and intestine between the two. You can train your bowel to work for you in preventing constipation, you can pamper your stomach by dieting carefully and using principles of good nutrition, and you can deal with hemorrhoids if they occur by using common sense approaches.

3. Even if your body is paralyzed or partially so below your waist, the problems this brings on can be coped with. You may need to empty your rectum and bladder by artificial means, but this can be done (with advice and tutoring from your medical advisor) at home as well as in a hospital.

4. Your digestive apparatus as well as your urinary system will be helped greatly to stay in good functioning order if you take ample fluids with and between meals.

5. The care of areas that are apt to be irritated from moisture and waste products—especially your perineum (crotch)—is highly important and best managed by materials that absorb moisture well and by frequent application of emollients.

6. Your heart and lungs need attention during disability and can be helped to maintain good function by general muscle toning (even in bed), wearing elastic support stockings while confined to bed and chair, and deep breathing and coughing frequently throughout the day.

10

The Care and Feeding of Your Bones and Muscles

We'll examine the effect of tone and rest on bones and muscles in this chapter and take a closer look at the affliction called osteoporosis. I'll show you what bone and muscle need to stay healthy, and the extras they may need to keep functioning.

Your upper limbs require different techniques of care and feeding than do your lower limbs. We'll have a look at the differences and talk about how you can ensure the best possible health for all four limbs under a variety of circumstances.

There are still a number of afflictions that do their damage in childhood, yet remain on into adulthood to plague your life. I'll describe some of these ailments and show you what others have done to help maintain function.

TONE THAT BONE

Earlier in the book, I mentioned that muscle toning brings along with it many bonuses of health, bonuses that reach even the inner recesses of your mind. You learned, too, that muscles are made of special tissue and are attached to bone with guy wires called tendons, yet another of your body's special tissues. Tendons are tough, resilient, and flexible. Some tendons, such as those that move your eyeball around in its socket, are even pulled through "pulleys"—tiny bony hooks and rings that furnish finely honed guides for the muscles of your eyes. Without them you wouldn't be able to move your eyeballs in virtually any direction around a complete circle.

Tendons, of whatever size and shape, have one thing in common: They're all attached at one end to a muscle, or group of muscles, and at the other end to bone. Some people have naturally "loose" tendon attachments to bone. That is, their tendons, though perfectly functional, don't have quite the pull on their muscles that some others do. The reason for the weaker pull is that their tendons aren't as firmly and rigidly anchored to the bony end of the attachment.

Toning exercise may help this tendency. It works two ways: It helps put toughness back into tendons, and it helps firm up the bony attachment of tendons—actually making the union of tendon to bone stronger.

In addition, toning gives bones a bonus as well, and when your bones improve, so also does your blood chemistry, your body's ability to rebuild virtually all its tissues (as they need to be rebuilt during the natural course of life—most certainly so after injury or disease), and toning even brings an important bonus to your mind!

How is this possible? What earthly connection could their be among all these different tissues, let alone your mind? Consider the following chain of events:

1. Constant muscle contraction (as with toning exercises) pulls on tendon.
2. Pull on tendon stimulates bony surface to which it's attached.
3. Stimulation of bone produces need for mobilizing calcium and proteins to strengthen tendon/bone attachment.
4. Virtually all calcium is bound to protein in your body. Increased mobilization of this calcium/protein complex travels throughout the length and breadth of your blood vessels, including those going to your brain.
5. The process of repair and replacement of the support cells in your brain is prompted by the increased calcium/protein in your circulation.
6. Your brain's support cell system keeps vital nerve cells (not replaceable!) in more efficient running order.
7. When your brain cells work more efficiently, your mind works more efficiently.

So there you have it, an indirect but definite connection between all those tissues you may have thought were completely self-reliant and independent of one another.

Olga P. finds new life

Olga P. is a woman in her late 40's. When she first came to my office, she looked more like a woman in her mid-60's and she had real problems.

She complained of feeling weak and tired all the time in spite of adequate rest, but what mainly concerned her was a rather definite tendency of late to be "hunched over," as she put it, and to have intermittent pain along her spine from her neck down to her tail bone. And her pain wasn't limited to her spine, she said. She also had spells of it in her chest, especially where her ribs met her breastbone in the front of her chest. She noticed occasionally that her hips also hurt, especially during motions where she twisted her torso to the right or left side. "I hurt right down to my bones, Doctor," she told me. And she was more correct than she knew in her description.

One of the first things I did was to X-ray her back—the lower part down near her sacrum, the large bone at the base of the spine just above the buttocks cleavage. I had a clue not only from Olga's symptoms, but also in the fact that she had gone through menopause only two years before—you'll recall from an earlier comment that osteoporosis is more prevalent among women at or just beyond menopause.

Sure enough, Olga showed the classic signs of osteoporosis: a definite thinning of the outside layer of the bones in her vertebral column, the part that the calcium is bound in. And a couple of her lower vertebrae were beginning to look much like Figure 5-4 earlier in the book, which shows the front end of the vertebra being narrower than the back (the so-called "wedging sign," because the vertebra resembles a wedge).

Olga was really worried when she heard the word "osteoporosis." She'd heard the term before and somehow associated it with some dread disease. However, I first reassured Olga that it might be a mistake to term osteoporosis a disease at all. I'd call it a departure from the normal way of bone, the reasons behind which are quite obscure, even today with the knowledge we have of bone metabolism. There were times, and some medical advisors insist even today that it's true, when it was believed that osteoporosis is strictly a matter of hormone balance in the system and that correcting this imbalance will correct the problem. However, this is only partially true. A good general diet with adequate vitamin and mineral supplements will do as well in all but the most severe cases of osteoporosis. By good diet I mean one that has adequate protein (derived from a variety of sources, not just one), adequate carbohydrate, and adequate fat. A good vitamin/mineral supplement should contain the minimum daily requirement of all the vitamins known to be needed by the human body, including vitamin A and vitamin D, as well as essential minerals, such as calcium and iron. Figure 10-1 summarizes osteoporosis control.

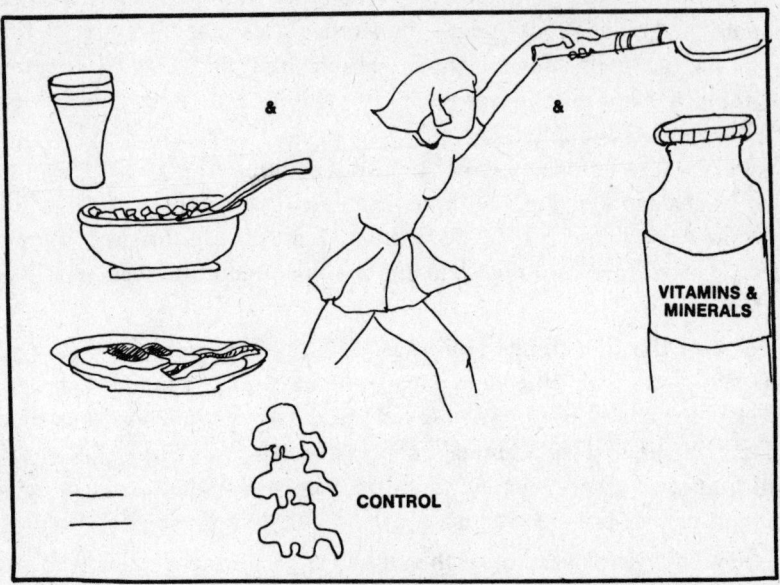

Figure 10-1

It does no good at all to load up on any one of the nutritional elements, as I've seen far too many people do, in order to "shotgun" cover the basic needs or on the assumption that if a little does good, then a lot more will do a lot better. Neither philosophy has any place in medical treatment, and may well do more harm than good.

A look into Olga's diet habits revealed that she did not get adequate protein, nor did she realize that since she was not a milk drinker and ate very little baked goods (such as bread and pastries) she was shorting herself on calcium. When both protein and a good source of calcium were restored, together with an ongoing toning routine (recall what I said about the effect of the pulling of tendons on their bony attachments) emphasizing her back muscles, Olga slowly and steadily got better, and after a year her symptoms did not come back.

If, today, I were to X-ray Olga's back again, I would still find evidence of osteoporosis—she did not cure the disorder, she merely got it under reasonable control. Will the fact that her osteoporosis still remains adversely affect Olga's good health or longevity? Absolutely not. She will

The Care and Feeding of Your Bones and Muscles

feel better and probably live longer, in fact, if for no other reason than that she is in better physical condition and nutritional balance than she was before. And Olga did *not* need hormones to accomplish this!

HEALTHY BONES AND MUSCLES

What is it that your bones and muscles need to stay in top shape? Olga already found that calcium and protein are needed. How much calcium and how much protein? It depends on what you do for a living, your overall size, and the general condition of your organism.

Carbohydrate (CHO)

CHO is the source of your organism's energy—the stuff that ignites inside your body's trillions of cells, burns and releases energy so that all those cells can function, doing the countless jobs that need doing all the time in the process of living.

If you did nothing but lie perfectly still in bed, you would still need a basic supply of CHO just to keep vital body functions going. Any activity above and beyond this—and I hope you're doing more than vegetating in bed—requires even more energy and, therefore, more CHO. Why? Because the minute you start walking, for example, well over half of your muscles become active against the force of gravity to move you around. This takes more energy than if all these muscles are at rest. If you work at a construction job all day, moving heavy forms, pouring concrete, loading and unloading heavy material from trucks, you need more CHO than someone who sits at an office desk all day and does accounting.

CHO is the prime source of this energy. It is not the only source. Both fat and protein can be metabolized by your body to yield energy—it takes longer to do it and it's not nearly as efficient, but it is possible. But what happens when you force your body to metabolize fat and protein stores for energy? You lose weight—and this is, of course, the idea behind a weight reduction program. I've covered this subject in my previous book, *The Biofeedback Diet: A Doctor's Revolutionary Approach*.

The idea in weight reduction is to *make* your body burn its stores of fat by eating somewhat less CHO than you actually need each day to accomplish what you're doing. But, if you don't need to lose weight, your CHO intake needs to be fairly level and reasonably constant day in and day out.

Most people discover what this amount is automatically, and eat according to what their appetite dictates. When you take in very much more than you need to burn as energy, your body has no recourse but to store it. A little can be stored for ready use in your liver, but for the most part your body will convert CHO to fat and that's how it's stored.

Protein (P)

Proteins are many hundreds of times more complex in their make-up than CHO or fats. They are built up of varying combinations of two dozen or so amino acids, about half of which are essential to your organism. If you are a vegetarian and take no other protein than that found in plants, you will *not* get enough of these essential amino acids. The same holds true for red meat, fowl and fish as well as for the grains and dairy products, all of which constitute the sources for nutritional protein. It is for this reason that it's unwise and unhealthy to go on a "milk diet" or to restrict your diet in any way such that one or more of these sources of protein are excluded from your eating habits.

Proteins go into the making of the matrix in which the calcium is deposited to form bones. Proteins are the basic building blocks for virtually all the cells in your body, including muscle cells. You might say, then, that proteins build muscle cells and CHO makes them move. In restoring tone to muscles, the cells enlarge. This takes even more protein.

Fat (F)

The third of the basic nutritional building blocks is fat. It is perhaps the most abused and misunderstood of all the elements in human nutrition. One hears so much about the excess of fat in the overweight state, and in such things as hardening of arteries, that fat's reputation has suffered a bit. Not that fat isn't the enemy of millions of people in our country who are overweight, but in their case they carry around much too much of it. Fat contains at least three essential fatty acids, and like the essential amino acids in protein, they are absolutely necessary for human nutrition. Fat, therefore, should constitute a constant portion of our diets (fats help form vital hormones), although not quite as large a portion as many people take in. See Figure 10-2.

Ben K. starves in cast

Ben K. was a young man I once knew who was injured in an auto accident and ended up in a right hip spica—a cast encircling his waist, lower back, right hip and thigh, knee and lower leg down to his right ankle. He'd sustained a rather tricky fracture very near his hip joint, high on the shaft of his thigh bone, and although his doctor fixed the fracture by driving a long metal pin down the thigh bone shaft through the fracture to keep it in

The Care and Feeding of Your Bones and Muscles 183

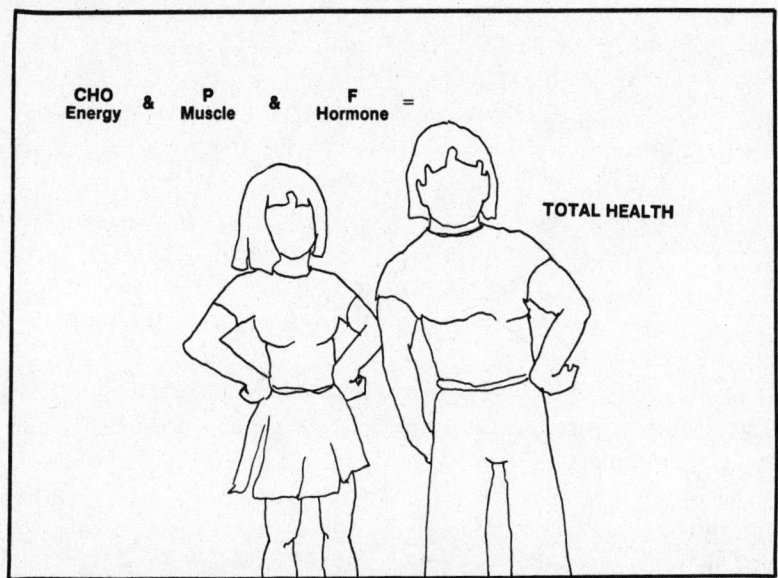

Figure 10-2

place, the cast prevented Ben from having to worry about motion of his hip joint during the crucial first weeks of healing.

Ben found himself in the predicament many active young men and women find themselves in when they must drastically alter their active life styles temporarily to fit in with what it takes to heal wounds, namely, to remain fairly quiet while their wounds heal. In Ben's case, he was a bit overweight to begin with, and when he came home under the loving care and attention of his wife and family, he was immediately besieged with as fattening an assortment of goodies as you would want to see. Cakes and pies baked by Mrs. K., candies and bakery sweets from Ben's mother and aunts, beer and assorted snacks from Ben's buddies. Within three weeks, Ben had added another 15 pounds to his already ample heft.

I happened to be making a house call on Ben's young daughter when I discovered to what lengths people will sometimes go when they let their frame of mind and "the fates" (Ben's accident) rule over common sense. There was Ben, all 205 pounds of him, propped up on a pillow in bed in mid-afternoon, working his way through a two-pound box of chocolates recently dropped off by one of his friends. When I'd finished with Ben's daughter, I began to chat with Ben about his gorging.

He confided that the monotony, among other things, was driving him up a wall. He didn't connect this right away with his obvious voracious appetite; in fact, he said he thought it would help him to heal faster if he ate well. I told him I thought so, too, but that what he was doing was simply eating too much, not at all well.

Finally, I was able to convince Ben that if he didn't do something about his diet, and soon, his doctor would have to make him a new cast since he'd just about outgrown the one he had.

I put Ben on a 2000 calorie a day diet with extra protein so that his healing right thigh bone would have ample foundation to form new bone and help heal his fracture. Since protein has only half the calories, weight by weight, of carbohydrate, Ben didn't have to give up *all* his goodies, just about three fourths of them.

I also had Ben start on a high potency vitamin and mineral tablet each day to further ensure that his healing processes had enough of these ingredients to work with. And, yes, Ben's diet had a small but consistent portion of fat in it as well. His uninvolved muscles were started on a toning routine three times a day. Figure 10-3 shows Ben doing some of these toners. Between some extra calcium in the vitamin/mineral tablet Ben took and the regular portions of dairy products in his new diet, he was assured of ample calcium to help in the healing of his broken thigh bone.

To further help Ben with his convalescence, I asked Mrs. K. to think about her husband's particular interests and to concentrate on getting him involved with one or more of them to occupy his time. This would help relieve his tension and would divert his mind from thinking so much about

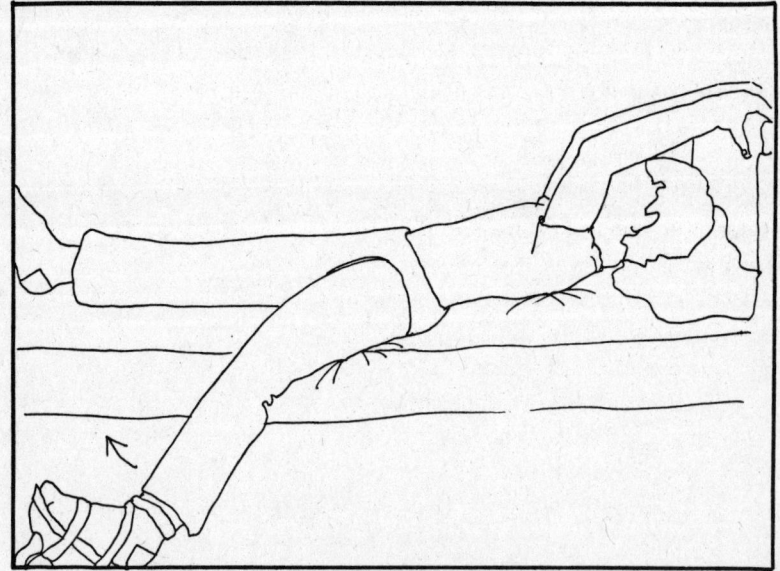

Figure 10-3

The Care and Feeding of Your Bones and Muscles

food all the time. Finally, I taught Ben some simple tricks of biofeedback that would help him to curb his hunger pangs. Ben was hard to convince at first, but he picked it up quickly and easily.

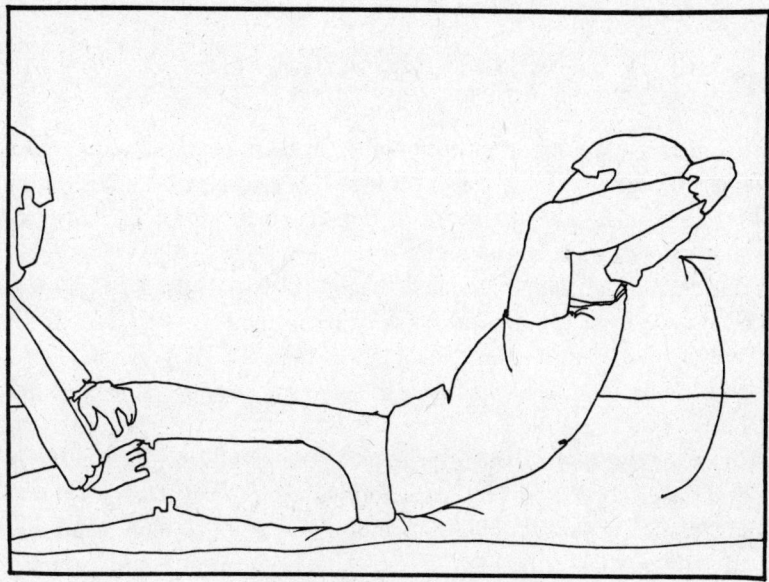

Figure 10-3 (continued)

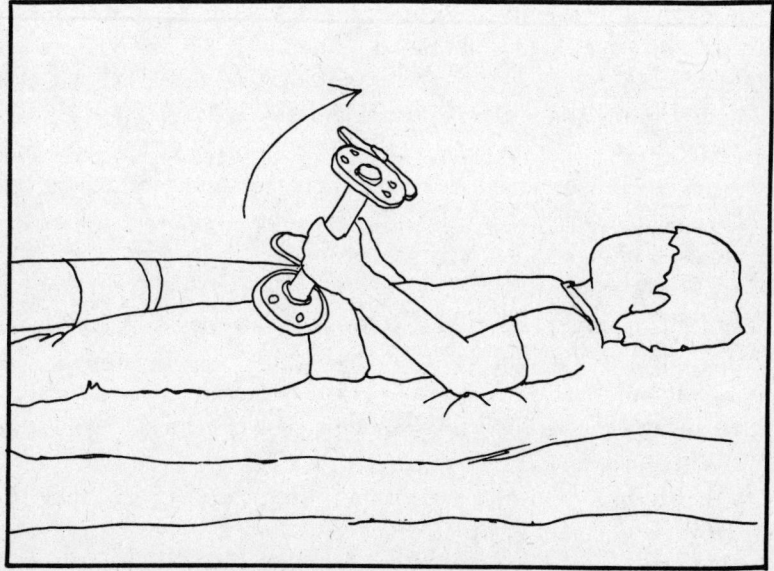

Figure 10-3 (continued)

The outcome was that Ben lost weight, felt better, and healed his injury quickly and solidly during his convalescence. And the new dietary habits Ben learned in this short span of time carried over well after he was back on his feet and back to work. Ben will live longer and be in better health for it.

CARE OF YOUR UPPER LIMBS

There are some important differences in taking care of and preventing problems with arms as compared with legs. These two extremities, your arm and leg, have basically different functions, and are trained from birth to perform entirely different tasks.

Your arms are basically the task masters of your body. That is, they are designed to perform the myriad tasks of living and coping. Your legs are your body's main support and locomotion system. They are designed to move you around and keep you upright so your arms and hands can get on with the business at hand.

Consider the main joint of your arm, the shoulder joint. Sure, it's a "ball and socket" type of joint as is your hip joint, but it is of a radically different type. The socket of your shoulder joint is much more shallow, and the ball bulges almost directly off the shaft of the arm bone, gaining the shoulder joint much greater mobility than is the case with the hip joint. Figure 10-4 shows the differences.

Not being concerned with weight bearing, your arm bones are smaller than those in your leg. Your elbow joint, besides bending and straightening your lower arm, rotates as well around its long axis—a motion your knee cannot duplicate.

Finally, your hand is the most highly developed organ of the muscle and skeleton system, being constructed to do so many tasks, in so many different ways with so much variation in delicate and sheer strength that books have been devoted to it. And although your foot can be trained to do some things your hands do, it can't hold a candle to your hand in the performance department.

Even with a single finger out of commission on just one of your hands, you feel helpless in the face of a good many routine functions you perform every day without thinking about it. This is one reason for the specialty in medicine today of surgeons who do nothing but treat malformations and injuries of the hand.

So this means that there are special things to learn and remember regarding your upper limb. I'll start at the top.

The Care and Feeding of Your Bones and Muscles

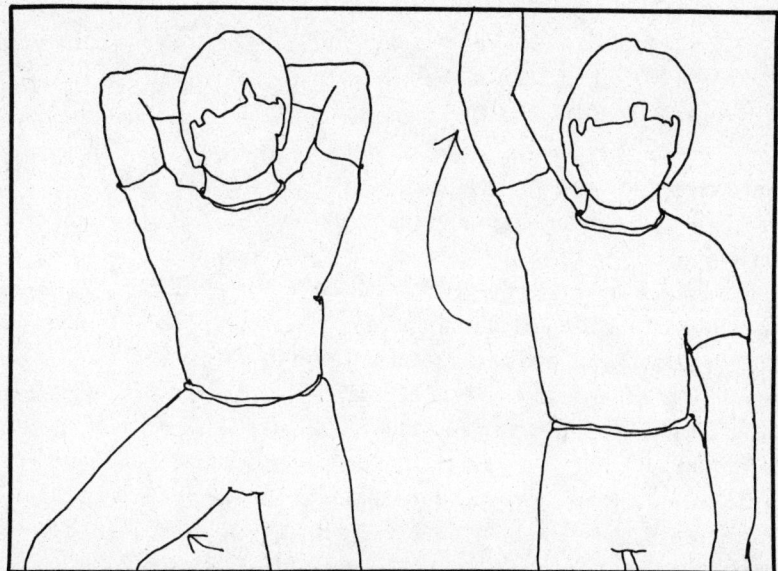

Figure 10-4

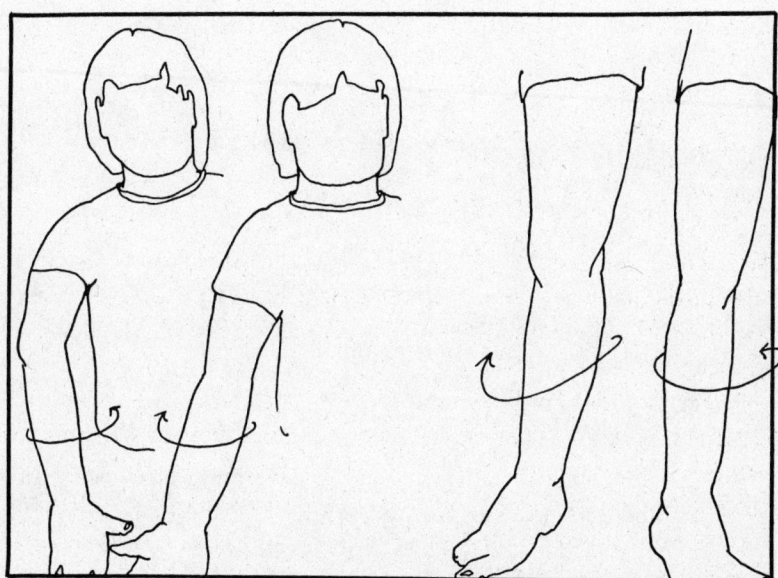

Figure 10-4 (continued)

ARM

Your arm is attached to your shoulder by means of a ball-like bulge of the bone of your upper arm that fits into a shallow hole in your shoulder blade called the socket. This ball is held in the socket by ligaments extending between it and the inner part of the socket, and by several sets of tendons attached to the muscles that move your shoulder.

Because a shoulder moves in six directions (flexion, extension, outward and inward, and internal and external rotation) and has many sets of muscle tendons and anchoring tissues within it, if it is not used fully each and every day in these motions, or at least partially in each of them, it gets stiff. Why? Like your thigh muscle that we talked about earlier, the muscles are large and tendons have a tendency to stiffen when they're not used.

If you place your arm in a simple sling for any length of time beyond a couple of days, your shoulder joint will stiffen, just as your thigh muscle will if it isn't used. This will happen even if your shoulder joint is perfectly normal! Therefore, the first rule with care of your arm is that, if at all possible, you should keep your shoulder joint limbered up every day *even if the rest of your arm is out of commission*. There are times when this isn't possible, but even then, some motion in the shoulder joint can be made until full range of movement is possible.

The following will help you to accomplish shoulder care:

1. Even if the strength of your shoulder muscles is diminished, use the pulley mechanisms already discussed to move it through all the possible ranges of motion. If a pulley isn't practical, ask someone to help you move your shoulder through its ranges of motion for ten minutes at least three times a day.
2. As strength returns, begin to put your shoulder muscles through active exercise routines. Use isometrics, weights, or the activities of daily living to accomplish this.
3. For prolonged stiffness and soreness, use hot packs or contrast hot and ice packs. Use before exercising and afterward if necessary.
4. Take advantage of anti-gravity methods to help you limber up a stiff sore shoulder. (Moving it while on your back in bed, or on the floor, or in a tub half full of water, for example.)
5. In some injuries and following too much vigorous exercise at the shoulder joint, it is possible to tear the attachment of one or more ligaments that attach to the ball of your upper arm bone. You'll

notice extreme pain when trying to rotate your arm at the shoulder joint if this happens. At any rate, if you notice special pain or discomfort when doing just rotation motions at your shoulder, seek the advice of your medical advisor; such tears can often be repaired.

ELBOW

Disease and injury around your elbow joint will likewise stiffen this joint unless you're careful to prevent it by the same principles of care that apply to your shoulder. When the acute stage of the disease (as in arthritis, for example) has subsided, and when healing of any injury has taken place, keep after that elbow until full range of flexion (bending up your lower arm) and extension (straightening out your lower arm) can be done.

WRIST AND FINGERS

It is never good if stiffness and inability to move joints occurs. In general and with most activities, the closer to the end of an extremity a joint stiffens, the easier it is to adapt to it—in other words, a stiff "frozen" shoulder joint is much more incapacitating than a stiff "frozen" wrist. One finger can be lost without the loss of most of your hand function. The loss of two or more is another story.

Although you can't always prevent deformity of a joint following its injury, you can often keep the deformed joint *limber* by paying careful attention to its use even though the joint may not be capable of moving through its former range of motion. For example, it's not unusual for knuckle joints to remain swollen and unable to extend (straighten out) the finger that attaches to them. This doesn't mean that you shouldn't *use* the involved knuckle joints to the fullest possible extent. On the contrary, you should use them even more than before so that they won't lose the remaining function they can perform.

TAMMY D. USES WHAT SHE HAS LEFT

Tammy D., a young woman in what appeared to be a miserable situation, having had a spinal cord tumor removed from high along her spine, illustrates the principle of taking good care of what is left after the devastation of such a problem.

Following successful surgery for the tumor, Tammy had lost most of the power in the muscles of her upper extremities. She could elevate her right shoulder a little and could move her fingers a little on her right side. Her left side was stronger, but generally weak. She became a "lefty" because her left side emerged as the stronger of the two sides.

But what about her right side? Was she doomed to a useless right arm? Here's what happened to help Tammy make use of what she had on her right side:

1. The muscle that elevates the shoulder—the "shrug" muscle—was strengthened through isometric toning, the movement of the muscle against resistance.

2. *All joints* of Tammy's right arm were put through daily movement, first by a physiotherapist in the hospital and then by her mother at home.

3. A special splint was fashioned for Tammy's wrist that held her hand and fingers up so that what little strength she had in her fingers and thumb could be used to their fullest efficiency. With her fingers held upward, she began to strengthen her grip—the squeeze power of her fingers. Figure 10-5 shows Tammy's special splint.

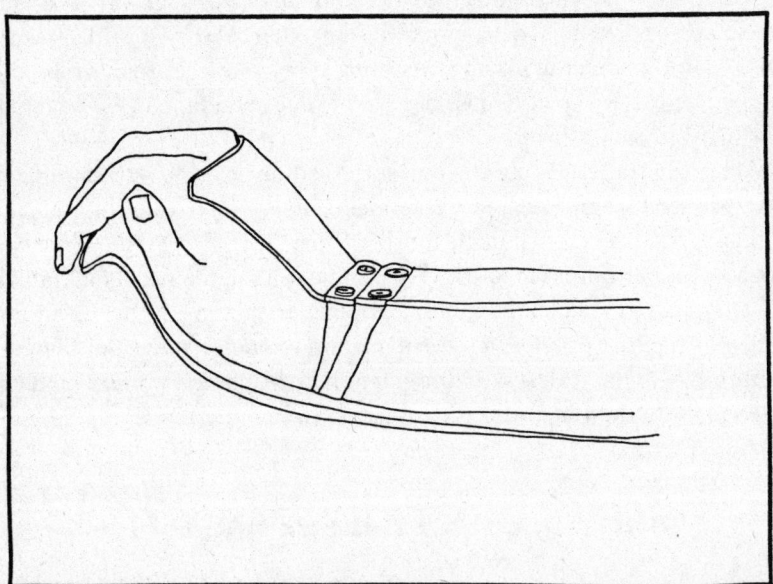

Figure 10-5

Eventually, Tammy could use a typewriter by using her shoulder elevator muscle to raise and lower her hand to the keyboard, and her cocked-up wrist to place her fingers on the correct keys. She also learned to hold a cup and silverware in her right hand to eat, and to hold a pen and pencil in her fingers to write. All this with only the partial use of two muscle groups—shoulder and fingers!

LOWER EXTREMITY

We've talked about the large muscle in front of your thigh—the quadriceps—that weakens so rapidly even when your leg is taken out of commission for a short time, and what needs to be done to restore this muscle's function. There are occasions when this isn't possible.

There are likewise occasions when you may have to work around a permanently stiff knee joint, one that just won't bend. And there are times when circumstances prevent the proper motion of your ankle joint. Either it won't bend upward enough to prevent your foot from dragging on the ground, or the pain and discomfort in the joint itself prevents all but minimal weight bearing on your foot just in the process of trying to walk.

HIP

When the front thigh muscle is weakened and can't come back, the side thigh muscles can take over and help you to use your leg. These are the muscles that pull your leg to the side, away from the center line. These muscles can be strengthened by supporting yourself with the side opposite the weak leg, and swinging the weak leg outward to the side, and back again as far as you can pull it across your good leg. The weighted shoe and wall techniques can also be used to great advantage with this toning. Sand sewn into a bag and fastened to your shoe, pressing your leg outward against a wall repeatedly, will help to add strength to these muscles. Walking—as far and as often as you possibly can—will help make a useless leg useful again, even though your gait may not look like it once did.

KNEE

If you are forced to live with a stiffened knee joint, the straighter the position your knee is stiffened in, the better it will be for you. If a thigh muscle is so weakened that it is impossible to straighten your knee joint so you can walk on it, don't despair—a brace can be made to hold it straight, and this, together with one (or two) crutches will enable your leg to be useful in walking again.

ANKLE

There are many diseases and injuries to the ankle joint that heal with so much traumatic arthritis in the joint that bearing weight on it is too painful to keep up for any length of time. When this happens—and sometimes all the care and skill in the world won't prevent it—your ankle joint can be fused. This is an operation that obliterates the joints (three of them) so that arthritis can't set in again. The surgery does take away the ability to move your ankle upward and downward because the joints responsible for this motion are gone, but it often enables you to walk or climb stairs *without pain*—a welcome relief in most cases.

FEET AND TOES

The main problem with the feet and toes following disease or injury is that they may not properly contact your shoe, and your shoe may not properly contact the ground when you walk. This causes pressure on areas that didn't have much pressure put on them before. So it is a matter of proper fitting, sometimes with special shoes that have built-in supports in the soles or heels. At other times, your toes may curl up and be quite uncomfortable when walking or even wearing ordinary shoes. This "hammer toe" effect can sometimes be relieved by simple padding inside your shoes. When this doesn't help, releasing the tendons that are curling your toes up (a surgical matter) will sometimes do the trick. I've seen toes that wouldn't respond even to this procedure and were finally removed (again, a surgical procedure) with relief of the problem.

VIC McC. GOES THE ROUTE

Vic McC. is a man who was born with cerebral palsy—a brain disorder that can affect the use of any or all of the limbs, and may even prevent normal speech development and general coordination of smaller muscles as well. He was unable to use his legs properly, but by utilizing his side thigh muscles to swing his legs, he could walk, though multiple surgeries when he was a youth to transplant lower leg tendons at his ankle and foot did prevent his having to wear braces or use crutches.

As he reached middle age, Vic noticed more and more trouble with his right hip, which bore the brunt of his unusual swing-out walk, and it finally degenerated the ball part of his right hip ball and socket joint.

The Care and Feeding of Your Bones and Muscles

Was this to spell the end of what was a heroic effort on Vic's part to get around from place to place? No! Surgeons implanted an artificial hip for Vic, and it worked. By eliminating his diseased hip joint and fashioning a new ball for the socket, the impossible pain of walking with his swing-out style of gait was eliminated.

It may be that Vic eventually will have to have the procedure performed on his left side as well, but knowing Vic's determination to stay with life's problems as they are dealt him, he'll do it willingly and without hesitation when the time comes.

So don't despair if one problem seems to follow another. Medical science is working in your behalf, even if it can't always restore things to their original order.

SUMMARY

1. The care of bones and muscles are interdependent: The toning of muscles also stimulates the toning of bone by pulling tendons that are attached to bone.
2. Osteoporosis can't be prevented entirely, but it can be alleviated by good habits of diet and exercise, and rarely does the condition require hormones. Newer drugs may prove to be helpful in difficult cases, but they haven't been fully evaluated at this time.
3. Proper care of muscles, bones and joints depends on a reasonable balance in your diet of protein, carbohydrate and fat. One cannot be neglected in preference to another. Proper nutritional balance controls weight, which in turn benefits you in reduced stress on joints and muscles.
4. Extra vitamins and minerals are a proper addition to your diet when you are recovering from any injury or surgery.
5. Upper and lower limbs perform different tasks for you, and their care in the face of injury or disease differs according to their different functions.

11

Coping with Problems of Nerve Damage to Muscles

One of the most seemingly difficult, if not impossible tasks confronting anyone afflicted with a debilitating injury or disease is dealing with damage to nerves and muscles. I want to talk here about how you may cope successfully with these afflictions. We'll see how damage to the spinal cord, the main electric cable connecting your brain with muscle, may be overcome even though the damage may be permanent.

You will also see how damage to nerves in limbs may be bypassed and the function of the limb in question improved and maintained.

There are many causes of such nerve damage to limbs and I'll examine some of the more common and important of them with you, and show that you can cope as others have.

I'll also talk about the tone of your nervous system—about times when it's important to tone nerves even when muscles aren't responding as well as they might, so that you can at least get from the ailing muscles all that can be expected under the particular circumstances.

SPINAL CORD INJURIES AND DISEASE

The great main nerve cable and switching mechanism that is your spinal cord is indeed a remarkable piece of apparatus. Not only does it carry hundreds of thousands of messages to and from your even more remarkable brain each day, during sleep as well as when you're awake, but it takes care of many of the "ordinary" reflex actions in your limbs and elsewhere that your brain doesn't have to be involved with. For example, a reflex action moves your fingers away from a hot surface even before the pain of the heat registers in your brain. Certain other nerves convey messages to

Coping with Problems of Nerve Damage to Muscles 195

your spinal cord while you're asleep concerning pressure and compression on, for example, your legs. A reflex action moves and changes the position of your legs (and the rest of your body as well) in response to such messages without your brain having to decide on such action.

Such reflex actions taken care of by your spinal cord can range from quite simple—involving, for instance, part of one hand—to very complex—involving all of your limbs and your head, neck, abdomen, and back as well.

In general, the longer the nerve tracts, or pathways traveling up and down your spinal cord, the more vulnerable they are to injury and disease that may affect such pathways at a given level of the spinal cord. This is why, for instance, a neck injury to the spinal cord is more damaging to total function than a similar injury at the level of the small of your back—an injury at your neck involves more pathways or tracts than an injury lower down along your spinal cord.

Nerve connections

After all of the fibers to the muscles and skin of your toes, ankle, lower leg and thigh have come together into the large nerve emerging from your upper leg, they enter your spinal cord at several levels at the lower end of this main cable. In general, the fibers that convey sensation to your lower

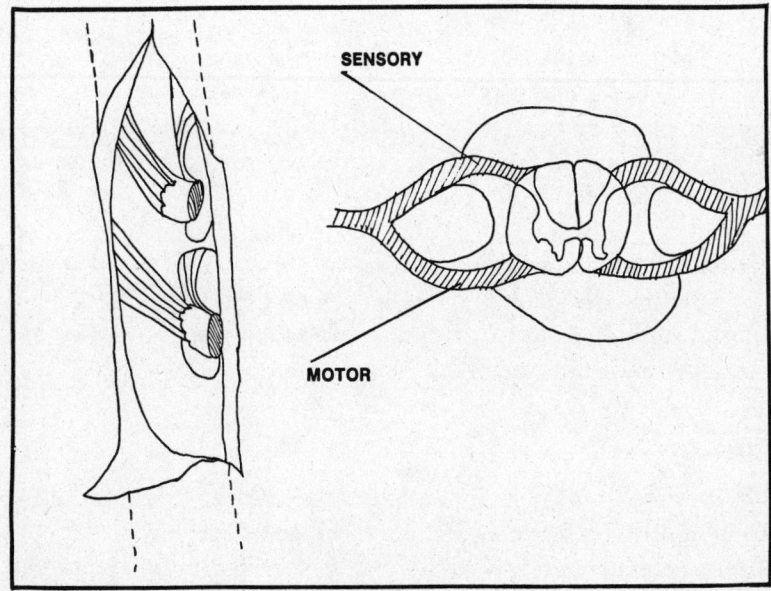

Figure 11-1

limb enter more toward the rear of the cord, and those fibers that convey messages to the muscles (to make them move) emerge more toward the front of the cord. This utilization of several levels, and at least two halves of the spinal cord with each main nerve trunk entering and emerging, usually spares some fibers of the main nerve trunk in injury or disease of the spinal cord. A fractured neck vertebra that damages the spinal cord, in other words, may weaken one or both arms, but unless the cord is completely destroyed at that level, it does not mean that *all* of the muscles in both arms, or *all* of the sensations in both arms necessarily vanish as a result. Nerve-spinal cord connections are illustrated in Figure 11-1.

Pain

Pain is an extremely complicated sensation, especially when it becomes chronic. I'll have more to say about pain as it relates to back problems in Chapter 12, but for now I want to point out that fibers conveying pain originate in bones and joints, in muscles, and in the skin and connective tissues of your limbs.

Your blood vessels also have pain fibers in their outer walls. These fibers are gathered together in the main nerve trunks and they enter your spinal cord toward the rear half. Having entered the cord, the fibers travel up the cord and enter several areas of your brain for "sifting" and any response that needs to be made to pain travels down the movement nerve pathways to the muscles involved.

The fact that pain enters the spinal cord at distinct *levels* is the basis for the so-called "gate theory" of pain relief that you may have read about in newspapers and magazines. According to this theory, if a low grade stimulus (usually mild electric current) can be set up above the part of the spinal cord where the pain fibers enter, such stimulus will act to block the pain from traveling any further up the spinal cord, and thus prevent its being felt by the brain. In some cases, this method seems to work quite well—for a time. But after the passage of time—a matter of weeks or a few months at most—the electric stimulus seems to lose its protective blocking ability, and the pain is again felt by the brain.

Injury

If a nerve is accidentally completely severed in your wrist, it can be sewn carefully together again with an excellent chance that it will "regrow" and that the muscles it was responsible for moving will move once again. This is not true of your spinal cord following injury or disease with destruction of nerve fibers. Your spinal cord nerves lack a special covering

Coping with Problems of Nerve Damage to Muscles

around them that limb nerves have. Lacking this cover, they cannot regrow when they are disrupted. The additional bulk of such outer covering around nerves *after* they enter the spinal cord would make it impossible for your spinal cord to fit into the relatively small bony tunnel that it occupies. For this reason, the human body has encased its spinal cord in a tough leathery layer surrounding the entire cord, and this is surrounded with hard bone for protection.

This is why you must retrain other muscles that are not involved with injury or disease in the case of spinal cord damage.

Sandra N. functions with quadriplegia

As illustrated by the story of Sandra N., a young woman in her late 20's, the tragedy of a fractured neck from a motorcycle accident is devastating in its effect on one's mind. A state of utter hopelessness and despair inevitably set itself into Sandra's personality as she lay there in her special bed in the rehabilitation hospital where she recuperated. At first there was nothing except facial movement and eye blinks. She could talk and swallow—these nerves arise in the mid-brain and were thus spared the destruction that occurred to her spinal cord at the level of her third and fourth neck vertebrae. And as a result, everything below this level was paralyzed.

Slowly, as Sandra's body recuperated from the "spinal shock" resulting from such a serious blow to the body's main nerve cable, some bits and pieces of movement began to return as the swelling and congestion around the site of the cord injury subsided and disappeared. A *few* fibers weren't destroyed.

This return of function allowed Sandra to be able to move her left upper arm (straighten at elbow), her right wrist and fingers, and her diaphragm (the diaphragm is your main breathing muscle). Sandra up to this time was also forced to have a portable respirator attached to her chest and upper abdomen to enable her to breathe.

With special help and bracing, the movements in Sandra's right upper arm formed the power lever necessary for her to learn to write with this hand again. Special braces held her wrist and fingers in a fixed position and a special attachment to her index finger and thumb held the pen or pencil steady while her triceps muscle—the one that straightens out your arm at the elbow—took care of the movement.

Sandra's left hand and wrist were weak, but she could move them a little. Enough, as a matter of fact, to enable her to learn to use a telephone, hold and page through reading material, and steady paper while her right arm wrote.

For the mechanics of eating, a special table was used to raise the food plate up to about chin level. With her left hand and fingers functioning on this table (her arm elevated and supported by a lift attached to the arm of her wheel chair) she could put food into her mouth. A long straw was used for liquids.

Eventually, Sandra, a bright young woman who had been a college student when she had her accident, finished her degree in accounting and was able to get a job with an insurance company in their accounting department. Her only dependency at this job, incidentally, was that she had to be taken to and from the building in which she worked. Her wheel chair was operated electrically from a control box fastened to the left arm support of the chair. Sandra still works for the same insurance company today, but at a much higher position; they trained her in actuarial work with the company and she is now head of that department!

I bring up Sandra's case not to focus on her obvious handicaps, but to point out that "being handicapped" is really a state of mind, that a catastrophic disabling injury such as a high spinal cord injury like Sandra's need not necessarily spell the day of doom. Nor does it mean that you need to retire from the world in which you find yourself. Sandra's partial recovery and going back to school and eventually to work took a period of over five years to accomplish—something that might be done by someone not so afflicted in a matter of months. But there was *determination* first and foremost, a feeling that was just the opposite of what set in shortly following her accident. And it goes right back to Chapter 7, in which I discussed mood and your outlook on what life deals you. If you let yourself continue to feel self-pity and begin to wallow in misery and depression during all your waking hours, naturally you will remain lost to the real world.

And what of the help it takes to achieve what Sandra did? Of course it takes help. I can't recount the hours upon weeks upon months of work by many others that went into Sandra's reconstitution, but Sandra accepted this help gracefully and gratefully, realizing that self-help results would eventually come along. And it's here that many people with spinal cord injury fail to respond to that which may help them: They don't want (or can't accept) help from others. Accept it simply because it's needed, and make up your mind to be the best person you can in return.

LIMB NERVE DAMAGE

There are many diseases and injuries capable of causing damage and destruction to the nerve trunks after they leave the spinal cord and course along into one of your four extremities. Any injury that cuts through or

Coping with Problems of Nerve Damage to Muscles

mangles a nerve trunk will put it out of commission. Nerves to arms and legs may be incapacitated from diabetes and alcoholism. Sometimes a toxic condition brought on by a virus or bacterial infection will damage nerves, as will a host of chemical "poisons" that may get into your system.

If limb nerve damage does occur, it may be of help to first consider how much better off you are with this condition than you would be with Sandra's, for example. Why? Because in the case of limb nerves, only the small group of muscles supplied by the nerve involved are affected—all the rest of your muscles and nerves are usually working.

And since Nature has equipped your limbs with more than one muscle to perform a given function, the malfunction of one nerve trunk, though it may involve several muscles, doesn't necessarily damage adjoining nerves that can be brought into play to do the movements prevented by the particular condition of the single nerve trunk, as illustrated in Figure 11-2 for wrist flexion.

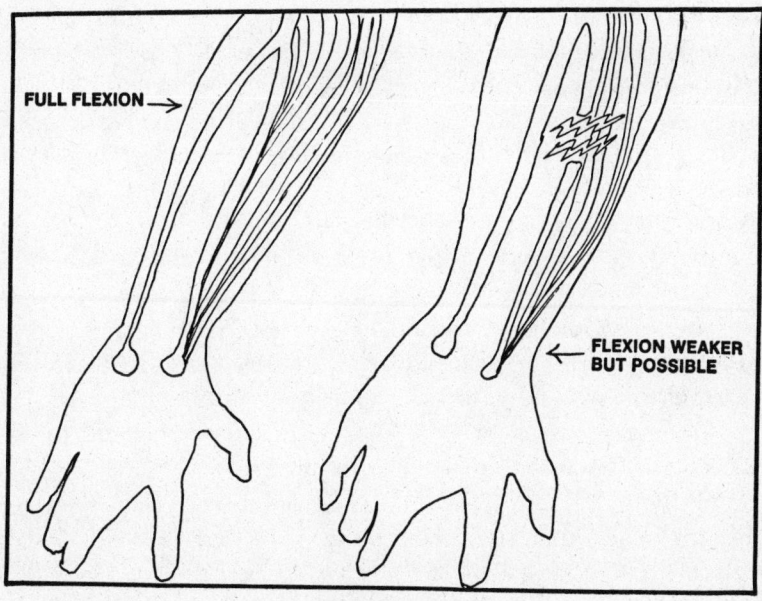

Figure 11-2

An example of such a problem appeared as a complication of diabetes in a patient named Simon E., a man in his late 40's who had had diabetes for about ten years, which required insulin to control.

Simon noticed that his feet and lower legs had "pins and needles" in them more and more often, like the feeling in your hands and feet when you sit in one position for too long with pressure on your elbow or the back of your knee and a hand or foot "goes to sleep" for a few minutes until the feeling of weakness and numbness is worked out by activity. In Simon's case, however, the numb feeling was never quite worked out.

After a couple of months of this, Simon noticed the same feeling in his right thumb, index and middle finger and in his right wrist as well. He was showing signs of what is called diabetic neuropathy, a poorly understood condition that sometimes complicates diabetes in spite of the best control with diet and insulin.

In Simon's case, however, he had let himself slip with his weight to the tune of having gained about 35 pounds of flab since I'd last seen him, and even though he watched his urine tests closely and adjusted his insulin dose accordingly, Simon could definitely *not* be said to be in good control of his diabetes.

So one of the first things I did with Simon, when I discovered his weak right wrist and fingers and the numbness of the skin of his fingers, hands and both feet, was to place him on a reducing diet and on exercises for general toning, especially for the muscles of his right hand and both feet.

He started by squeezing a firm ball with his right hand for 15 minutes three times a day—he used a tennis ball to start with. The next thing was isometrics for his wrist—with his forearm flat on a table, his left hand clasping his right hand and pushing, he flexed his right wrist upward against the pressure from his good left hand.

The second toning routine consisted of Simon holding a sponge mop against either one of his feet as he sat on a high stool or chair, and forcing his weakened ankle upward against the pressure of the mop. This, too, was performed religiously three times a day for 15 minutes. At first, of course, Simon found that his ability to move against even the slightest resistance from his good hand and the mop was poor, but I cautioned him that he would easily become discouraged by this for a time. I told him to make himself keep it up anyway because the other flexor muscles of his right wrist and of both his ankles would be strengthened and would begin to take over more and more of the function that had been lost by his ailing nerves. In addition, I told him that I thought that the ailing nerves themselves would improve with time, though I didn't hold out any promises that the involved nerves would ever regain normal function, and that the involved muscles might remain weak.

Within three months Simon lost 18 pounds, and within six months he lost 24 pounds. In this same time, through diligent attention to the muscles not involved by the partially destroyed nerves, Simon regained about 50 percent of the strength in his right wrist, and about 35 percent of the lost strength in both ankles—enough to be able to walk fairly normally without his feet dragging (a common first sign of weak ankle flexion).

About a year later there was continued numbness in the thumb of Simon's right hand, but he had almost full muscle power in his fingers and wrist. His ankles remained weak, but he continued to be able to walk normally for average distances. He had also managed to reduce his weight by 38 pounds and needed 15 less units of insulin each day to control his diabetes. He felt better than he had at any time in the past five years (about the time he began to put on weight) and he had prevented perhaps a lifetime of having to switch to being left-handed. Not a bad bonus for his investment of time and trouble with toning and weight loss!

Creeping paralysis

I think we're seeing this disease more and more, especially as the virus diseases—the true influenza-like diseases—sweep the country in waves every few years. The true name of this affliction is Guillain-Barre syndrome (pronounced "Geyon-Barray"). There were a number of cases, you may recall, following the swine flu vaccination program a couple of years ago.

The disease may follow an infection with virtually any virus and is thought to be a peculiar allergic reaction to the virus on the part of the nervous system.

At any rate, the disease begins much like Simon's did, except that it usually involves the limb nerves equally on both sides, and usually starts in the legs and rapidly works its way up the body. It may even affect the nerves responsible for breathing and finally the arms and hands as well.

After the acute phase, usually treated with injections of high doses of cortisone drugs, the patient may find himself at home in bed with one or more muscle groups weakened, if not paralyzed, like Simon. And in this case, it is even more important that you bring home the tenets of good, constant, hard-working physiotherapy and put them to use on the affected limbs by doing isometrics, putting the entire limb and its joints through daily motion and exercise at least three times a day for at least 30 minutes. It's the only way you're going to get those limbs partially or wholly functioning again.

Alcoholic limbs

Yet another rather common source of limb nerve damage is booze. I don't think most people with alcohol problems realize the wide-spread damage that can be done to the human organism from excessive drinking. Alcohol is quite capable of damaging the nervous system, including your brain; it often destroys your stomach and intestinal tract, including your liver; and it can damage your most precious resource—your mind—beyond salvage.

I have seen the entire gamut of such damage much too many times to recount in my experience in medicine, but the one thing that has impressed me about the limb nerve damage caused by alcohol is that *it is generally reversible if the person who has it is willing to give up booze entirely and work at retoning his damaged nerves and weakened muscles!*

Take the case of Ella A., a patient I first came in contact with in a mental health center where she had been admitted for the fourth time in two years with the DT's—another common complication of prolonged alcoholic binge drinking. I'd seen Ella on two previous occasions when she had been admitted, and she'd pulled through the DT's with vigorous therapy and good care. Unfortunately, she didn't learn the lesson about the threat of permanent damage to her central nervous system, not to mention the deterioration of her family life. Ella began to recover from her most recent binge, but it was obvious that she was having problems with her legs—her balance was off and her leg muscles remained weak. She had to spread her legs outward to walk, and they were unsteady.

Ella was in the first stage of alcoholic neuropathy—damage to limb nerves—as a result of toxic effects from alcohol.

Ella and I had a long chat shortly before she was due to leave the hospital program. I told her that if she got herself into a state like this again, she might well be unable to walk at all, and even if she were able to walk, she might be unable to maintain an upright position because of impaired balance.

She asked if there was anything she could do. I replied that the only way to begin in such situations was with *complete and total abstinence from alcohol* from this point on.

Ella had begun to get a good idea about why she was drinking from the people responsible for her therapy in the alcohol program at the center. It wasn't that she didn't, or couldn't understand why she was drinking heavily. She just hadn't been ready to stop before. Now, with vital elements of her health threatened, she was ready to take that final hard step—and for the alcoholic, it is the toughest one of all.

The first thing I did was to put Ella's leg muscles through their entire range of motion, using my arms and hands to resist their movement as she forced them to move. It was quite obvious to her that her hip flexors, knee flexors, and ankle flexor muscles were all functioning below par to varying degrees. Hip flexors move the leg forward in walking, knee flexors bend the knee and stabilize the knee joint as the leg is swung forward and operate the

Coping with Problems of Nerve Damage to Muscles

leg as stairs are climbed, and ankle flexors keep the foot from dragging (foot drop).

The following is the routine I put Ella on at home:

1. First, sit-ups to add strength to abdominal muscles. Lying flat on the floor and doing sit-ups helps tone up your hip flexor muscles as well.

2. Second, scissor kicks to directly tone hip flexors. Lying flat on the floor and elevating both legs about a foot or so off the floor, knees straight, not bent, makes your main hip flexors contract. Swinging the legs first out as far as possible, then in until they cross also tones up thigh muscles.

3. Third, thigh toners using an object such as a sand bag fastened to her shoe (as previously described). While sitting on a high stool or table edge, thighs straight on the stool or table, and lower legs dangling down, slowly lifting the lower leg up until it is level (fully straightened) with the thigh, then back down again and repeating.

Deep knee bends also help, hands on hips and standing with legs slightly apart, squatting down until knees are fully bent, then straightening back up, using the thigh muscles to do the work, to an upright standing position again, and repeating.

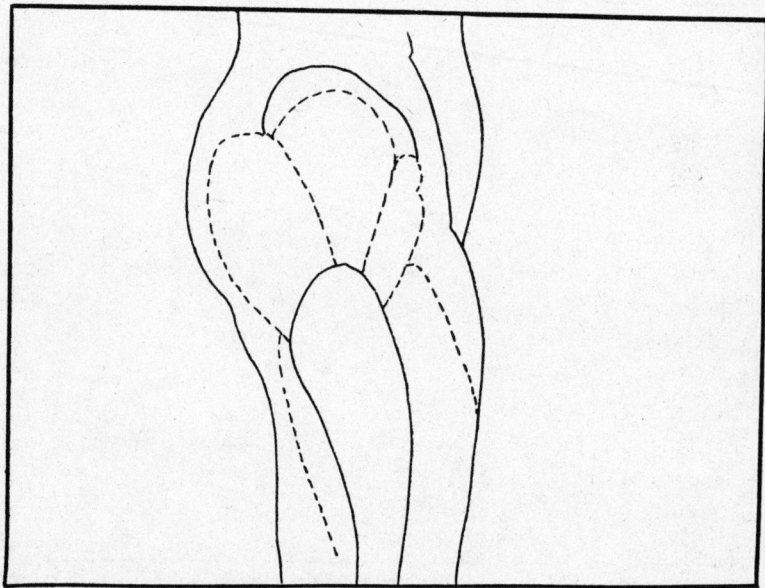

Figure 11-3

204 Coping with Problems of Nerve Damage to Muscles

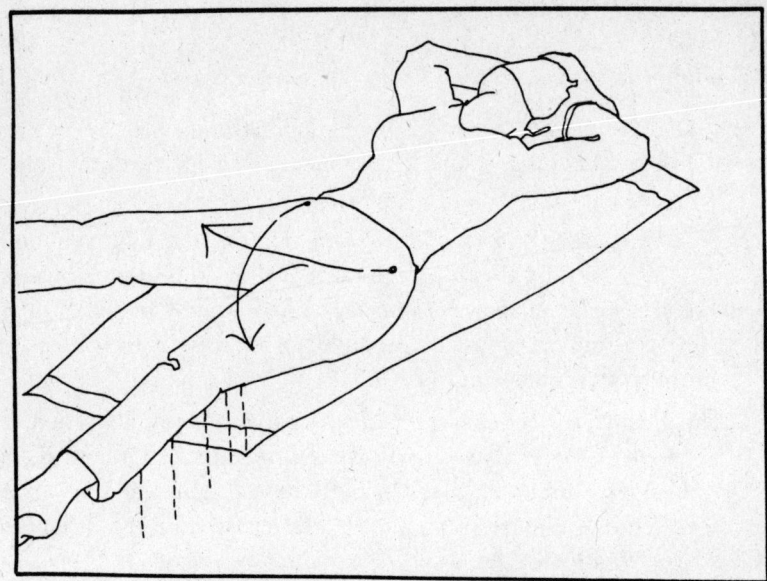

Figure 11-3 (continued)

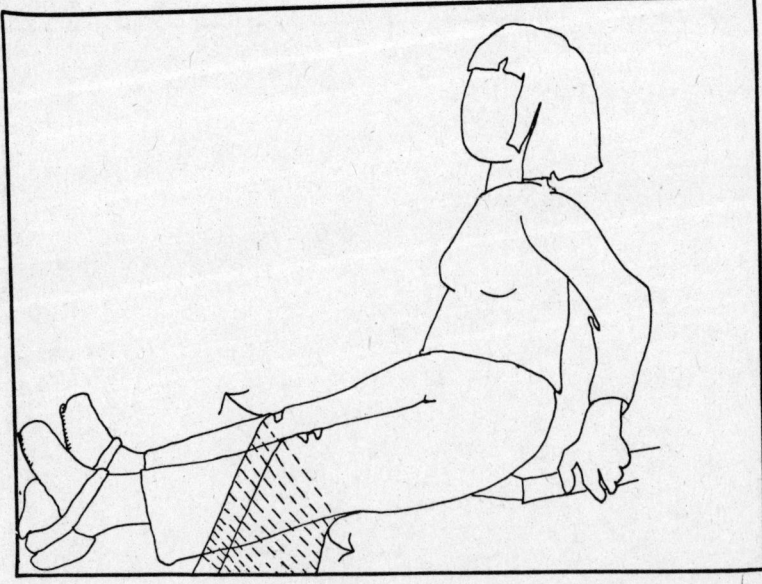

Figure 11-3 (continued)

Coping with Problems of Nerve Damage to Muscles

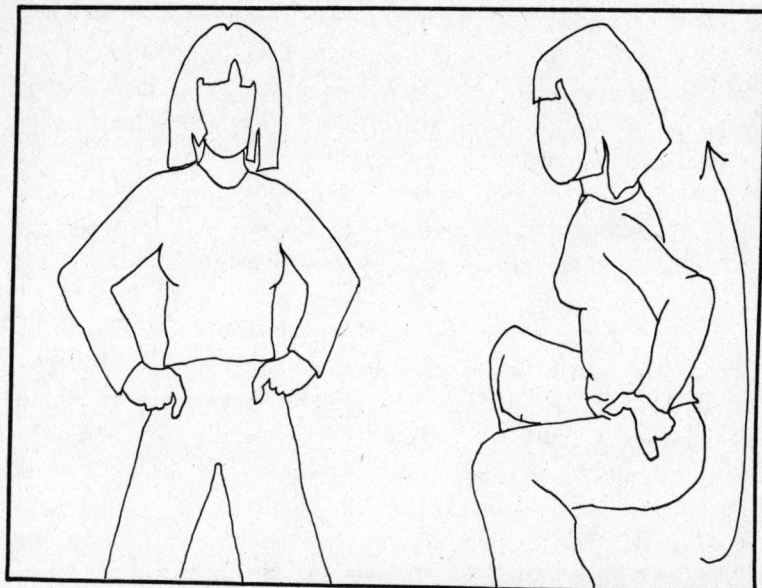

Figure 11-3 (continued)

4. Finally, again sitting on a table, lower legs dangling, or lying down, legs straight, flexing her ankle up with the muscles of her lower leg against the resistance of a mop (previously described) or against the resistance of the opposite foot positioned across the top of the foot being exercised. Figure 11-3 shows Ella's efforts and the muscles involved in doing them.

5. I then put Ella on a diet, not to reduce her weight so much as to supply adequate amounts of CHO, P, and F each and every day. Her system would need these vital nutritional elements in plentiful amounts to heal the damage to nerves and liver she had caused by excessive alcohol intake.

6. I also started Ella on extra vitamin B tablets daily—four of them to be taken with each meal and at bedtime. Every week, in addition, I injected Ella with a solution of pyridoxine, one of the B vitamins essential to proper functioning of nerves.

At first, Ella rebelled. This is understandable, since her legs and abdominal muscles were not only out of tone, but weakened from the nerve damage. She was able to do only two or three of the toning exercises at a time, and she became discouraged early on in the situation. But I prodded her frequently with encouragement and, yes, even admonition of what would come if she pulled back from the routines. I had her doing the routines faithfully three times a day, even if it took an hour to do them, and even if she could only do two of each—but I also insisted that she add at least one more of each toner every week. If she could do only two scissor kicks, for example, she added one more, even if she had to rest for a time after doing two. And when she could do three sit-ups, she was to add a fourth, even if she only got her torso halfway to a full sitting position.

It was a long tough haul for Ella. The therapists for her alcohol problem gave her marvelous support while she was getting a real physical work-out from me. It really paid off! In three months, Ella had tripled the number of toners in each category. She had begun to return strength to her weakened muscles. She could walk without the peculiar wide-based stance she once had, and could do so without dragging either foot on the ground. Her damaged nerves did come back—not completely, but enough to restore her confidence and faith in her abilities. This in turn helped her to stick to her pledge of no more drinking. She has remained dry since then, and has become an enthusiastic advocate of physical conditioning. In the role of alcoholic counselor, she now helps others to recover from her original problem.

TONING YOUR NERVOUS SYSTEM

Most people don't realize it, but when they're exercising their muscles, they're also toning their nervous system in the process.

Whenever you send a message from your brain down the nerves responsible for walking, for example, the following events take place:

1. Impulse travels down nerve from brain to muscles via the motor (locomotion) branches.

2. Muscles move in response, sending messages back up nerve pathways that convey various sensations from your limbs (position, pain, touch, vibration, etc.).

3. Brain modifies the messages according to this "feedback" and your limbs respond accordingly.

4. The messages are in effect toning your nerves. Sometimes a nerve or group of nerves can't carry complete messages to limbs because of damage or disease. But *some* part of the message may get through. It's important to encourage even some messages by making it a point to send them along with toning exercises daily.

Coping with Problems of Nerve Damage to Muscles

Fibrositis and myositis

Fibrositis and myositis are rather common afflictions. The disorders usually come on gradually, and may or may not follow a bout with a cold, the flu, or a relatively mild injury.

The pain is usually fairly well localized in a small area, but it may spread to involve a wider area and may pop up at a location distant from the one where it was first noticed. The back, especially the area between the shoulder blades and the neck, and the low back are common sites, but any large muscle group such as the calf of the leg, the thigh, or the chest can be involved as well.

With these afflictions, as with many others, it is easy to fall into the habit of overprotecting the sore areas, by not using the muscle groups around the sites of pain and aching so that they won't hurt so much.

This can be a mistake, as a patient named Ross Y. learned. As a result of having relatively mild fibro-myositis involving his neck and upper and lower back, he avoided activity that involved the use of his neck, shoulder, and back muscles. He was in his mid 50's, and eventually was granted a transfer from the shipping department of the trucking company he worked for to the dispatching area, to give his aching back a rest.

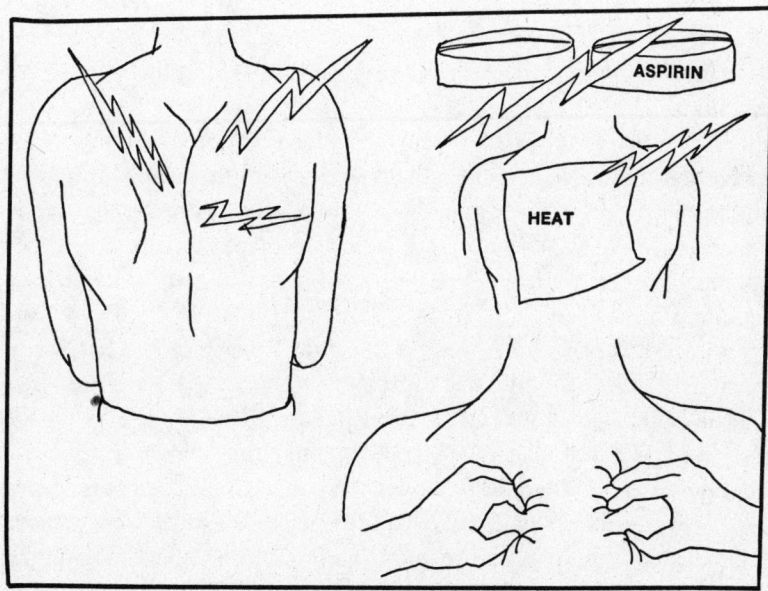

Figure 11-4

This super-caution pampered his neck, shoulder and back muscles to the point of almost complete non-use. The symptoms of pain, aches and irritation over his neck and back finally brought him in for treatment. By carefully searching his neck and back area with my finger tips, exerting pressure over his areas of pain, I located four "trigger points"—definite areas where pressure with my finger tips brought on sharp, very uncomfortable pain as compared to the wider areas of his neck and back that were touchy but not really as painful as the trigger areas.

I injected these trigger areas with a simple local anesthetic to interrupt the pain. Immediately following the injections, Ross noted almost complete relief from all the areas that seemed to be involved with pain and aches, and I then demonstrated to him that he could exert any of his neck and back muscles as much as he wanted without having much discomfort at all.

When I convinced Ross that the use of high constant doses of aspirin (up to eight a day with meals), and local heat to the trigger areas I'd found together with massage (his wife came in with him and I showed her where to massage), Ross was able to restore tone to his neck and back muscles through exercising and eventually completely overcame his symptoms. Figure 11-4 summarizes this home care.

Even in brain tumors

I treated another patient, named Angela F., a young woman who had a tumor successfully removed from the left side of her brain but was left with paralysis of the right side of her body (remember that the left side of the brain controls the right side of your body, and vice versa). She had neglected to notice the *partial* return of *some* function in her right arm and leg because no one at home was putting her paralyzed limbs through their daily routine of full ranges of motion. When I discovered some function in both her ability to flex her arm and bend her knee, proper toning (her front thigh muscles and the front upper arm muscles) with help at home from her husband returned enough strength in these muscles so that eventually Angela could walk with a brace on the right lower leg, and could use her right arm to help lift and carry objects.

The point is that even if there is just a quiver of action in a muscle whose nerves have been damaged, it must be encouraged and later *demanded* to go through all the activity it can with the idea of restoring the fullest tone possible. Neglect of even the slightest movement may cause it to disappear forever and will cause you to miss out on the potentially important return of partial function!

SUMMARY

1. Spinal cord injuries involve more damage to nerves in direct proportion to the level of injury or disease—the higher in the cord the damage, the more nerves may be involved. Even so, some function may remain in the limbs involved, and such function, slight though it may seem, needs to be encouraged and strengthened for maximum use of the limb later on.

2. With care and very hard work, even quadriplegia (paralysis or partial paralysis of four limbs) may be overcome to the point where you can be a useful and necessary part of life again.

3. Limb nerve damage can be overcome by surgical repair of the damaged nerve, or, if this isn't possible, by retraining other muscles, not affected, to take over the function of the damaged nerve. Careful, painstaking exercise to restore tone is essential in this retraining.

4. Even damage to nerves from diseases such as diabetes and alcoholism can be helped by general attention to control of the disease (insulin and abstinence from alcohol), nutrition (ample carbohydrate, protein and fat plus extra vitamin B), and restoring tone to muscles.

5. Fibrositis and myositis are conditions that can lead to overprotection of nerves and muscles because of pain and aching. Since control of these disorders is relatively successful with simple treatments, muscles and nerves that are allowed to weaken because they aren't used can be restored with little effort.

6. Even with brain tumors, there is often some residual function of some muscles and nerves from the affected areas. Following removal, these areas must be watched for carefully and, if found, they should be toned up to their maximum.

12

How to Manage a Problem Back

In this chapter, I will talk about the problem of your back—a problem that has become an enigma of this century. I'll have a look at the fiction as well as the facts concerning problems with your back, including the subject of "the disc," what it means and how it is dealt with.

We'll look at the chronic back syndrome—what causes it, why, and how you can deal with it effectively. And certainly no discussion of the back would be complete without an examination of the so-called "whiplash" injury, common in these days of traffic congestion. We'll see how it's brought about, what structures are involved, and what you can do when you have such an injury.

Finally, I will present some special approaches to tough back problem situations so that you will see how such problems are sooner or later bound up with states of mind as well as with physical aspects of the back. And we'll look at some approaches to handling both sides of this puzzling structure—the back.

YOUR BACK AND ITS CONTENTS

The human back is really quite remarkable. It is the main "strut" for your body's support. It is composed of bone (24 separate bony vertebrae plus a large bony base called the sacrum), ligaments that hold the vertebrae together and span the spaces between sacrum and hip bones (called iliac bones), cartilage as in all other joints (the joints between vertebrae and between the sacrum and the two iliac bones), and, of course, muscles and nerves.

In addition, a large part of your upper back is fashioned by your rib cage, against which your two shoulder blades are held in contact by muscles.

How to Manage a Problem Back

What makes a back remarkable is not so much that it contains so many of all the elements I've just listed, but rather that it manages to work so well in spite of the abuse it receives from its owner.

Injuries—truth and fiction

There are many people who believe that since man hasn't always walked upright through the ages, he necessarily hasn't adapted to this position yet. The evidence shows that man has probably walked upright for at least three million years, and that his evolutionary adaptation has been very successful regarding the back, regardless of what some may think.

That your back is subject to injury and disability, more so than any other part of your anatomy, is nevertheless true, and this is because most people take their backs for granted and haven't learned how to take care of them.

Consider this: Your back is not anatomically built to bend like your arms or legs. If you fall into the habit of many, you actually make your back do the work that your legs should be doing almost every day. How could this be? You housewives almost always bend over at your waist, when picking up a laundry basket full of heavy wet clothes, as you dust the furniture in your house, in cleaning out the bathtub, or as you pick up your child (or grandchild) from the floor or playpen. And you men are just as guilty as you remove the grass-catcher from your lawn mower, lift up a corner of your dining room table to replace a caster in one of the legs or lift a thousand different heavy objects that you must pick up from the floor at work.

Now consider this: What do virtually all these activities, performed by both men and women every day, have in common? *They all involve bending over at your waist to get the job done quickly and easily. And this is just what you should NOT do if you have the health of your back in mind!* Figure 12-1 illustrates this point.

When you bend at the waist, not only are you putting all the weight contained in the object you may be picking up at the end of a lever involving your torso, back, upper extremities, head and neck, but you are also bending this lever at least 90 degrees (at your waist), and then you are asking your back to straighten up with all this weight and carry it wherever it may need to go. This is comparable to using a five-foot broom handle as a lever to move a refrigerator! Something has to give, and your back will be that something sooner or later.

The remedy is very simple. All you have to do with any chore that involves lifting an object from floor level is to *squat down, bending your legs and keeping your back reasonably straight all the while!* In this position, you can clean the bathtub or lift the object from the floor *with your legs doing the lifting or weight bearing*. Then your back is free to do what it does best: support and stabilize your body as you work, *without* doing all the lifting!

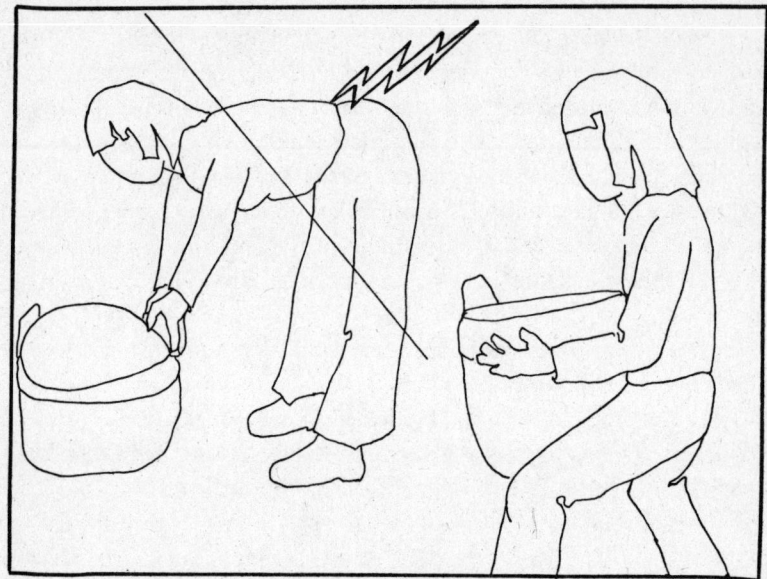

Figure 12-1

Injuries at work

Ninety-five percent, or more, of all back injuries are brought about through carelessness, generally on the part of the person who is injured. The reason for this is that you and I are not alert to what we're doing when we go about our day to day work. A patient named Brian R. found this out the hard way.

Brian came to me after he was sent home by his boss because of a back injury he got at work in a warehouse. When I asked how he'd received the injury, he said that he was shifting heavy cartons of merchandise on a pallet, and his working partner dropped one of the cartons suddenly. Brian had grabbed it, and the sudden heavy weight caused an excruciating pain in his mid and lower back.

Fortunately, Brian hadn't done anything serious to his back, but of course all the pain made him feel as though he had broken it. And his boss mentioned the possibility of a serious disc problem. This made Brian even more apprehensive about the situation, and the more Brian fretted about this, the worse his back pain got.

How to Manage a Problem Back

The following things were done for Brian's back:

1. I carefully examined his back with my hands and fingers, having him go through the various motions at his waist—bending slightly to the right and left, and forward and backward. I could assure him that some of his large back muscles had been strained, but that no evidence of serious damage was present.
2. I did X-ray Brian's back. I did this mostly because of his deep concern—suggested by his well-meaning boss—that something might be broken. Nothing was. I reassured him of this fact. His mind and his tense back were eased.
3. I instructed him to do four things for the next couple of weeks:
    A. Place something solid between the mattress and springs of his bed, such as a piece of plywood or bed slats laid side by side from the level of his pillow to his hips. Alternatively, I asked him to sleep on the floor for a few nights if he couldn't find the plywood or slats for his bed.
    B. I told him to avoid stooping or bending at the waist for any reason. If something had to be done at floor level, lifting or otherwise, he should squat on his legs to do it, and he should not lift an object heavier than 25 pounds, squatting on his legs if it was on the floor, keeping his back perfectly straight at all times.
    C. Three 15- to 20-minute hot soaks to his sore back area daily, either in the shower, the tub or via hot moist packs applied by his wife would also help.
    D. He was also to take two or three aspirin every three to four hours around the clock while awake, also at night if he awakened with back pain.

Within a week, about 75 percent of Brian's back pain was gone, and in two weeks his back was completely well.

I'd always been interested in what causes back injuries, so I later quizzed Brian about the day of the accident. He confided that he had family problems on his mind when he went to work that day, and that he had become so engrossed in thinking about them that he was doing his pallet loading almost by mere reflex. His partner expected him to be ready to take the heavy carton, but Brian's mind was wandering. He suddenly realized that the carton was falling and grabbed it by reflex. He was a good deal more careful from then on.

The case of Dottie McD. is typical of the "housewife back." In this case, Dottie, a young woman in her late 20's with a baby toddler, told me she was bent over her baby's crib picking up toys, and took hold of her baby to lift him out. She said she felt something snap in her lower back and couldn't straighten up. She had to call in a neighbor to help her with her youngster while she lay down, the only position in which she found relief from the pain. Again, Dottie feared the worst. She knew that the snap she'd heard and the severe pain in her back and one buttock meant disaster: the dreaded disc problem. She was, fortunately, wrong.

Dottie's was a rather common disorder of backs when they are put in awkward positions. It can occur in anyone, but tends to be seen more in people who are on the overweight side, as was Dottie's case.

What happened was that one of the lesser "facet" joints of Dottie's vertebral column had slipped out of position and was the cause of the pain, the muscle spasm, and the apparent radiation of the pain into one buttock. Figure 12-2 shows these facet joints in the lower back.

In Dottie's case, an injection of a local anesthetic directly into the area of the facet joint (not a difficult procedure), and exactly the same instructions as in Brian's case, cleared up her problem within five days. Weight reduction, attention to back muscle tone and avoidance of waist-bending positions will save Dottie from any more such episodes.

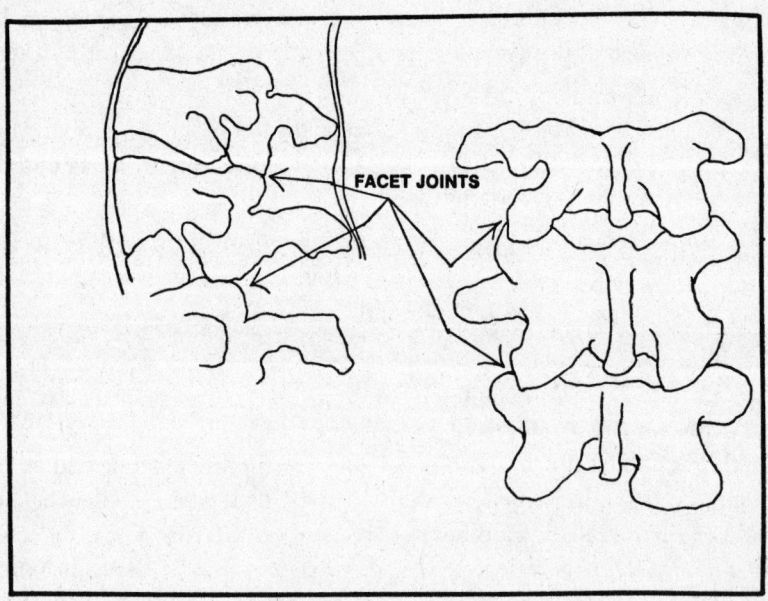

Figure 12-2

THE DISC SYNDROME

Orthopedic surgeons, neurologists and others dealing with the disc problem over a span of more than 35 years have learned from experience that some factors are worth consideration.

The first is that "ruptured discs" do indeed occur—not as often as they are given credit for, but they do cause problems. The second is that the presence of an "out of place" disc does not necessarily mean that surgery is the only thing that can or should be done. The third, and most important of all, is that because a disc problem is or has been present does not mean that you're condemned to live the life of a handicapped person, unable to stress your back from that time forward.

A disc causes problems of two kinds: a sudden forceful wrenching in which your low back takes the brunt of the injury, and a slowly developing degeneration of one or more discs in which the gradual loss of the cushioning space (the disc) between two vertebrae is the source of trouble rather than the slipping out of place of part of the disc cartilage.

The discs that can cause problems are generally one or more of the three lumbar (last of the vertebrae) discs and the disc between the last of the lumbar vertebrae and the sacrum (the large solid base of your spine). The following list is typical of disc problem signs and symptoms:

1. The pain is constant, starting in the region of the lower back, and usually extends into your buttock, thigh, and sometimes your lower leg. The pain is usually on only one side. It may be relieved by lying down on the side opposite the painful one.
2. The discomfort is often aggravated by coughing, sneezing, and having a bowel movement.
3. Some weakness of thigh, leg, or foot muscles may be evident.

Figure 12-3 shows how the cartilage discs may press on a nerve trunk.

Treatment of discs

Every effort should be made at conservative treatment of a disc problem. Such an approach may include hospitalization with traction on the pelvis, physiotherapy with local heat and massage and gentle manipulation of muscles and lower spine, medicines to reduce pain and decrease swelling—including at times one of the cortisone drugs to decrease the inflammation that always occurs around the area of the protruded disc—and of course, rest for the spine.

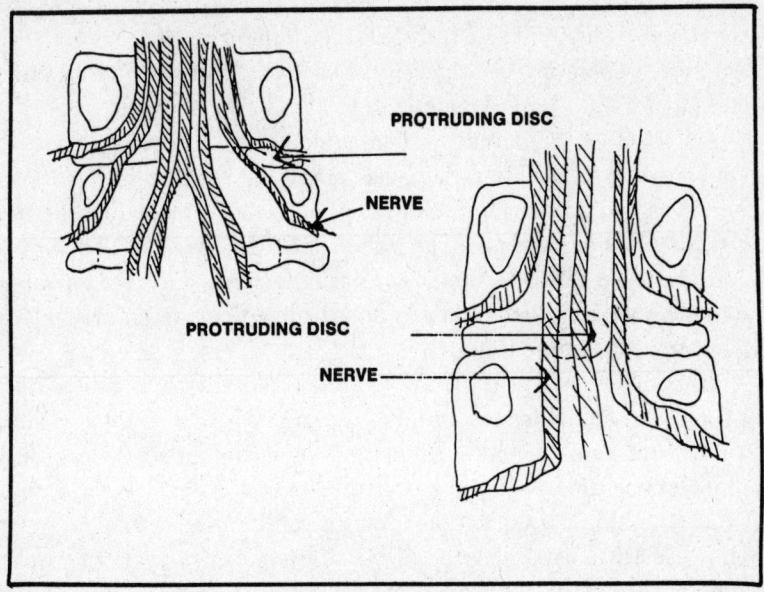

Figure 12-3

If done carefully and diligently, such conservative therapy will relieve the distress and incapacity of the damaged disc in a high number of cases. The time this takes varies a good deal with individuals, but improvement ought to be seen within a week, and by four to six weeks there should be fairly complete relief of symptoms with full activity in progress.

If such improvement is not forthcoming at this time, surgery for the involved disc, or discs, is definitely in the picture; the necessary diagnostic X-rays and examinations to precisely locate the area of the problem should be done, and the errant disc or discs should be removed. There are important reasons for proceeding without undue delay after a thorough trial of conservative therapy with a disc problem.

The first is obvious: If the piece of disc that is pressing on the nerve trunk is not removed, the nerve may suffer permanent damage, and the muscles it supplies may never work as they should. A second reason is that the longer the delay, once it is seen that conservative therapy is not going to work, the more your psychological defenses against fear of crippling—a quite natural fear in all of us—are broken down, and the more apt you are to slip into the rut of believing that you are indeed "ruined" for the rest of your life.

How to Manage a Problem Back

You need faith and confidence in your medical advisor in this situation, as in all crucial medical circumstances. If there is something that causes this confidence to be less than you would like, whatever it may be, it is easy enough for you to ask your advisor for another opinion. And you should not hesitate to do so.

Recovery from disc surgery

There is nothing really different or unusual about recovery from disc surgery. Nor do you have to remain immobilized in bed for any extended period, and you don't have to look forward to giving up most of the activities you pursued before the surgery. There are some limits imposed on heavy physical exertion for a time, but such limits are no more than what is reasonable for any surgical recovery, given the areas involved in healing.

The main thing to remember is to get back into all the activity and physical motion that your medical advisor instructs, and at the times he gives you. But be active up to those limits. Sure, your low back will hurt for a while, just as your abdomen would hurt for a while after a hernia repair or a gall bladder removal. This normal sensitivity of the muscles and ligaments involved in surgery takes several weeks to diminish, and of course, the restoration of strength to muscles weakened by inactivity depends strictly on how you follow your medical advisor's instructions as to what you must do at various stages after surgery.

If you work at a job that involves heavy lifting and straining, he may say that you will have to avoid such work for a specified amount of time. But he will, or should, also tell you which things you *can* do in the way of physical activity, and you should do them faithfully. Your boss at work may find something for you to do for a couple of weeks following your return to work that fits such limits on a temporary basis. Or your boss may ask you not to come back until you're ready, until your medical advisor says you may return to your former job. And it is just at this point that a good deal of the trouble starts for someone who has had surgery to correct back trouble.

Lou T., victim of over-response

I'm sorry to say that the case of Lou T., a man in his early 40's who found himself in just such a position as I've described, is an altogether too common one, and a situation we must all strive to correct in our society if such problems aren't to get completely out of hand.

Lou worked for a trucking firm on the loading dock, a job he'd had for several years and at which he had done well. He injured himself at work, developed a disc in his lower back, and had surgery to relieve the pressure on one of the nerve trunks going into his right leg. The surgery was performed well and it was timely (no long delays when conservative methods didn't work).

His company put him on Workman's Compensation following his injury—this is the insurance that employers are required to have on their employees to cover accidents and injuries sustained on the job. Lou's recovery was excellent in every respect, and he received a paycheck right on time during his recovery phase.

When it came time to start work again, however, Lou's boss called him into his office at the trucking firm and told him that a somewhat younger man in good health had taken over Lou's job, that he didn't think Lou could return to his job in the future (even though his doctor had released him to do so), and that there was nothing "at present" in the firm that the boss could assign to Lou at a less physically demanding job. Lou couldn't believe it. When he pressed his boss on the "can't return to his usual type of job" statement, the boss said that it "wasn't his fault"—that "his compensation insurance premium would go up if they found out about it," and he frankly couldn't afford it. Lou was now in a real pinch. Several weeks later, after several unsuccessful applications for similar jobs elsewhere, a change was seen in Lou's personality. And the scars from the change proved to be far more serious than those from his back surgery. The following set of circumstances in Lou's case are typical of thousands in similar situations.

1. A good measure of control over his situation was lost by Lou when the company sent him to their "surgical specialist who deals with compensation cases." Lou's own doctor was removed from the picture "by regulation."

2. Like most, Lou got a lot of attention from his family while recuperating—they took over many things that Lou had done before his injury, they pampered Lou by doing things for him that he could do for himself without problems, but it is natural to try to make things pleasant for anyone recovering from serious illness.

3. The rejection by his firm and by the others he had applied to was somewhat the same as saying, "Look, we don't want cripples working for us. If you ever had another accident, we might not be able to afford the cost of our insurance." In addition, the rejection seemed to lend an atmosphere of doubt to Lou's apparent recovery. "Maybe," he thought, "I'm not in as good a shape as I've been led to believe."

4. Finally, aided and encouraged to a degree by the sympathy and help of well-meaning family and friends, and by the way employers are compelled to act by stint of rules and regulations, Lou settled into the rut of the chronic invalid—with devastating results.

How to Manage a Problem Back 219

Lou continued to draw compensation and applied for Social Security disability. He got it. And he got a chronic back syndrome—he'd been convinced he was an invalid, and he became one.

The postscript to Lou's case is equally sad. He applied for Vocational Rehabilitation when his Workman's Compensation was about to run out. But his frame of mind at the time was so geared to the invalid state, and the people at Vocational Rehabilitation were so wary of his "bad back" history, that they tried to train him in something that wasn't geared to Lou's skills or interests. And Lou didn't make the grade in three more retraining attempts.

Such is the way of the chronic back syndrome. Figure 12-4 illustrates improper and healthful attitudes.

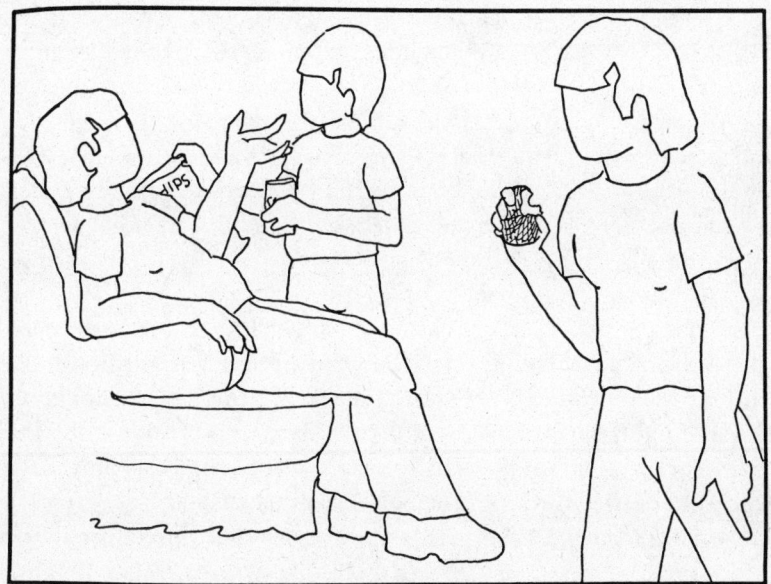

Figure 12-4

Does it always happen this way?

No, not always, but entirely too frequently. I think of the case of Tom C., a man in much the same situation as Lou, but who had not one, but two separate disc surgeries—both bona fide and both necessary to prevent nerve damage. Tom was out of work for a total of five years. He had worked in a foundry and had trouble with the first disc as a result of an accident at work. Problems with the second came about while he wasn't working. He went much the same route with compensation and Social Security disability as did Lou, but it wasn't quite enough for Tom. He wasn't content in his own mind to become "an invalid for the rest of his life" even though that was what government officials and those in his field of work seemed to be telling him.

Fortunately for Tom, he'd always had a way with figures, and he was retrained in the accounting field. He subsequently got a job with the same foundry he'd worked in five years previously, but this time in the foundry's accounting department—an irony of fate, but one which has stood Tom in good stead to the present time. Tom is no longer regarded as an invalid, but as a productive member of his family, the foundry, and society as a whole.

THE WHIPLASH

If there is any more emotionally laden injury than whiplash, I haven't seen it. Whiplash, so-called because it usually occurs when one is in a car that's struck from the rear by another car, is much overdone as an injury, though no one would pretend such an injury is a push-over either.

As a passenger in a car that's struck from the rear, your head and neck are first snapped backward, and then jerked forward by the reflex action of the muscles in your neck that oppose the backward motion. The head and neck are put through much the same motions as the cracking of a whip.

Personally, I have never seen a serious aftermath from whiplash, though I've seen a lot of people who have convinced themselves and others that serious permanent injury has been the result of it. I suppose one thing that brings on such a feeling on the part of the injured party with whiplash is that, first and foremost, it is a maddening thing to be pulled up to a stop at a red traffic light, for example, and then to have someone plow into the rear end of your car. Obviously, the driver of the car behind was either asleep at the wheel or misjudged the situation a good deal.

Anyway, your neck hurts if you're the one that gets hit from the rear. And someone's going to pay if you have anything to say about it. Often, the someone will be an insurance company.

Another point about such an injury is that your neck is involved—and if you injure your neck it's got to be serious.

What happens in whiplash is that the ligaments and flexor muscles of your neck are overstretched. And since most of these muscles and ligaments are attached on the bony vertebrae near where the nerve trunks come out, there is often tingling, numbness and pain conveyed down these nerves into one or both arms for a time after whiplash, though the nerves themselves are rarely injured.

But all this doesn't mean permanent damage. In fact, most of the time nerves are not damaged, merely irritated, but the distress convinces many that much trouble is at hand, and judging from the way some medical

How to Manage a Problem Back

advisors treat the injury, your suspicions of grave injury may be greatly increased. Figure 12-5 shows the structures involved in whiplash.

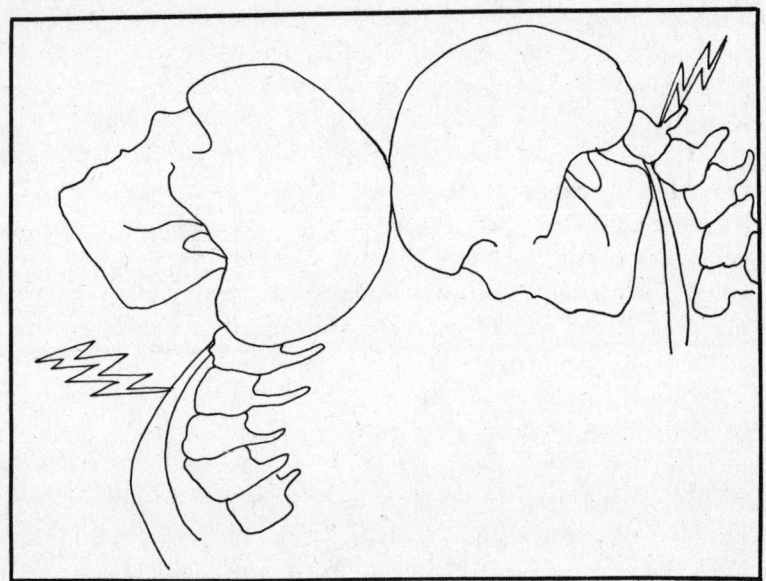

Figure 12-5

Treatment of whiplash

After a whiplash injury, almost any motion you make at your neck—flexion, extension, rotation—may hurt like the dickens. It may hurt even if you don't move it. Therefore, the initial treatment is to put your neck at rest as far as possible. This can be done by you—you simply don't make the moves that hurt. If this is difficult, a so-called cervical collar may be helpful. A cervical collar can be anything that is stiff, yet flexible enough so it can be wrapped in place around your neck like a collar, extending from the lower part of your skull down to the points at which your neck joins your shoulders.

Cervical collars can be purchased at your pharmacy or surgical supply house, or they can be homemade fairly easily by using a piece of cardboard covered and padded with gauze or muslin—or any soft material—and fastened in place around your neck with lacing or safety pins. It is a good idea to measure the distance around your neck beforehand with plain paper. Then cut the cardboard from this pattern and carefully mark where the ends come together. Allow for a margin of overlap and cut the cardboard so that the fastened ends can be adjusted for comfort and a snug fit. The collar should rest comfortably beneath your chin and extend underneath your lower jaw to where the back of your neck and your head come together. It should fit snugly enough to help splint the movements of your neck, but not so tightly as to be uncomfortable when you're looking straight ahead.

It seems popular to treat whiplash by means of cervical traction, especially when the discomfort persists for very long. This is a method applied by means of fitting a harness under the jaw and around the neck to the base of the skull. The two sides of this harness are fitted with small ropes or cables that extend above the head of the person being treated, who is seated in a chair. The ropes or cables are joined to a single rope, passed through a pulley and brought down to where weights of varying sizes may be attached. This has the effect of pulling up and stretching the neck—precisely what is *not* needed in a whiplash injury. If you have bruised, overstretched muscle and ligaments to begin with, it doesn't make too much sense to stretch them some more. In my opinion, this method of treatment—cervical traction—only worsens the problem.

Because ligaments attaching muscle to bone and to muscles are injured in whiplash, it takes from six to twelve weeks to heal completely. A cervical collar, if worn, should be used for two or three weeks. Then it should be removed so that stiffness can be gradually worked out.

Marlene R. proves a point

The case of Marlene R., a middle-aged lady who had pulled up at a stop light at a busy intersection in a large city, comes to mind as an example of unusual neck trauma. The driver of the car following hers must have been daydreaming as well as exceeding the speed limit by at least 15 miles an hour when he collided with Marlene's car. At any rate, he hit her car going at least 35 miles an hour, according to skid mark calculation by police officers later.

As if this weren't trouble enough, after the car hit Marlene, Marlene's car was pushed over the rear bumper of the car in front of her, which in turn was pushed into the next car until the first car at the intersection light was involved. Then the car behind the one striking Marlene's was hit again by the car behind it, and like dominoes falling in a row, this continued back until seven cars behind Marlene's were also involved!

Each time another car behind her rammed into one in front, Marlene got her neck jerked, after already having it snapped twice—once after the first collision and again with the forward collision with the car in front.

Yet in spite of this trauma—and it did produce a good solid whiplash injury at least four or five times worse than the usual single neck jerk accident—Marlene recovered significantly in three weeks, and completely

How to Manage a Problem Back

in eight weeks following the injury, using only a cervical collar, aspirin, local heat and a biofeedback technique in which she simply concentrated on her bruised swollen neck muscles and fed into them through her mind a command to relax, to return to normal size and function, and to be less irritable. She used biofeedback in the same setting as I've described elsewhere in this book. Figure 12-6 shows Marlene's cervical collar.

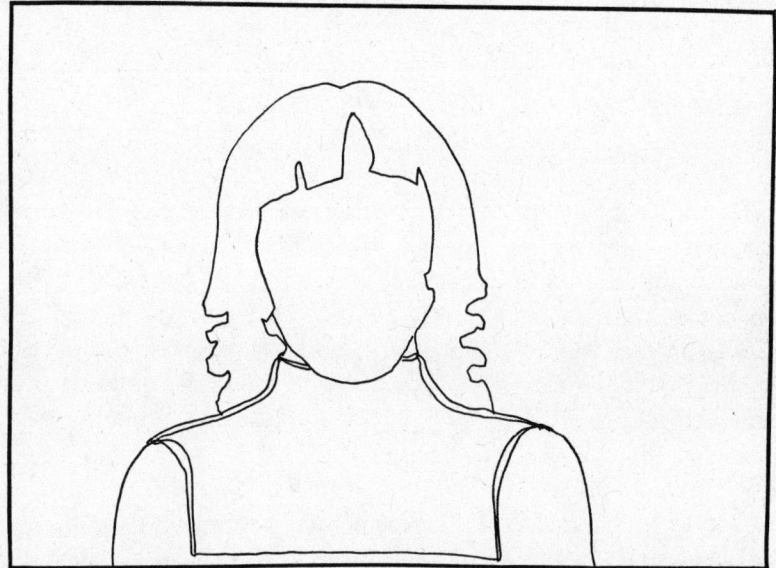

Figure 12-6

SOME SPECIAL BACK PROBLEMS

Rheumatoid arthritis

There is a particular form of arthritis of the spine known as ankylosing spondilitis (or Marie-Strumpell's disease). It is a severe form of rheumatoid arthritis, and almost always begins in the sacro-iliac joints—the joints between your sacrum (the large bone at the base of your spine) and the iliac bones of your hip. Although sacro-iliac joints are falsely accused of causing a multitude of back problems, they are usually innocent in cases of back pain except in this condition.

Although capable of slowly involving your entire backbone, rheumatoid arthritis of the spine behaves in much the same way as it does anywhere else in your body and can sometimes be entirely confined to your sacro-iliac joints. When these joints are involved, pain is the first symptom.

The pain is located on either side of the sacrum, or on both sides, as it was in a patient of mine named Clint L. Clint noticed his pain was chronic—worse at some times than at others, and not particularly brought on by back strain or relieved by rest. It takes X-rays of these joints to diagnose Marie-Strumpell's disease, and when it was clearly shown on Clint's X-rays, I injected each sacro-iliac joint first with a local anesthetic agent, and then with a cortisone derivative. Local injection, when possible and practicable, is very much preferable to giving cortisone drugs by mouth or as injections into a muscle for reasons I have already discussed. Clint needs such injections into his sacro-iliac joints about once or twice a year, and the disease has not progressed to the rest of his spine.

Poor tone and sway back

This is a common condition, more so in women than in men, mostly because the child-bearing functions in women cause a weakening of abdominal muscles from overstretching and inattention to retoning following pregnancy.

Weak, poorly toned abdominal muscles cause the lower back to "sway" in, increasing the normal in-curve at the lower back. When this happens, all the vertebral joints of the lower and midback, their hundreds of ligaments and tendons, and their nerve trunks are pulled beyond their ability to comfortably adjust. The consequence is, as in the case of a young woman patient named Carla D., chronic back pain.

When I first saw Carla in the office, she told me a typical story: She'd had three youngsters over the past six years, was overweight by about 25 pounds, and spent most of her time running around after her small kiddos, aged nine months, one and a half years, and three years. Her abdominal muscles were thinned out and flabby, allowing her pelvic organs and upper abdomen to push out almost as if she were pregnant again. Her back was really giving her fits. I explained the problem and told her that it was going to be primarily up to her to remedy the situation. She started doing sit-ups, and scissor kicks at first. When she became comfortable with these two exercises at home (after about three months) I put her on pelvic toning in addition. This consisted of contracting her vaginal and rectal muscles while sitting on the toilet or lying down in bed. It's hard to describe pelvic contraction, but it occurs when you tighten up or close your rectum following the expulsion of a bowel movement—you can feel your pelvic muscles pulling up in your vaginal and rectal areas. The idea is to pull on the muscles (all the major pelvic sling muscles work together in this movement), to hold the contraction for longer and longer periods—up to two or three minutes—and to slowly relax them, repeating the process for a total of 15 minutes when the initial weakness is gradually overcome. It is

How to Manage a Problem Back

amazing what this simple exercise toner will do, not only for the sway back, but also for helping to keep your uterus and bladder in place.

Carla restored tone in her back muscles within three months with this toning routine. She then took up tennis and swimming to maintain her muscle tone and has been free of back pains since. Figure 12-7 shows Carla's abdominal and low back curve before and after the toning routine.

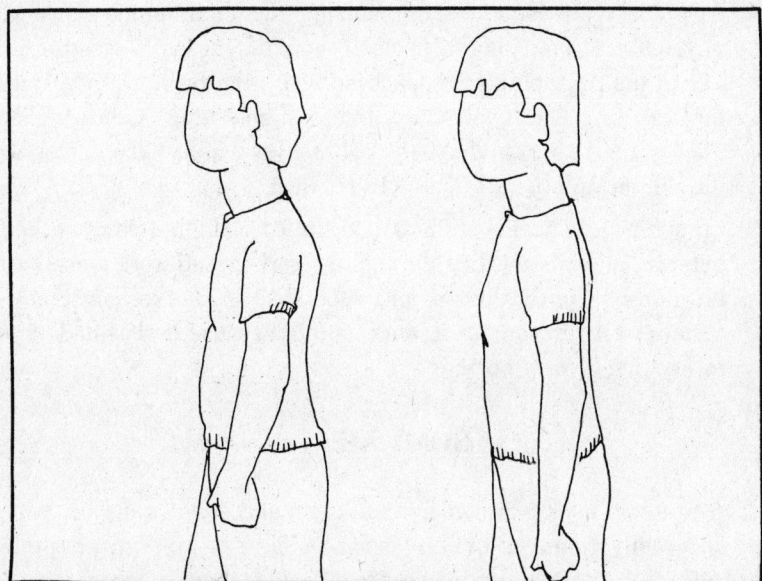

Figure 12-7

The chronic, chronic back syndrome

Tom C., described earlier in this chapter, was an example of the very longstanding back syndrome. He represents a surprisingly large segment of our population who get into a rut as a result of what is usually a bona fide injury at the outset, but because of the way the whole thing is handled—by doctors, employers, insurance compensation, lawyers, and family—becomes a chronic and difficult problem, resting as much on psychological considerations as on physical ones. I believe that at least the following things must happen after back injuries to avoid having them become chronic situations:

1. Initial involvement of the injured person's own doctor is essential, regardless of his specialty or interests, and irrespective of company "injury specialists."

2. The timely and accurate diagnosis of the problem—if a serious problem (disc protrusion) is present, it should be treated as quickly

and expeditiously as possible, with vigorous physical rehabilitation of the back as soon as practical after surgery, if an operation is necessary.
3. The family should be brought in to help with management at home—not to wait hand and foot on the injured person, but to get him to *help himself with his problems* as soon as possible.
4. A special team capable of approaching the family problems and the physical and emotional aspects of the pain should be used if in 12 weeks the pain problems concerned with the back are not well on the way out. There are pain clinics which handle such problems. They cannot work, and usually will not work unless the person with the chronic problem seeks help in time.
5. Compensation agencies in all states must make quicker and better determinations regarding the injured worker, and work closely with his family, family doctor, and specialist. A worker must not be penalized regarding future work merely because he has had a back injury that is now healed.

SUMMARY

1. A problem back is a common affliction and can usually be quickly and easily managed by the principles of rest, support, pain relief, and most importantly by using good sense about how you use your back from day to day, even if it's apparently well and strong.
2. Not all pain that starts in your back and runs into your buttock and leg is caused by a protruded disc. Such ailments are usually simpler problems and can often be relieved by the above principles plus the timely injection of simple local anesthetics into the proper areas.
3. If a protruded disc does occur, it should be treated for a period of time conservatively, and if not relieved, it should be removed surgically without further delay.
4. Rehabilitation of a back after surgery, or an injury not requiring surgery, is built around similar principles: toning, care of the back, getting back to work as soon as sound advice will allow, and no prolonged babying or inactivity.
5. Whiplash need not be a disabling injury that will cause trouble for the rest of your life. Its treatment usually involves six to twelve weeks, and such injuries generally do nothing to harm vital nerves to your arm, nor do they injure your spinal cord.

6. Back problems need to be correctly diagnosed by your medical advisor, and good sense must be used in treating them. Prolonged bed rest and prolonged avoidance of anything that might strain your back is not what is needed. In fact, the sooner you are up and doing what you normally do, if at all possible, the more likely you will be to overcome the critical situation that will make the backache permanently disabling to you psychologically, if not physically.

13

How You Can Get Back to Work

In this chapter, I will give you some ideas on how to get yourself back to work—how you can make contact with people whose job it is to help you do just that. Your state has special agencies that deal with such problems, and you should at least be familiar with who they are and what they do, as well as how they operate.

There are things you can do right in your own home if it's impossible for you to get to a place to work. I'll talk about some of them and show what some other people have done in this situation.

There are times when you must have help because of your incapacity, whatever it may be. There are local and federal agencies that can help. You should know who these agencies are, where you can find them, and what they can do.

STATE AGENCIES

I suppose it's because our country is so big, and there are so many sections of it to be represented, that there exist programs—most of them excellent ones—that were originally set up to help people with a variety of needs, yet about which relatively few people know.

Sometimes, this general lack of knowledge about what the agencies do is the individual program's own fault—they just don't think about getting their message out to the people who might well be able to use their services. Sometimes, too, the services and agencies involved just don't have the time or the money to spend on public relations as they'd like.

Vocational Rehabilitation

This agency above all others, over 55 years old, is designed to help handicapped people find work that is consistent with their particular affliction. And it is one of the few governmental agencies (managed by each state) that actually predates all the Social Security laws and titles of the country, having been originally set up by congressional decree to help returning veterans of World War I who were injured or diseased to find employment. Gradually over the years, Congress changed the direction of Vocational Rehabilitation to cover others not connected with the war, until finally the agency was tailored to meet the needs of all handicapped people, regardless of the nature of their infirmity, and irrespective of how or where they were made unable to work.

Today, Vocational Rehabilitation has agencies in every state, including Hawaii and Alaska, and in addition their agency is decentralized—that is, the agency has offices in many towns across your state so that you may reach one without traveling to your state capital. They exist to help you with virtually any handicapping medical or emotional condition—in fact, *you must be disabled* in some way in order for them to help.

Even if you are threatened with the loss of your present job, but have not yet been forced to quit, Vocational Rehabilitation can help.

The first thing Vocational Rehabilitation (V.R.) needs, of course, are the medical records that substantiate your problem. The more detailed these records, the better. If the records you have access to are old—say, more than a year or two—the agency will have experts in the field of medicine or psychiatry examine you for up-to-date information at its own expense; it won't cost you a penny!

When the records are assembled, V. R. doctors, all familiar with the problems of handicapped people, review them to help the counselors with whom you'll be dealing to build up a vocational plan most likely to succeed, given your particular problem.

If it means sending you to trade school to learn a skill that you can handle with your remaining capacity to work, then that's what V. R. will do. If it means sending you to school to take special courses designed to make you functional in an occupation—accounting, for example—then that's what V. R. will do for you. And even if it appears that your aptitudes and personality are compatible with going to college for a degree to serve you at a job, then V. R. will handle that as well.

In between assessing your handicap and helping to get you back to work, V. R. also performs an important job: restoration. If there are ways in which your particular ailment can be made better, can be further improved so that you may have a better capacity to function, V. R. will undertake this task at no expense to you. Like anybody else, the people who work in V. R. have limits. They are, after all, human just like the rest of us. They cannot make you into something that you haven't the potential to be. Nor can they cause you to function beyond your best capacity. But V. R. *can* help and assist you to reach you maximum potential, with your cooperation and motivation!

Seeing is believing

I've been a medical consultant to a state V. R. agency over a span of five years, and there is no end to the complicated situations I've seen unraveled by the V. R. people in behalf of clients who wished to become self-sustaining and productive citizens once again.

I recall, for example, Hal T., a middle-aged man confined to a wheel chair because of vascular complications in his brain. The problem had done away with much of Hal's mental abilities as well. He had trouble remembering things and visualizing things in his head. And, of course, knowing he was not quite the person he once was made Hal depressed.

However, with V. R.'s help, Hal managed to pick up his life again. There were several concerns in town that used the telephone for sales and promotional purposes. In bringing Hal and these concerns together, V. R. was able to set up a business in Hal's own home. They helped to build an office with a special telephone that Hal could use with his partially functioning arms and hands and developed a special indexing and customer list program for Hal's special use.

Things got off to a slow start at first, but Hal had the persistence it took to make a success of whatever he did. In a span of three years, he'd saved enough money to start thinking about what he might do to get back to his original occupation, which had been custom tailoring.

Again, V. R. entered the scene. Some special patterns for clothing were found that Hal could cut out at home, several at a time, with a special machine purchased by V. R. Along with several other special tools designed especially for people like Hal with only partially functioning arms, legs and hands, Hal began slowly and painstakingly to get back into his own field once again.

Today Hal has a thriving business in custom tailoring. He is happy with what he's doing. And most importantly, Hal is contributing, to himself, to the family income (three fourths of it comes from his business), and he is contributing to society in a productive manner. It has bolstered his self-esteem—something that was lacking before and was the main reason for his previous depression.

I also recall the case of Richard S., a man plagued since early childhood with heart valve damage from rheumatic fever. He was never able to run and play like other kids, and in fact his whole life was built around the restrictions imposed by his damaged heart.

As Richard grew up, married, and tried to find a job, there were many things his heart prevented him from doing. Finally, he did find a job as hotel manager in a small town.

Unfortunately, the job required Richard to climb stairs a good deal, and although at first he found he could do it if he took plenty of time and was careful to pause for rest part way up, it wasn't long before he just couldn't keep his breath long enough to continue.

Fortunately for Richard, it was about this time that the technique for open heart surgery came into its own. Richard sought V. R. help and one of the first things that happened was that Richard was sent to a cardiac diagnostic center and thoroughly worked up. The experts at the center thought they might be able to help him with surgery, and Richard was willing to try anything at this point. He had his surgery, requiring an artificial valve replacement and the surgical opening of a second valve. Within six months of his surgery, Richard became literally a new man. Finally, after more than 30 years of exile from life, Richard could now be about as physically active as he wished. This opened up vistas he'd never dreamed of. He ended up running a bonded furniture moving business that was an outstanding success.

But fate had other plans. Six years later, Richard suffered a massive stroke from complications of his artifical heart valve. He lost consciousness one day at work, then awakened paralyzed on one side and mentally quite confused. One would think that after two such serious personal set-backs, Richard might be justified in just giving up. But not so! In spite of speech difficulties and problems doing mental arithmetic, together with a practically non-usable right arm, Richard once again began a climb back to productivity and seeking V. R. help a second time.

This time, different plans and strategies had to be used. First, when physiotherapists had returned his ability to walk with a cane, Richard returned to school—to drafting school, as a matter of fact. V. R. ordered drafting tools and equipment made especially for people who can only use one hand. And Richard was a top student in his class, according to the school director.

Today Richard has a job utilizing his new skill as a drafting engineer. He is good at it and the job supplies him with an income well above average. Fortunately, his heart remained strong throughout this second major physical and mental ordeal, and today he enjoys as good health as anyone can following a stroke and major heart surgery.

Of course, Richard had help with all this. No one can succeed against such odds without help. But V. R. knows how to help such people, and though no one would say they are perfect or that success always results from their efforts, V. R. does amazing things to help people like Richard and Hal.

Locating Vocational Rehabilitation

I mentioned earlier that V. R. is decentralized. This is true in every state. They have offices throughout your state to make it easier for you to get to one for help. The particular state department in which V. R. operates does differ from state to state, however. In some states, V. R. is located in the state welfare department; in others, in the department of vocational education, and in still others, V. R. is a separate department reporting directly to the governor.

To find your nearest V. R. office, talk to the county welfare people nearest your home. And remember, unlike all the other welfare offices, V.R. attempts to get people *off* welfare and working again, even though the two offices may work closely together in the effort. If the people at county welfare can't direct you to V. R. call your *state* welfare department. They will put you in contact with the state V. R. people, and they can easily direct you to the V. R. office nearest your home.

Other state agencies that can help

Your state has another agency, called the State Job Service, that can help you if you're disabled (the agency is required to have at least one employee who deals solely with handicapped people) and you need work.

This office used to be called the State Employment Service, but has changed its name. The people in this office also work closely with veterans' organizations to place veterans of the various wars into jobs. But their work isn't confined just to veterans.

You should call your State Job Service directly in your state's capital since not all state job agencies are decentralized. They can tell you what you may do to receive help.

The State Job Service also administers the WIN program. WIN stands for Work Incentive Program. Their purpose is to help men, women, and youngsters past the age of 16 to find permanent, suitable jobs—people with handicaps and disabilities caused by emotional or physical ailments. They, like V. R., supply training where necessary and job placement services. They can help you find work!

Your state welfare department also administers a fairly new plan—called Title XX—a federally financed plan to perform certain services involving families and young children. Among other things, Title XX can help secure jobs for disabled people and furnish financial help while those people are being trained for jobs, or while they are looking into job openings. Title XX may also assist with day care for your children. Again, your county welfare office can put you in touch with the Title XX people in your area.

Finally, there is CETA—the Comprehensive Employment and Training Act. This agency is a product of the National Manpower Commission, and is generally decentralized in most states.

The purpose of CETA is to promote job training and employment opportunities for all people who are economically disadvantaged and/or disabled (the two usually go together!). They also help people who are underemployed; that is, people working at jobs that are not sufficient to earn them a living, or that are below their potential.

CETA offices can be found locally, in your counties and cities, and in your state capitals.

NATIONAL AGENCIES

The Veterans Administration is interested in seeing that disabled veterans are substantially employed. It is usually easiest to contact your state VA at the capital, or in any larger city in your state since the VA is not usually as decentralized as other agencies.

The VA maintains another office called the Veterans Reemployment Rights commission, especially designed to help veterans who have just come off a tour of duty with any of the armed forces, whether during wartime or not. If you may be in this particular category, don't hesitate to contact this agency for help.

The Federal Civil Service Commission supervises government employee personnel. They are like your state's civil service agencies, except, of course, they are concerned with federal government employment. Recently, the Federal Civil Service agency has taken a very serious look at incapacitated and disabled people with the idea of helping them seek part-time and permanent employment in thousands of federal jobs.

A good thing about their concern is that they are willing to try to place people who are the most severely handicapped—people with severe brain damage, for example, or those with advanced sight or hearing problems or mental retardation.

To reach these people, you must call your state's regional federal office, located in your state's capital city, and inquire of them the phone number of the Federal Civil Service Commission. If you have a phone directory of your state's capital, or of any major city in your state, you can find this agency listed under U.S. Government.

Yet another national agency is NAB—the National Alliance of Businessmen. This is a cooperative organization composed of private businessmen, government people, and labor unions who have banded together to help provide training and jobs for disadvantaged people, veterans, and disabled persons.

NAB is not generally housed with city, county or state government offices, but they have offices of their own. To find them, you should consult your telephone book or call the telephone information service in your nearest large city.

Finally, to ensure that the most severely handicapped people are able to work, the Employment Standards Administration (a federal government bureau) supervises sheltered workshops—places where very simple tasks can be learned by the severely disabled. This agency allows such workshops to pay below minimum standard wages to employees where the work doesn't merit standard wages. But disabled employees do get pay, and in many cases it is the only thing left for them to do.

This agency operates under the U.S. Department of Labor, and to contact them regarding workshops, you should look under the U.S. Government listing in the phone book.

WORK IN YOUR HOME

There are a good many things you can learn to do right in your own home.

I am thinking, for example, of Jenny W., a patient with severe arthritis of the hips and spine, who even with stiff deformed fingers was someone who would not allow her sewing ability to diminish because of her health problems. Jenny simply opened up her sewing room for business when her husband died. She did custom sewing of clothes, draperies and furniture slip coverings. In Jenny's case, she never saw the furniture for which she sewed the slip covers. She talked to the customers on the phone and gave them instructions on how to measure for the new coverings they wanted. The customers purchased the material and delivered it to Jenny's house where she did the work. Yes, there were a few mis-fits at first, but Jenny guaranteed her work, and she corrected her mistakes without charge. As a consequence, she had very few dissatisfied customers.

Morris T., a man afflicted with a rare nerve disorder which paralyzed his legs and confined him to a wheel chair, learned TV repair work by correspondence (paid for, incidentally, by his local Vocational Rehabilitation agency), and when he finished, he opened up a TV repair service right in his own home.

Another man I know, Michael D., had a hobby of collecting and restoring antique furniture. After suffering a stroke, which left him with a paralyzed right side, speech problems and difficulty with memory, he

How You Can Get Back to Work

opened up an antique appraisal service in his home, and continues to do quite well at it today with the help of his wife.

Lujean B., another acquaintance of mine, was a school teacher before her confinement to a wheel chair following a bout with poliomyelitis, only two months before the protective vaccine was made available! She is today a successful writer, having raised her family and made all her contacts with her publishers from her wheel chair right in her own home.

WHY WORK?

I've known many people who have been content to retire from the outside world after a disability—just sit around on their duffs at home, day in and day out, while the government checks, the compensation checks, or the medical retirement checks continued to come in. This is one way of looking at an affliction that takes you out of the mainstream.

Another way is to look at it as a challenge. So you can no longer do the work you once did, or even anything close to it. Is this a good reason to quit? To give up completely? To roll over and cry "Uncle"?

Considering the cases I've mentioned thus far (and I could go on and on with them), are they any better or more talented than you are? Sooner or later with whatever disability you may have, you're going to have to come to grips with the question, "Am I going to let all this beat me, or am I going to fight?"

I hope you still have spirit enough left, regardless of your particular problems, to want to fight. Because if you haven't, you have lost something vital. You have given up the right and privilege of being that highly unique and specialized entity called human.

SUMMARY

1. There are a number of local, city, county and state agencies whose job it is to aid you in your return to work when you are disabled.
2. Vocational Rehabilitation has done at least as much as most agencies to return incapacitated persons to work in jobs consistent with what they have to work with.
3. Vocational Rehabilitation, as well as most of the agencies that can help you with your back-to-work problems, may be located through your local social welfare office. If you need to, you can phone your state Social Security department at your state's capital to locate one of several agencies that can help.

4. CETA, WIN, Job Service, and Title XX are other agencies designed especially to help you get back to work. They can be located through your social welfare offices or in your phone book.

5. The Veterans Administration, NAB, and the Federal Civil Service Commission are national agencies that you can go to for back-to-work assistance.

14

Special Help with Special Bone, Muscle and Joint Problems

SPECIAL EXERCISES

You'll find this discussion helpful in a variety of ways. The exercises listed here under specific categories will help you maintain tone in your muscles that are functioning well, and will show you how to use your weakened muscles so that their tone can be restored.

As I've repeatedly pointed out in this book, your toning exercises form an absolutely essential part of your home care for bone, muscle and arthritic disorders. However, when you start to put together your routines—and they'll be specific to your particular afflictions—remember that it is far better to start out very slowly at first, and then *gradually* increase the *time* you spend doing your toning, *gradually* increase the *numbers* of times a day you set aside for toning, and *gradually* increase the *difficulty* of the exercises.

This is important even if you find you are only able to do a minute or so of an exercise—*at least do that minute*! Then, after a time—a couple of days or a few weeks, if necessary—add another toner to your routine or add another minute to the exercise time. Try to improve your best effort, even though it may seem ever so slight an improvement.

Fingers and hands

Finger toning and strength are gained by anything that makes you use a "grasp," or fist clenching movement. We've seen how this is easily accomplished by merely repeatedly squeezing on a ball—a rubber ball, a tennis ball, a baseball, or a softball. The ball will be a more effective toner

238   Special Help with Special Bone, Muscle and Joint Problems

for you if it "gives" a little—that is, if it is compressible, but not so soft that you can easily bend both sides in until they touch. Something in between is what you want.

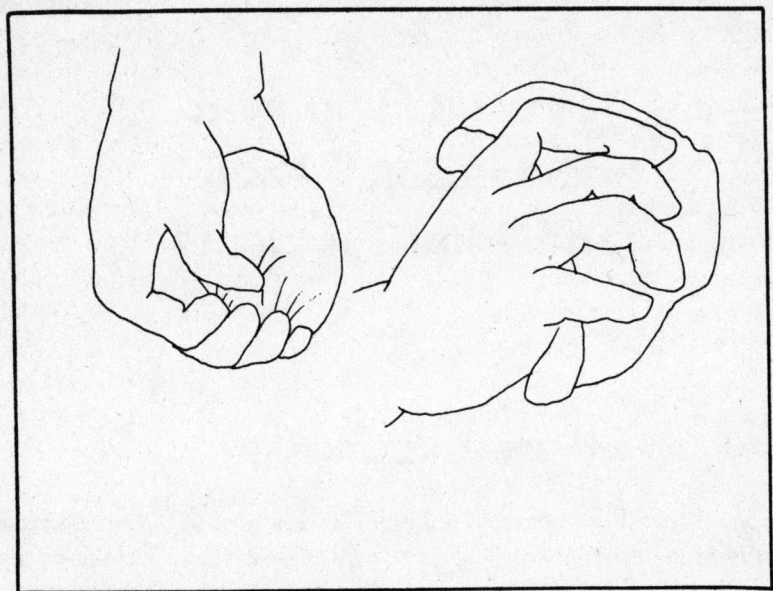

Figure 14-1

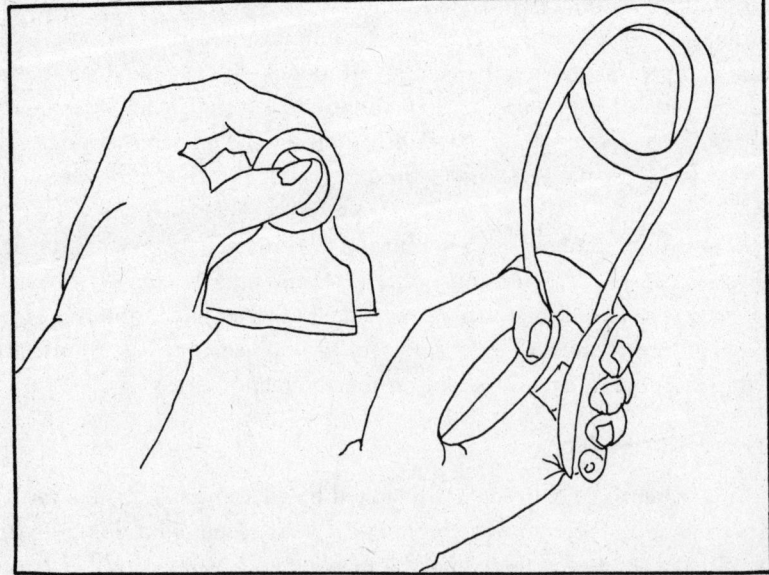

Figure 14-1 (continued)

Special Help with Special Bone, Muscle and Joint Problems 239

If a ball isn't handy, you can squeeze almost anything for the same effect—the rubber end of a drain plunger, a metal clip of the kind used to hold papers together (one with a strong spring, good for individual finger toning since clips are usually operated with the thumb and one or two fingers), or even a special "hand gripper" you may buy at most sporting goods stores. Clay and "Silly Putty" also work. Figure 14-1 shows the various squeezing toners.

Finger dexterity is another thing. In addition to strength (restored by gripping or squeezing), your fingers that are stiff and perhaps deformed, as in arthritis, need to be kept *limber* as well. For this, I've had many a man with such problems do activities such as rug-hooking, and even knitting and crocheting. It's amazing how limber you can keep your fingers by doing some of any of these activities for a while each day, as shown in Figure 14-2.

Of course, if you are musically inclined, playing most instruments is excellent finger therapy, particularly the piano. I've started dozens of men and women on beginner's piano lessons for this express purpose: to encourage limber, flexible fingers. And I've seen several people become quite good at it who had never played before in their lives!

The use of a typewriter is an excellent finger limbering routine. You can learn the keyboard in a very short time, and the habit of typing letters, grocery lists, short stories, or just in keeping a daily journal or diary can do wonders for those stiff fingers.

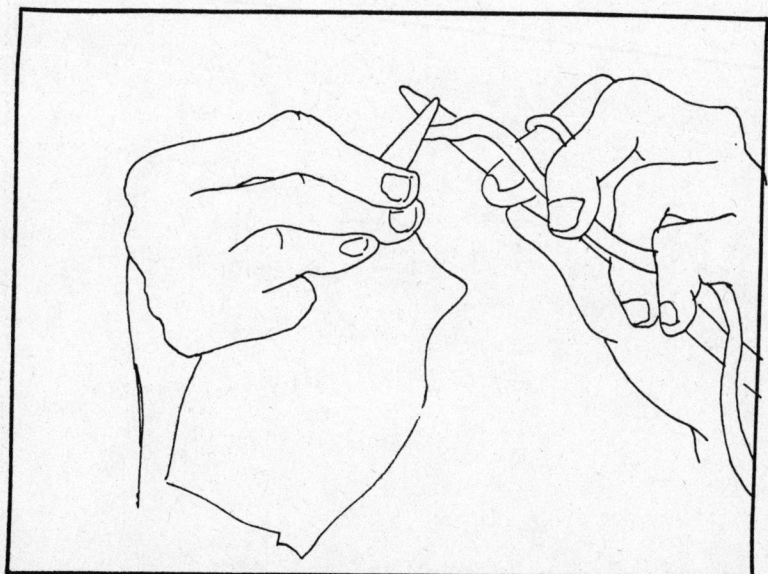

Figure 14-2

240 Special Help with Special Bone, Muscle and Joint Problems

To preserve good hand and finger function, the movement that pulls your thumb across your palm and your little finger toward your thumb (called the "opposing" motion) is quite important. Practice this motion along with grasping toners. Use your opposite hand to help your thumb and

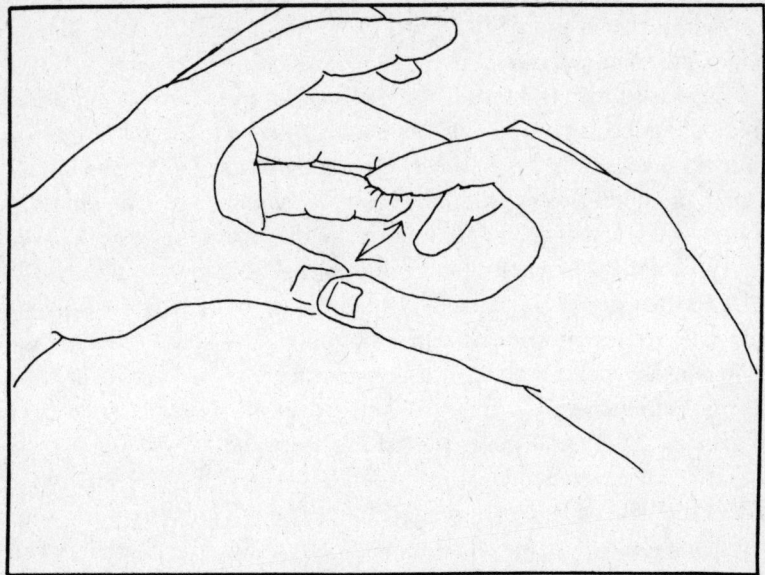

Figure 14-3

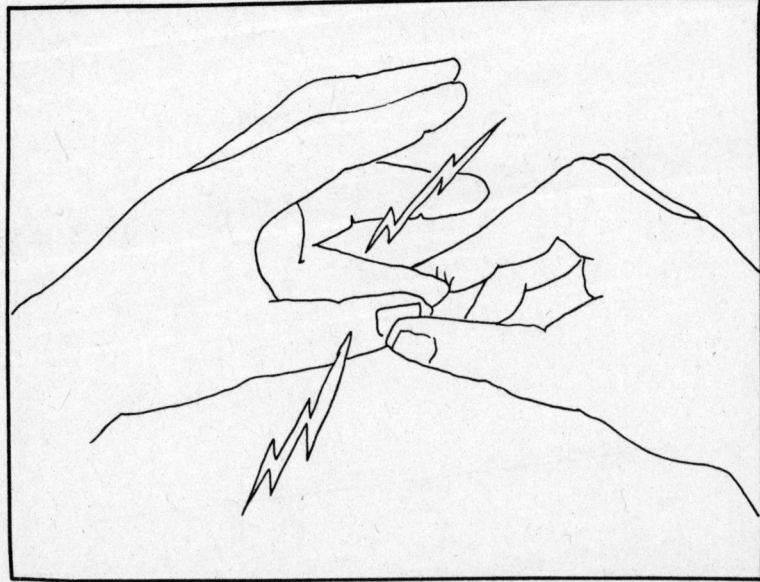

Figure 14-3 (continued)

Special Help with Special Bone, Muscle and Joint Problems   241

little finger touch, but notice I didn't say *force*—no force to the point of real uncomfortable pain is ever proper in exercise.

Discomfort, yes. But not pain. So never force anything to this point, but do encourage motion (between fingers, thumb, or in any joint or muscle group) right up to the point where it gets uncomfortable, as illustrated in Figure 14-3.

Keep repeating the motion up to this point, and you will usually find that in time you can comfortably go past the point that was, at the start, painful.

Bouncing a ball on the floor may seem rather unproductive and unglamorous, but there is nothing like bouncing a larger ball—volleyball or basketball—repeatedly, using your hand and wrist, to limber up a stiff wrist. The same applies to turning a wheel, as with driving a vehicle, and to opening and closing a window—a handy object available in most homes. The harder the window is to open, the better for wrist strength. And a door knob is a good substitute for driving if you can't operate a car. Just the repeated act of turning the door knob, opening and closing the door as you do so, will help limber and strengthen fingers and wrists. See Figure 14-4.

Elbow and forearm

Remember that your elbow has movement in four directions: flex, extend, rotate with palm up, and rotate with palm down. We've talked about

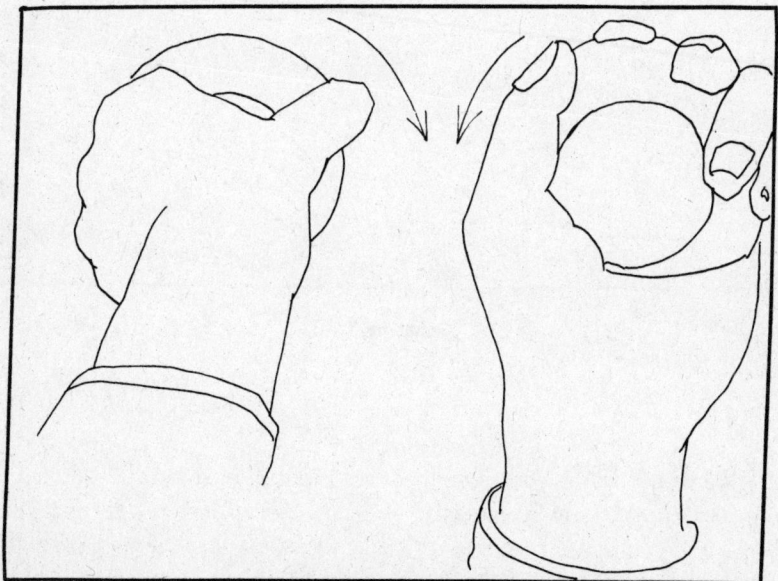

Figure 14-4

242   Special Help with Special Bone, Muscle and Joint Problems

various ways to help limber up and strengthen the flex and extend motions, flex being forearm pulled up, and extend being forearm straightened out. Gradually increasing weights grasped in your hand will add difficulty and thence strength. Sand bags, skillets, steam or dry irons, and buckets partly filled with sand or water will work.

But twisting motions at your elbow are also important. One of the simplest methods to accomplish elbow twisting is to take a wooden board an inch or so thick, make several nail holes on the flat surface of the board (not clear through it, just start the nail holes) and then use a screwdriver to insert screws of varying lengths into the holes and then remove them, as in Figure 14-5. If the screws prove too difficult at first, borrow a cork screw and a scrap of cork board, or even some large corks, and work the cork screw into the board or cork, then remove it. The motion it takes to do this will give that twisting motion at your elbow.

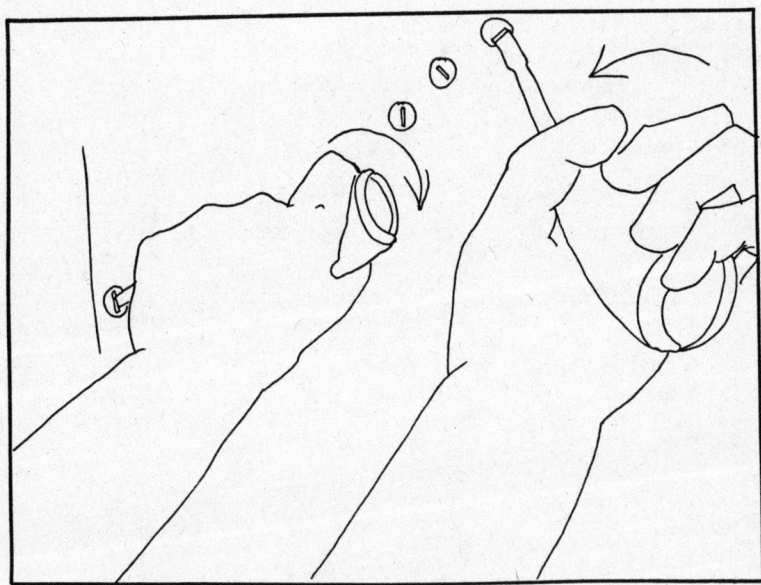

Figure 14-5

Shoulder

We've seen how your shoulder joint is the most mobile joint in your body, and how easily it can stiffen if not used. Most people forget that, although it's important to get motion at the shoulder whereby your arm is pulled up parallel to the floor, it's also important to get motion that elevates your arm to a vertical position above your head.

Special Help with Special Bone, Muscle and Joint Problems 243

Swimming does this as well as anything, but so does bending forward at your waist, allowing your arms to swing freely in front of you. This has the effect of letting gravity pull up your arm without having to use muscle power to get that far. Then, with arms swinging freely, moving your arms straight out in front gets full motion at the shoulder, as in Figure 14-6. You can do this shoulder joint toning with weights held in your hands once your shoulder begins to limber up. Another good limbering exercise, especially for arthritis in one or both shoulders, is wall-climbing. This is done by standing next to a wall (use both a stance where you face the wall, and one where your body is at right angles to it) and using your fingers to "climb" up the wall as far as your shoulder joint will allow. You may only be able to get up the wall about even with your chest the first time, but try over a period of time to climb a little past your usual level. Mark your best climb with a pencil or a piece of tape on the wall; then set your goal to exceed the level even if it's only by an inch or so.

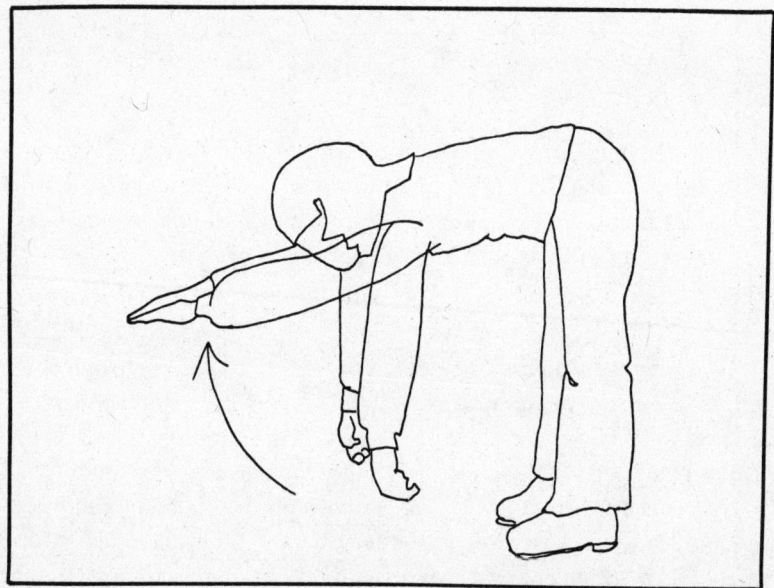

Figure 14-6

This should be continued, four times a day for 10 minutes, until you have limbered your shoulder so that you can climb to the fullest height your shoulder will allow, your arm being almost straight above your head. Climbing is shown in Figure 14-7.

If you are confined to a wheel chair or in bed, this same exercise can be done with a little modification—your goal should be the ability to clasp your hands behind your neck.

244 Special Help with Special Bone, Muscle and Joint Problems

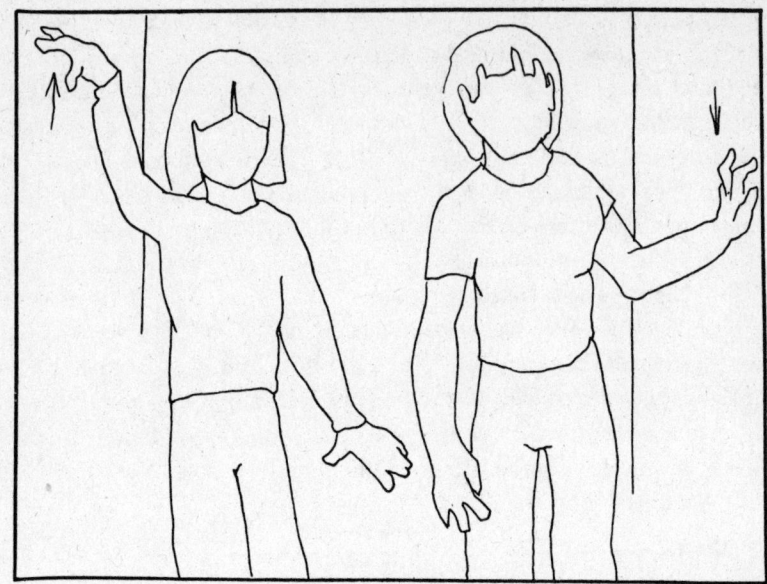

Figure 14-7

And remember, too, that if you have to take the fullest advantage of gravity for your shoulder toners, lie down on your stomach on the floor or bed and let the floor or bed support your arms as you move them from your sides to straight out, then to alongside your head.

Neck

Your neck is generally neglected in toning, but you can tone your neck while sitting or standing up by clasping your hands behind your neck and pressing your neck back against your clasped hands. Then shift your clasped hands to your forehead, and force forward against them.

For side flexion at your neck, simply place one hand alongside your head and ear, and press; first to the left, then to the right sides, alternating hands. For rotation toning at your neck, place your right hand alongside your right forehead (head turned to your left side), and rotate against your right hand. Reverse sides and hands and repeat.

Back

We've seen how sit-ups tone up your abdomen. They also help tone your lower and midback muscles because they are the natural antagonists of your abdominal muscles. As you lie back down on the floor, having done your sit-up, your back muscles are toned.

Special Help with Special Bone, Muscle and Joint Problems 245

Another way to help your mid and low back is with "bend-ups," done standing (or sitting on a stool or table), hands on waist, bending your upper torso forward about 90 degrees and then returning to the straight position. Do this in three directions—to your right as you bend forward, to the middle, then to your left side as in Figure 14-8.

Then, arms extended straight out at your shoulders, parallel with the floor, bend far to your right and left sides alternately, using the muscles that extend from your side ribs down to your hip bones to bend.

The "cradle" can be done standing or lying down on your stomach—we've seen how it's done standing. Lying down on the floor, bend up both legs and reach around to grasp each of your ankles with your hands. Then rock yourself forward so that your chin touches the floor, and pull back with your legs and back muscles to rock backward, pulling your torso off the floor in repeated movements. This will tone up your entire back.

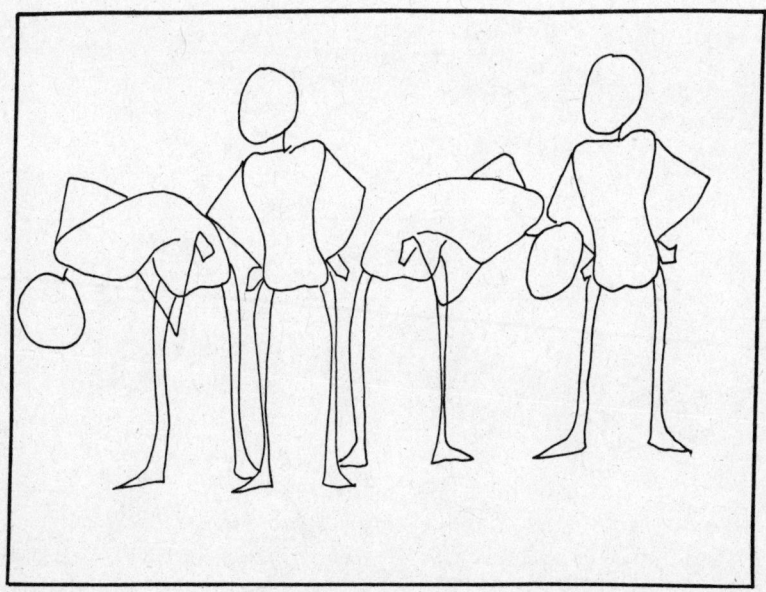

Figure 14-8

Hips

We've had a look at scissor kicks. They do wonders for both your abdomen and your hips. In the same position on the floor, pick up both legs and pull them up, knees straight, and continue to pull them all the way back as far as you can, then back to the floor again, and repeat. Set your

246   Special Help with Special Bone, Muscle and Joint Problems

goal to be able to touch your toes to the floor in back of your head. Figure 14-9 shows you how.

Standing with support (for example, hands resting on a table or chair back edge), swing each leg (alone) first out to the side as far as you can,

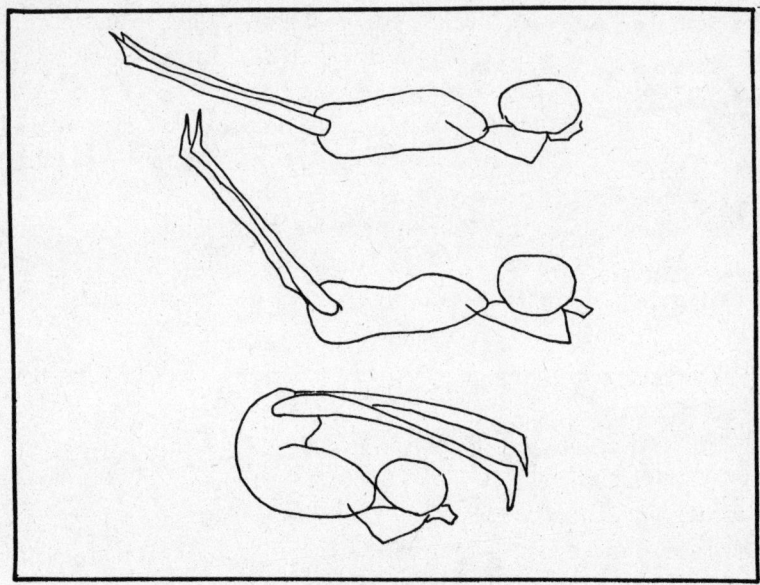

Figure 14-9

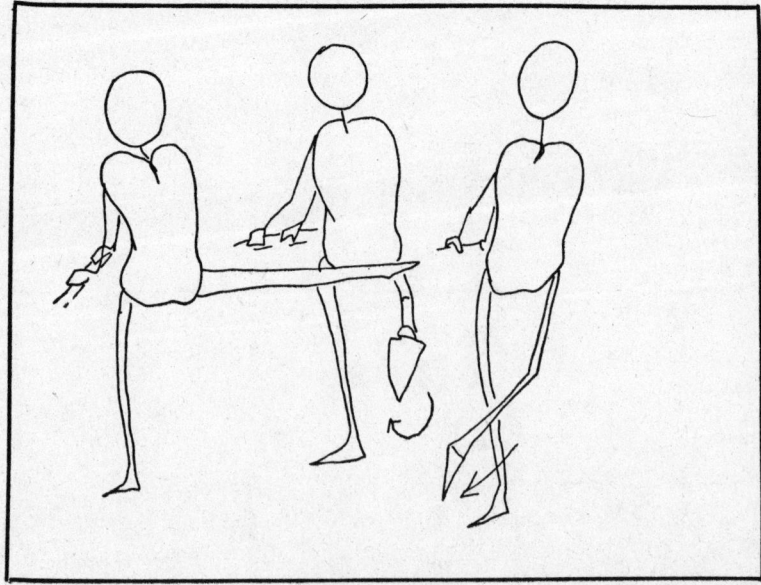

Figure 14-10

Special Help with Special Bone, Muscle and Joint Problems 247

then to the rear as far as you can, and then to the opposite side, crossing in front of your stationary leg and continuing as far as you can. This toner is also good for toning your rear end muscles. Figure 14-10 illustrates this exercise.

Knees and thighs

Squat stands are good thigh and knee exercises. The toner is done standing, hands on hips, feet spread a little apart. Squat down all the way, knees fully bent, and thrust your arms forward, straight out, at the same time. Then make your thigh muscles pull you back up to standing again. Repeat.

If you're confined to a chair, but have some power in your thighs, practice straightening your lower legs at the knee, one at a time. If possible, add some weight to your feet with sand bags, an iron, or a skillet tied to your shoe.

Lying in bed, you can do this toner by allowing one leg at a time to dangle over the edge of your bed and straightening your lower leg at the knee so that it's parallel with your bed; then repeat.

Don't be discouraged if you can't get your leg fully straight, or can only do it once or twice before you have to quit. You may only be able to do this toner once or twice for two or three weeks, but *keep it up—you will begin to regain strength!*

Lower leg and feet

If you can stand, try walking for a short distance, first on your heels, then on the balls of your feet. This strengthens the front lower leg muscles as well as your feet.

Then try walking on the sides of your feet for short distances for ankle and foot muscle toning. For foot arch toning, stand straight and rock back and forth in one place, first up onto your toes, then back on your heels.

GENERAL CONDITIONING

The following drawings in Figure 14-11 will illustrate general conditioning exercises from which you can select to make up part of your daily toning routine. Remember to start out slowly and then work up, both with the numbers of the movements you make and with the time spent with each one. The exercises shown here are progressive; that is, the least "energetic" toners are first. Then they progress a little each time so that the ones at the end are the most vigorous. Try to progress along the scale of difficulty, but

248　　**Special Help with Special Bone, Muscle and Joint Problems**

don't become discouraged or hesitate to go back to the less vigorous ones if you don't make it—*time* is what is important. And you've got plenty of it.

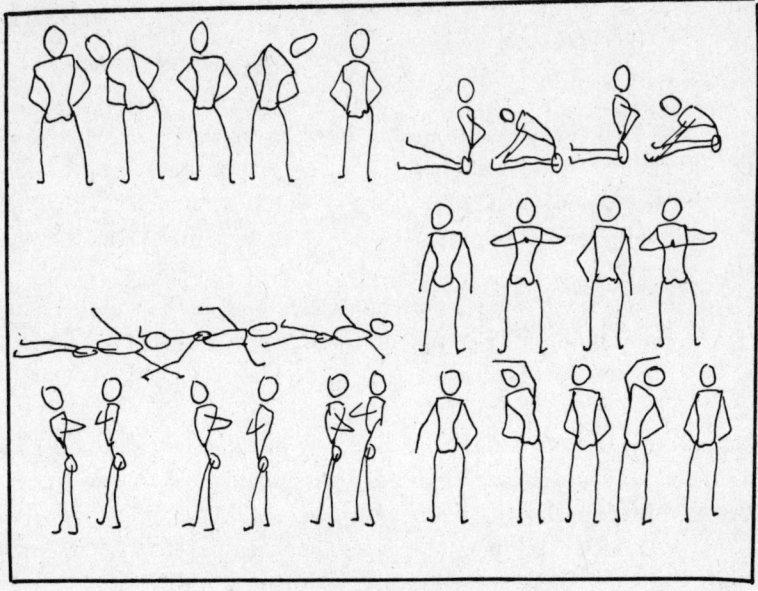

Figure 14-11

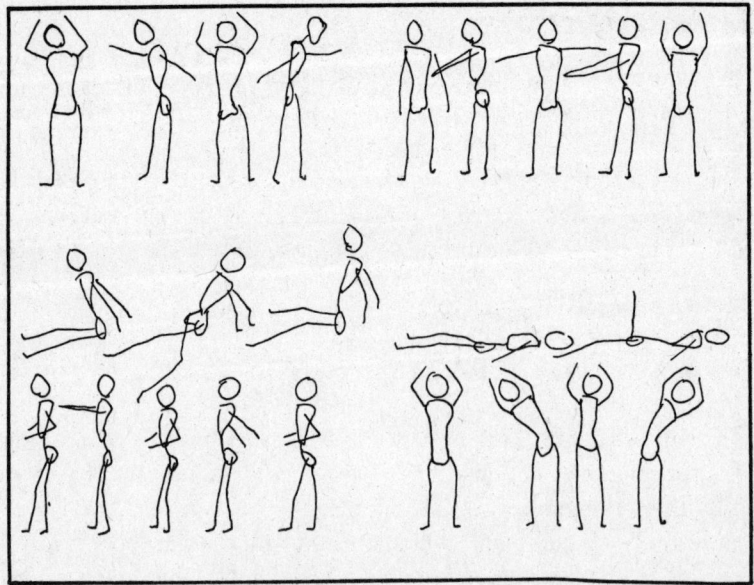

Figure 14-11 (continued)

Special Help with Special Bone, Muscle and Joint Problems

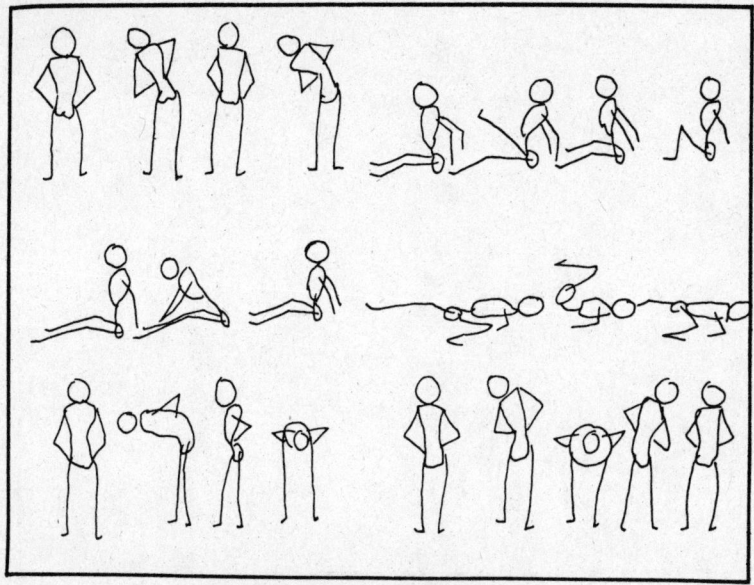

Figure 14-11 (continued)

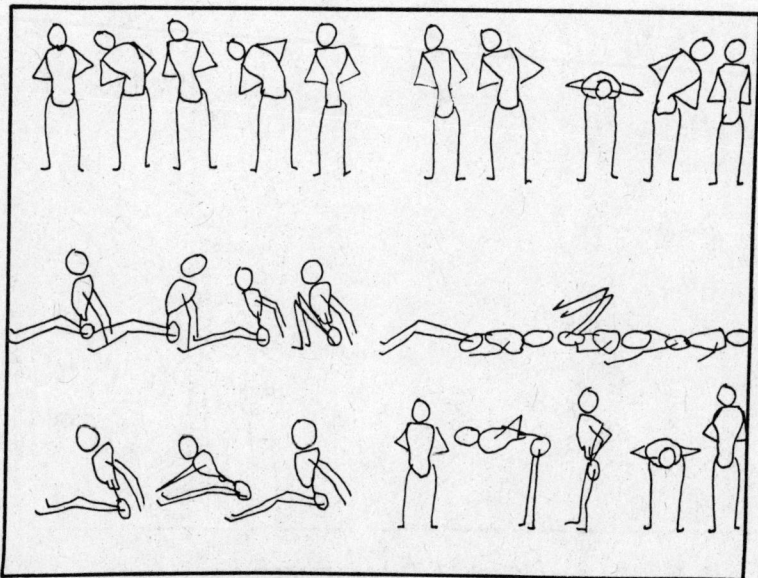

Figure 14-11 (continued)

250 Special Help with Special Bone, Muscle and Joint Problems

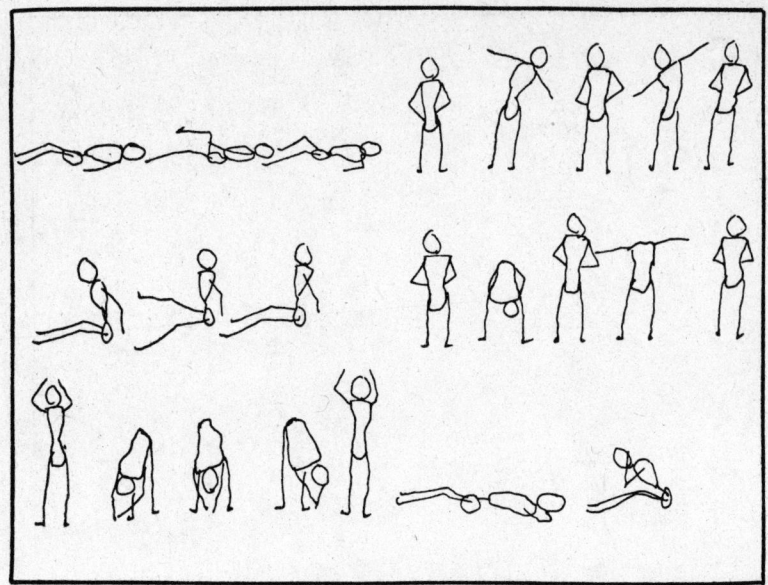

Figure 14-11 (continued)

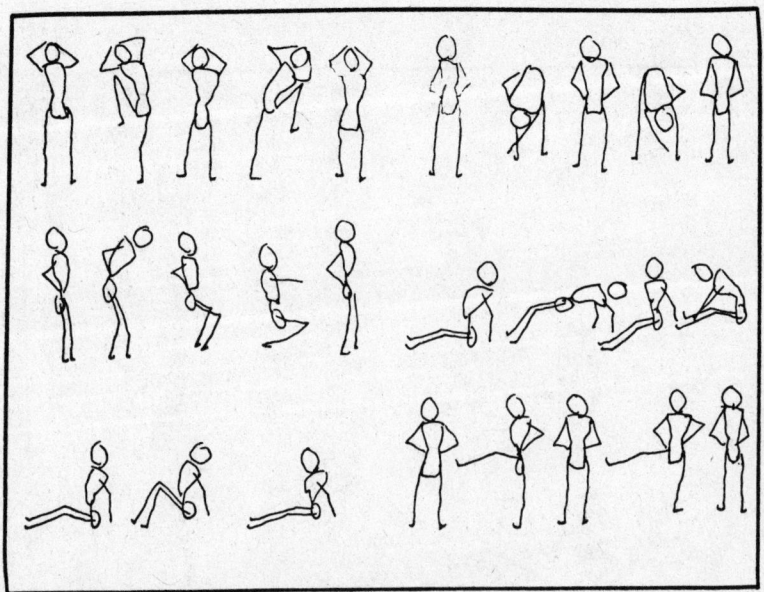

Figure 14-11 (continued)

Special Help with Special Bone, Muscle and Joint Problems 251

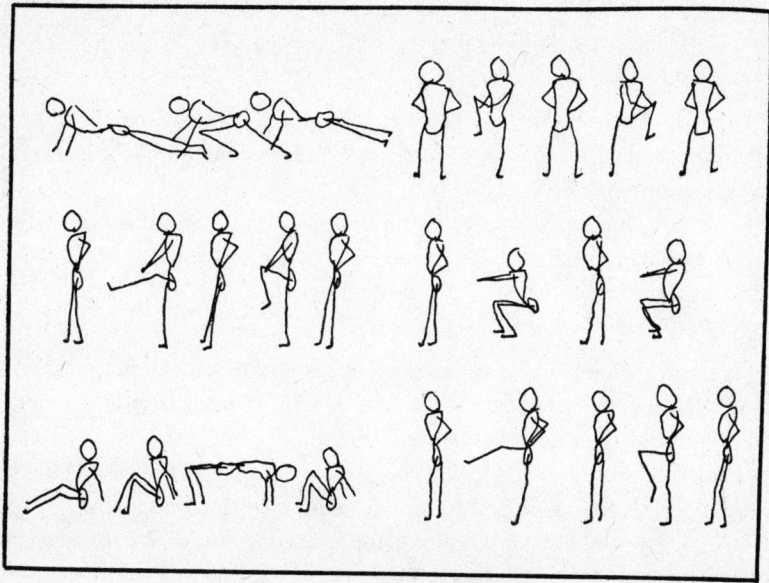

Figure 14-11 (continued)

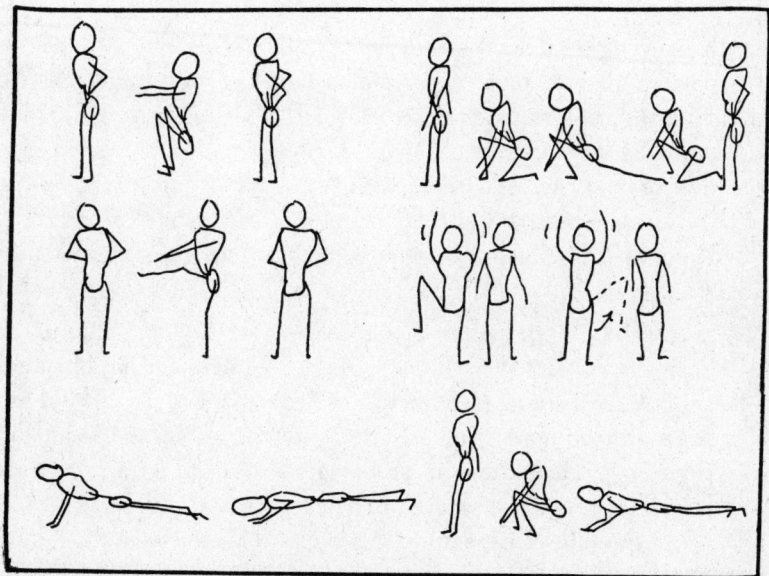

Figure 14-11 (continued)

SPECIAL SKIN PROBLEMS

There is nothing that can plague a disabled person quite so much as the development of skin ulcers, sore pressure points, corns, bunions and other skin ailments.

Any skin problem you may develop is potentially a trouble-maker, so it will help to know what you can do when they appear.

Pressure problems

Pressure problems first develop on areas of your skin that are asked to bear constant or repeated pressure from weight or from friction caused by constantly rubbing your skin over a surface.

As a rule, pain and redness of the skin over the affected area is the first sign of trouble, but for those of you who may have lost your ability to feel pain (over the buttocks, for example, following paralysis of your legs), you must either use constant vigilance on your own (if you can see the areas that take the pressure or friction) or caution those who help you at home to constantly inspect areas you can't see.

Skin can be toughened, if it presents an area that reddens and pains easily, by applying rigorous methods of skin care. The following list summarizes these methods:

1. Keep your skin clean and dry especially over pressure points like palms, elbows, back of shoulders (where they contact chair or pillow), buttocks, back of knees, heels, feet and toes. This is best done by washing *gently* with a bland soap (no perfumes or deodorants), gentle rinsing with warm water, and drying with a thick absorbent towel. After drying, apply a skin cream or lotion—plain Vaseline or plain mineral oil are satisfactory for this purpose.

2. If areas of skin persist in being easily reddened and painful, but have not broken down as yet (have not ulcerated or blistered), apply liberal amounts of tincture of benzoin (available at your drug store without a prescription) with cotton, and allow the area to dry. Benzoin protects the skin and also causes it to form extra tough layers of outside skin over irritated points of pressure. Do *not* apply tincture of benzoin to any open or oozing wound.

3. Protect reddened, painful areas of skin with a lightly wrapped padding like cotton, mechanics waste, Kerlix (a commercial non-irritating gauze that comes in rolls), or any non-irritating material.

Special Help with Special Bone, Muscle and Joint Problems

Do *not* wrap tightly or allow adhesive or plastic tape to contact irritated, red or painful skin.

4. Adjust your position, whether it be in bed, wheel chair, or straight chair, to move frequently during the course of each day. If you can shift to get pressure completely off such areas of skin that look as though they might be trouble-makers, do so, and frequently. If buttocks are involved, turn over on your stomach and sides. Shift weight, if you're sitting, to the least sore side. And take every precaution to remove any constant source of irritation. This may mean removing shoes, socks and slippers altogether, for example, if the problem skin involves your heels, feet or toes.

    Sometimes this can be done by proper padding with sponge rubber that can be purchased in varying thicknesses. A common place for a problem is in back of your knee joints where they chafe and rub on chair edges.

5. If the skin over such an area breaks down and becomes raw, oozing, or infected, it demands immediate and special attention. You will want to consult your medical advisor as a first step. He will instruct you in dealing with and preventing infection. This may involve using antibiotics taken by mouth and/or applying an antibiotic ointment locally to the open area.

    Treatment may also involve the use of special pillows or seat covers for your wheel chair—ones that inflate with liquid or air—to reduce pressure. It may involve the use of special shoes, or padding added to the arms of chairs in your home.

6. Sometimes, in spite of the best efforts to prevent it, serious deep ulcers will develop from such skin problems. These are called "decubiti" and may well require surgical skin grafting to clear them up.

    In a few cases of deep decubiti that simply won't heal, and in which surgery is not possible or practical, I've had some success with an old-fashioned method seldom used nowadays. It involves packing the wound with plain table sugar, and bandaging carefully over the wound to hold the sugar in place. Generally this dressing is applied fresh each day. I don't know exactly how or why it works, but it does in some stubborn cases.

7. If friction of ordinary bed sheets seems constantly to aggravate hands, arms, legs, and back, switching to blanket sheets sometimes helps a good deal. Blanket sheets are made of soft, non-

irritating cotton blends and will often stop friction irritation where muslin or percale sheets will only make them worse.

8. If you know you're going to be confined for some time, think of the pressure problems over your bony knobs—knuckles of hands, knobs of wrists, elbows, collar bones, shoulder blades, spine, hips, knees, ankles, and toes. The skin over these areas is thin and hasn't as good a blood supply as skin over broad flat areas of your body. Protect these areas *before* they become irritated or troublesome. You'll save much grief with such preventive measures.

9. Corns on your feet and toes can be handled if you're careful about how you do it. Protruding hard skin overgrowths (corns) can be carefully shaved with a razor blade (after soaking in warm water), being careful *not* to go too deep and draw blood. Just keep it shaved down a little every few days, and use corn pads with holes in their centers for protection in between.

    Bunions are overgrowths of bone, usually occurring at the junction of your big toe and your first foot bone. Bunions can be chiseled away at surgery, but what is simply needed is a *much wider shoe or slipper* to stop the exquisite pressure pain they cause.

10. Your skin folds may chafe and become irritated simply from inactivity and the action of sweat. The rules of thumb with skin folds (armpits, groins, crotch, back of knees, for example) is to keep them clean and dry, and keep them lubricated—Vaseline, mineral oil, lanolin, or any good skin cream should suffice. For excess sweating, use a plain talcum powder liberally applied after washing and frequently at other times during hot weather.

When in doubt, or if your skin problem seems at all out of hand, don't be afraid to consult a medical advisor about it. If you live in an area where there are local or county visiting nurse services, call them for help—their services are often free and they can come as often as the situation calls for.

Remember, too, that if you are someone who does not seem to tolerate ordinary soaps too well (they are all alkaline), there are some brands of soap available that are "acid" soaps—they can usually be used on skin that is sensitive or irritated by ordinary soaps.

BOWEL AND BLADDER

The most common and aggravating problems associated with disability, especially where confinement is necessary, revolve around the bowel and

Special Help with Special Bone, Muscle and Joint Problems

bladder. People with spine problems and paralysis are particularly vulnerable to malfunction in these two organ systems.

Bladder

I've discussed with you the advisability of always drinking plenty of fluids, and this is particularly important during prolonged periods of wheel chair or bed confinement. You must keep your urinary system functioning in top condition during disability because of certain changes that occur in your system which aren't under your control.

For example, one of the most important things a person confined to a bed or wheel chair must do—and this is urgent for those suffering from paralysis in the lower parts of their bodies—is to assume an upright position several times a day, if at all possible. Proper renal function demands that this be done, even if it takes two people to aid and assist you to this position, and even if it requires you to be strapped to a "tilt table" to accomplish it.

In addition, it is important that such afflictions (paralysis) come under the attention of a urology specialist or a medical practitioner who can use a cystoscope well. A cystoscope is an instrument used to look inside the bladder wall, and it can also be used to remove bladder stones that may accumulate in your bladder, of which you may not be at all aware. Bladder stones are quite common in people who are paralyzed, and should be removed when found.

Visits to have this done can be arranged through visiting nurse services or your medical advisor. It should be done twice yearly. You will save your urinary system much potential damage if you pay careful attention to making such visits a routine. The procedure can be done on an out-patient basis in a properly equipped hospital or clinic.

If it appears that you will need to wear a catheter (a plastic or other tube remaining in place inside your bladder to drain urine), your medical advisor will instruct you on its care and attention. Pay very close heed to his advice as there is increased incidence of urinary infection with catheters, even with the best of attention.

Bowel

We talked earlier about constipation and rectal problems with hemorrhoids. Sometimes you will find that altering your diet to leave as little residue (bulk) as possible in your intestine will go a long way in helping you through periods of bulky hard stools, straining to empty your rectum, or if you must use your finger to empty your rectum, difficult lengthy sessions on the toilet.

The following are the essentials of a low residue diet:

Food Group	Foods Allowed	Foods to Avoid
Beverages	Coffee, tea, Sanka, carbonated beverages, cocoa, milk—one pint daily, including that used in cooking.	Milk in excess of one pint a day.
Breads	Toasted white bread, melba toast, soda crackers.	Coarse grain breads, hot breads, whole wheat breads, graham crackers.
Cereals	Cream of wheat, cream of rice, Malt-o-Meal, corn flakes, rice crispies, puffed rice, most refined cooked or dry cereals.	Ralston, Roman Meal, Wheatena, Wheaties, All Bran, Bran Buds, all other whole grain cooked or dry cereals.
Cheese	American and Swiss cheese used in cooking only, cottage cheese, cream cheese.	All strongly flavored cheeses.
Desserts	Plain puddings, ice cream, sherbets (these from milk allowance), gelatin; white, yellow and sponge cakes; sugar, vanilla and arrowroot cookies.	Pastries and desserts with nuts, coconut, raisins, seeds and berries.
Eggs	All except fried.	Fried.
Fats	Butter, margarine, cream, white sauce, mayonnaise, bacon, plain gravy or milk, gravy from milk allowance.	Nuts, coconut.
Fruits	Canned or soft cooked fruit cocktail, peaches, pears, apples (peeled), apricots, bing cherries, royal anne cherries, pineapple, fruit juices, baked apples without skins, ripe banana, sectioned orange and grapefruit.	All other fruits, berries.

Special Help with Special Bone, Muscle and Joint Problems

Food Group	Foods Allowed	Foods to Avoid
Meat, Fish or Poultry	Tender ground beef, lamb, veal, poultry, glandular meats, lean roast pork or ham, fish. All to be roasted, broiled or baked.	Highly seasoned meats such as frankfurters, salami, bologna, all pickled meat, cured and spiced meat, clams, oysters and sausage.
Potato and Substitute	White potato, rice, macaroni, noodles, and spaghetti.	Fried potatoes, potato skins, potato chips, sweet potatoes.
Soups	Broth, strained cream soups made from milk allowance, vegetable soup if made with allowed vegetables.	Commercial vegetable soup, onion and other highly seasoned soups.
Vegetables	Cooked asparagus tips, green or wax beans, beets, carrots, canned or pureed peas, pureed corn, chopped spinach, summer or mashed squash, tomato juice.	All raw vegetables, lettuce, celery, tomatoes, peppers, and onion.
Sweets	Moderate amounts of sugar, clear jellies, honey, syrup, marshmallows, hard candy, gumdrops, milk chocolates, plain creams, (if diarrhea is present, all sweets to be eliminated).	All others.
Miscellaneous	Salt, smooth peanut butter, paprika, parsley, vinegar, vanilla, cinnamon and mint.	Popcorn, pickles, spices, all seed-containing jams, pepper, mustard, catsup, sesame, poppy and caraway seeds.

If you find that your stool and rectum are excessively dry, add more fluids to your daily intake. You may also find that mineral oil will help. It is best to use mineral oil in doses of one to three tablespoons at bedtime since some of the vitamins in your food are fat-soluble—this means they are dissolved in fats and oils, and taking mineral oil near mealtime or in the morning might short you on needed vitamins. If you take extra vitamins and minerals, take them first thing in the morning.

Your bowel is not paralyzed even if none of your muscles are working below your waist. Your bowel will, therefore, respond to exercise just as readily as if you aren't paralyzed. There are many toning procedures that you obviously can't do, but you may be able to do some involving your abdomen. Just the forceful sucking in of your abdominal muscles, and holding this position for a few seconds, then letting them relax and repeating, will help your bowels immeasurably. If you can do sit-ups, or even partial ones, by all means do them as well.

There is a class of medicines (called dioctyl sodium sulfosuccinates) that have the property of attracting water to your stool without any laxative effect whatever, without causing cramps, and which is not habit-forming as are most laxatives. Your medical advisor can see that you have a supply of one of these very helpful medicines, especially useful if you use the digital (finger) method of emptying your rectum.

DIET

People who are disabled and confined tend to have more trouble maintaining their weight than normally active people do. However, being overweight is just as harmful to your health as it would be if you weren't disabled, and as retarding an influence on the efficient control of your disability as any I can imagine.

In the first place, you don't need complicating health problems on top of your affliction, whatever it may be. In the second place, no matter what the nature of your arthritis, bone or muscle disorder, you can count on its being severely complicated by an overweight state.

The following table is a reasonable guide to your ideal weight as compared with height and frame.

IDEAL WEIGHT FOR HEIGHT TABLES

Men

Weight in pounds according to frame in indoor clothing.
Height (with shoes on—1-inch heels)

Feet	Inches	Small Frame	Medium Frame	Large Frame
5	2	112-120	118-130	126-141
5	3	115-123	121-133	129-144
5	4	118-126	124-136	132-148

Special Help with Special Bone, Muscle and Joint Problems

Feet	Inches	Small Frame	Medium Frame	Large Frame
5	5	121-129	127-139	135-152
5	6	124-133	130-143	138-156
5	7	128-137	134-147	142-161
5	8	132-141	138-152	147-166
5	9	136-145	142-156	151-170
5	10	140-150	146-160	155-174
5	11	144-154	150-165	159-179
6	0	148-158	154-170	160-184
6	1	152-162	158-175	168-189
6	2	156-167	162-180	173-194
6	3	160-171	167-185	178-199
6	4	164-175	172-190	182-204

Women

Weight in pounds according to frame in indoor clothing.
Height (with shoes on—2-inch heels)

Feet	Inches	Small Frame	Medium Frame	Large Frame
4	10	92-98	96-107	104-119
4	11	94-101	98-110	106-122
5	0	96-104	101-113	109-125
5	1	99-107	104-116	112-128
5	2	102-110	107-119	115-131
5	3	105-113	110-122	118-134
5	4	108-116	113-126	121-138
5	5	111-119	116-130	125-142
5	6	114-123	123-135	129-146
5	7	118-127	124-139	133-150
5	8	122-131	128-143	137-154
5	9	126-135	132-147	141-158
5	10	130-140	136-151	145-163
5	11	134-144	140-155	149-168
6	0	138-148	144-159	153-173

For young women between 18 and 25, subtract one pound for each year under 25 from weights given in tables.

It is also good to remember that there are differences in calorie requirements in people who are active and people who are not. A calorie is a unit of heat energy derived from various foods. All foods, with a few exceptions, contain calories. Protein and carbohydrates contain half the calories of fats, weight for weight. Using the following table you can determine what your calorie requirements may be based on your activity.

Ideal Weight	Calories Per Day For Maintaining Weight	Calories Per Day For Reducing Weight	Calories Per Day For Unusually Active People
100	1400	900	1800
110	1550	900	1800
120	1700	1000	2200
130	1800	1000	2200
140	1950	1200	2500
150	2100	1200	2500
160	2250	1400	3000
170	2400	1400	3000
180	2500	1400	3000

There is an easy way to figure out how to diet according to the calories you need, and still get what you need in the way of protein, carbohydrate and fat in your diet. In the following tables, the amounts (weights and measures) of various foods are given, together with their calorie content per measurement. Use it to guide you in weight loss or weight maintenance:

List 1—Vegetables

Group A

*Asparagus
*Broccoli
*Brussels sprouts
Cabbage
Cauliflower
Celery
Chard
*Chicory
Collards
Cucumber
Dandelion
Eggplant
*Escarole
*Greens and
  beet greens
Kale
Lettuce
Mustard
Mushrooms
Okra
*Parsley
*Peppers,
  green or red
Radishes
Rhubarb
  (without sugar)
Romaine
Sauerkraut
Spinach
Squash, summer
String beans,
  young
*Tomatoes
Turnip greens
*Water cress

*These vegetables have a high vitamin A content; at least one serving a day should be used.

Special Help with Special Bone, Muscle and Joint Problems

You can eat any amount of the vegetables from this list, if they are uncooked, in addition to 1 serving from Group B. If cooked, a single cupful is permitted in addition to 1 serving of Group B. If you wish, you may have an additional cupful of Group A in exchange for your Group B serving.

Group B

One serving = ½ cup; 7 grams Carbohydrate, 2 grams Protein, 36 Calories.

Beets	Pumpkin
*Carrots	Rutabagas
Onions	*Squash, winter
Peas, green	Turnips

*These vegetables have a high vitamin A content; at least one serving a day should be used.

List 2—Bread, Vegetables and Ice Cream—*15 grams Carbohydrate, 2 grams Protein, 68 Calories.*

Bread, 1 slice
    Buscuit, roll, 1 (2″ diam.)
    Muffin, 1 (2″ diam.)
    Cornbread, 1½″ cube
Flour, 2½ tbsp.
Cereal, cooked, ½ cup
Cereal, dry flakes or puffed, ¾ cup
Rice or grits, cooked, ½ cup
Spaghetti, noodles, etc., ½ cup
Crackers, graham, 2
Crackers, oyster, 20 (½ cup)
Crackers, saltine, 5
Crackers, soda, 3
Crackers, round, thin, 6-8
Vegetables
    Beans (Lima, navy, etc.), dry, cooked, ½ cup
    Peas (split peas, etc.) dry, cooked, ½ cup
    Baked beans, no pork, ¼ cup
    Corn, ⅓ cup
    Parsnips, ⅔ cup
    Potatoes, sweet or yams, ¼ cup
    Potatoes, white, baked or boiled, 1 (2″ diam.)
    Potatoes, white, mashed, ½ cup

Sponge cake, plain, 1½" cube
Ice cream (omit 2 fat servings), ½ cup

List 3—Meat—*7 grams Protein, 5 grams Fat, 73 Calories.*

Meat and poultry (beef, lamb, pork, liver, chicken, etc.),
   1 slice (3" × 2" × ⅛")
Cold cuts, 1 slice (4½" × ⅛" thick)
Frankfurter, 1 (8-9 per lb.)
Codfish, halibut, etc., 1 slice (2" × 2" × 1")
Salmon, tuna, crab, lobster, ¼ cup
Oysters, shrimp, clams, 5 med.
Sardines, 3 med.
Cheese, cheddar, American, 1 slice (3½" × 1½" × ¼")
Cheese, cottage, ¼ cup
Egg, 1
Peanut butter, 1 tbsp.
   Limit peanut butter to one serving per day unless carbohydrate is allowed for in diet plan.

List 4—Milk—*12 grams Carbohydrate, 8 grams Protein, 10 grams Fat, 170 Calories.*

Milk, whole, 1 cup   *Milk, skim, 1 cup
Milk, evaporated, ½ cup   *Buttermilk, 1 cup
Milk, powdered, ¼ cup

*Add 2 servings from List 6 (fats) if milk is fat free.

List 5—Fruits—*10 grams Carbohydrate, 40 Calories.*

Apple, 1 small (2" diam.)   Grape juice, ¼ cup
Applesauce, ½ cup   Honeydew melon, ⅛ (7" diam.)
Apricots, fresh, 2 med.   Mango, ½ small
Apricots, dried, 4 halves   *Orange, 1 small
Banana, ½ small   *Orange juice, ½ cup
Berries (blackberries, raspberries, Papaya, ⅓ med.
   *strawberries), 1 cup   Peach, 1 med.
Blueberries, ⅔ cup   Pear, 1 small
*Cantaloupe, ¼ (6" diam.)   Pineapple, ½ cup
Cherries, 10 large   Pineapple juice, ⅓ cup
Dates, 2   Plums, 2 med.
Figs, fresh, 1 large   Prunes, dried, 2
Figs, dried, 1 large   Prunes, 2 med.
*Grapefruit, ½ small   Raisins, 2 tbsp.

Special Help with Special Bone, Muscle and Joint Problems

*Grapefruit juice, ½ cup
Grapes, 12
*Tangerine, 1 large
Watermelon, 1 cup

*These fruits are rich sources of vitamin C; one serving a day should be used.

List 6—Fats—*5 grams Fat, 45 Calories.*

Butter or margarine, 1 tsp.
Bacon, crisp, 1 slice
Cream, light, sweet or sour, 2 tbsp.
Cream, heavy, 1 tbsp.
Cream cheese, 1 tbsp.
French dressing, 1 tbsp.
Mayonnaise, 1 tsp.
Oil or cooking fat, 1 tsp.
Nuts, 6 small
Olives, 5 small
Avocado, ⅛ (4" diam.)

Variations for 1000 Calorie Diet

If you desire, for example, a 1000 calorie a day diet for sharp weight reduction, the following plan will provide it:

Breakfast
1 fruit exchange (List 3)
1 bread exchange (List 4)
2 meat exchanges (List 5)
½ milk exchange (List 4)
Coffee or tea (any amount)

Lunch
2 meat exchanges (List 5)
1 bread exchange (List 4)
Vegetables as desired (List 1)
½ milk (skimmed) exchange (List 4)
1 fat exchange (List 6)
Coffee or tea (any amount)

Dinner
2 meat exchanges (List 5)
1 bread exchange (List 4)
Vegetables as desired (List 1)
Coffee or tea (any amount)
1 fruit exchange (List 3)
1 fat exchange (List 6)
1 vegetable exchange (List 2)

To add or subtract calories, use the exchange list to increase or decrease your daily intake. Remember, too, if you're dieting to lose weight, you'll notice that a fairly big chunk of weight will come off right away at first. Then it will level off—as it should—to three or four pounds a month, if you're careful to follow your diet. This is plenty fast enough. It may take you a year to accomplish your total reduction, and even if it takes longer, don't despair. It's safe this way, and it's contrary to your good health to "crash" diet.

BIOFEEDBACK

In Chapter 7 of this book, I discussed the use of various biofeedback techniques and showed you how others have used this interesting and successful method to help them. There are unlimited ways to utilize biofeedback to help you when you are homebound with various ailments.

For muscles

Perhaps one of the most common sudden incidents occurring in anyone with a muscle problem, and this includes paralysis as well, is muscle spasm—the sudden appearance of hardness and pain in a muscle. It can be your foot, your leg, your abdomen, your chest, your back or neck, or even your face. For reasons that are not always clear, muscles will suddenly undergo a severe spasm, a contraction in which the pain is excruciating and the muscle is hard as a rock.

Biofeedback can help. Just concentrate on the sore muscle. Form a picture of the tight painful muscle in your mind and don't allow anything else to enter your thoughts. Then command the muscle to relax—repeat the command several times, trying not to allow the pain to distract your concentration. You'll find that it works, no matter where the muscle is or what causes the spasm. Also remember that sometimes a low concentration of calcium in your system can bring on muscle spasm. Make dairy products (milk, bread, cheese, and ice cream) a regular part of your diet.

For pain

Biofeedback can help with pain as well. Concentrate on the painful area. Visualize that painful leg, back or neck. Concentrate on the anesthesia of the nerves going to the area causing your distress. Repeat to yourself several times that the nerves going to that area will become numb, that the pain will vanish. You won't get results the first time you try biofeedback. It takes practice just like everything else that is worthwhile. I only ask that you keep practicing this technique for your own benefit. It will help. It may work only partially many times, but when you have become

Special Help with Special Bone, Muscle and Joint Problems 265

convinced that it will work at all, then you'll begin to experiment with ways to make it do better for you.

For side effects

Consider weight loss. There is always a certain amount of stomach distress when you first start on weight reduction—hunger pangs, cramps, nervousness, unsettling mental effects. Biofeedback can help with all these side effects. You make it work by sending or "feeding back" counter orders to the part involved.

For example, hunger pangs are caused by the overactivity of your stomach when there is a reduced supply of food in it. The walls of your stomach rub together and sometimes it churns around like a machine. Concentrate on your stomach. Concentrate on slowing its motion, on relaxing it (it is, after all, only a bag of muscle), on making the pangs disappear. Sooner or later, you'll be able to bring hunger pangs under control.

Can't get moving with your exercises? Try using biofeedback to help. Give yourself an order, when you climb into bed for the night, that you won't be able to accomplish anything before you go through your exercising toning the next morning. Repeat this message several times to yourself, and then push everything from your mind and sleep. You will soon be able to perform your morning toning without fail. And you'll feel very uncomfortable if you don't.

Index

A

Abdominal muscles, 34
Activity:
  abdominal muscles, 34
  ankle, 34
  biofeedback switch, 47–48
  breaking cycle of indolence, 33–37
  chair, 37–46
    making most of it, 37
    things you can do, 38–46
    two-leg paralysis, 41–46
  determination, 46
  disability, 46
  disuse effect, 33
  drive, 46, 47
  fatigue factor, 29
  full ambulation, 46–48
  impairment, 46
  inactivity, 31–37
  key to mobility, 28–31
  mental blues, 33
  nervousness, 33
  osteoarthritis, 32
  poor tone, 33
  put-off, 31–37
  scissors-kicks, 34
  shoulder, 34
  sit-ups, 34
  urinary tract infection, 41
  weight gain, 33
  when?, 52
Agencies:
  national, 233–234
  state, 228–233
Alcohol, 75, 199
Alcoholic limbs, 201
Allopurinol, 56
Amputation, 157
Ankle:
  arthritis, 141
  care, 192
  exercising, 34, 35
Antibodies, 73
Arm, 148, 186–189, 241

Arthritis:
  ankle, 141
  aspirin, 139
  hips, 143
  knee, 141–143
  packs or baths, 140
  pain, 139.
  rest, 139–140
  sling, 140
Aspirin, 55, 56, 139
Attention, 133–135
Attitude, 20–22

B

Back:
  cartilage, 210
  chronic syndrome, 225–226
  contents, 210–214
  disc syndrome, 215–220
    over-response, 217–220
    recovery from surgery, 217
    treatment, 215–217
  iliac bones, 210
  injuries, 211–212
    truth and fiction, 211–212
    work, 212–214
  ligaments, 210
  muscles and nerves, 210
  muscle toning, 68
  poor tone and sway back, 224–225
  rheumatoid arthritis, 223–224
  rib cage, 210
  sacrum, 210
  special exercises, 244–245
  vertebrae, 210
  whiplash, 220–223
Baths, 140
Biofeedback, 81–82, 129–133, 264–265
Biofeedback Diet: A Doctor's Revolutionary Approach, 19, 181
Biofeedback switch, 47–48
Bladder, 255
Bladder stones, 169

Blood supply, 16
Blues, mental, 33
Body:
  bowels, 163–165
  cardiopulmonary tract, 170–175
    at bed rest, 170–174
    sitting up, 174
  digestive tract, 160–167
  hemorrhoids, 165–167
  mouth, 162
  stomach, 163
  swallowing apparatus, 162–163
  teeth, 160–162
  urinary stones, 169–170
  urinary tract, 167–170
Bone graft, ununited fractures, 63–64
Bones:
  exercise, 65
  tone, 177–181
Bones and muscles:
  ankle, 192
  arm, 188–189
  carbohydrate, 181–182
  care and feeding, 177–193
  cerebral palsy, 192
  elbow, 189
  fat, 182
  feet and toes, 192
  healthy, 181–186
  hip, 191
  knee, 191
  lower extremity, 191
  osteoporosis, 179
  protein, 182
  tone that bone, 177–181
  upper limbs, 186
  wrist and fingers, 189
Bowels, 163–165, 255–258
Brain tumor, 208

C

Calcium, 94
Canes, 118–121
Carbohydrate, 181–182
Cardiopulmonary tract, 170–175
Cartilage, 15–16, 210
Causalgia pain, 99–101
Cerebral palsy, 64, 192
Cervical collar, 17
Chair, activity, 37–46
Cold, 54–55
Common sense, 20–22

Comprehensive Employment and Training Act, 233
Conditioning, 94, 247–251
Congenital dislocation of hip, 62
Country Doctor's Common Sense Health Manual, A, 19
Creeping paralysis, 201
Crutches, 117–118

D

D, vitamin, 94
Death of loved one, 72, 77
Depression, 125–126
Determination, 46
Devices:
  household aids and hints, 121–123
    dressing, 123
    house generally, 122
    kitchen, 123
  more immobilization methods, 110–113
  paralyzed limbs, 113–115
  splints, 103–110 (*see also* Splints)
  walking, 115–121
    canes, 118–121
    crutches, 117–118
    walkers, 115–117
Diabetes, 199
Diet, 59, 256–257, 258–264
Digestive tract, 160–167
Disability, 46
Disc syndrome, 215–220
Dislocation of hip, congenital, 62
Disuse effect, 33
Dressing, 123
Drive, 46, 47
Drugs, 18

E

Elbow, 189, 241
Elbow joints, replacement, 61
Employment service, 232
Employment Standards Administration, 234
Exercise:
  bones, 65
  joints, 65
  losing flab, 59
  muscles, 65
  sometimes it cures, 65–68
  stress, 76

F

Face, 148
Fat, 58, 182

Index

Fatigue factor, 29
Federal Civil Service Commission, 233
Feet, 151, 192, 247
Fibrositis, 207
Fingers, 189, 237
Flab, losing, 58–61
Foods, 256–257, 258–264
Foot-drop, 26
Forearm, 241
Fracture:
  compound, 64
  deal with, 89–90
  main lower leg bone, 20
  term, 86
  ununited, bone graft, 63–64
Frustration, stress breeds, 82–84
Fuel, locomotion system, 16–17
Fusion of joints, 63

G

Gouty arthritis, 50, 51, 55, 71, 75–76
Guillain-Barre syndrome, 201

H

Hands, 237
Heat, 54–55
Hemorrhoids, 165–167
Hips:
  arthritis, 143
  care, 191
  congenital dislocation, 62
  replacement of joint, 61
  special exercises, 245
Home care:
  activity, 52
  aspirin, 55–56
  diet and exercise, 59
  exercise cures, 65–68
    bones, 65
    joints, 65
    muscles, 65
  full mobility, 53–54
  heat and cold, 54–55
  losing flab, retaining tone, 58–61
  pain relief, 55–56
  prevention, 56–58
  rest and mobility, 51–52
Household aids and hints, 121–123

I

Iliac bones, 210
Immune system, 73

Impairment, 46
Inactivity (*see* Activity)
Indolence, 33–37

J

Job service, 232
Joints:
  exercise, 65
  fusion, 63
  replacement, 61

K

Kidney stones, 169
Kitchen, 123
Knee:
  arthritis, 141–143
  care, 191
  replacement of joints, 61
  special exercises, 247

L

Legs:
  lower, 247
  muscle tendon transfer, 64
  paralysis, 41–46
  physiotherapy, 151
Ligaments, 15, 63, 210
Limbs:
  alcoholic, 201–206
  nerve damage, 198–206
  paralysis, 113–115
Low back pain, 82–84
Lumbago, 78

M

Medicines, 78
Meditation, 76
Menopause, 93
Mental blues, 33
Mental stress, 70–84 (*see also* Stress)
Mind:
  activity at rest, 125–129
  biofeedback, 129–133
  depression and shock, 125–126
  rehabilitation, 127–128
  remorse and self-pity, 126–127
  too much attention, 133–135
  using what's left, 135–136
Mobility, 22–24, 28–31, 51–52, 53–54

Mouth, 162
Multiple sclerosis, 52
Muscles:
  biofeedback, 264
  care and feeding, 177–193
    (*see also* Bones and muscles)
  exercise, 65
  relaxant, 18
  tendon transfer, 64
  tone, 19–20
  working of organism, 14–15
Myositis, 207

N

National agencies, 233–234
National Alliance of Businessmen, 233–234
Neck, 244
Nerve damage:
  brain tumors, 208
  fibrositis, 207
  limbs, 198–206
    alcoholic, 201–206
    creeping paralysis, 201
  myositis, 207
  nerve damage, 194–209
    (*see also* Nerve damage)
  spinal cord, 194–198
    injury, 196–197
    nerve connections, 195–196
    pain, 196
    quadriplegia, 197–198
  toning nervous system, 206–208
Nerves:
  alcoholism, 199
  diabetes, 199
  going to muscles, 16
Nervousness, 33
Nutrition, 19–20, 94

O

Organisms:
  cartilage, 15–16
  ligaments, 15
  muscles, 14–15
  power and fuel, 16–17
  tendons, 15
Osteoarthritis, 32, 51, 55, 57, 71, 78–81
Osteoporosis, 90–94, 179
Osteotomy, 63
Oxygen, 17

P

Packs, 140
Pain:
  biofeedback, 264–265
  low back, 82–84
  relief, 55–56
  spinal cord, 196
Pain killer, 18
Paralysis:
  creeping, 201
  limbs, 113–115
  two-leg, 41–46
Phantom limb, 96–99
Phenylbutazone, 55, 56
Physical Medicine Department, 24
Physiotherapy, principles, 148
Pity, self-, 126–127
Polio, 64
Power, 16
Pressure problems, 252–254
Prevention, 17, 56–58
Protein, 94, 182

Q

Quadriplegia, 197–198

R

Recuperation, 17
Rehabilitation, 127–128
Remorse, 126–127
Renal stones, 169
Replacement, joint, 61
Rest, 51–52, 139
Rheumatoid arthritis, 51, 55, 57, 71, 72–75, 141, 223–224
Rib cage, 210
Ruptured discs, 215

S

Sacrum, 210
Sand, 155–157
Scissors-kicks, 34
Sedative, 18
Self-pity, 126–127
Shock, 125–126
Shooting pains, 100

Index

Shoulder, 34, 148
Sit-ups, 34
Skin problems, 252–254
Social services agencies, 24
Speech, 25
Spina bifida, 20
Spinal cord:
    injuries and disease, 194–198
    tumor, 189
Splints:
    ankle pain, 109–110
    cold or painful feeling, 110
    fingers, hand, wrist, 104
    lower joints, 108–109
    padding, 110
    painful toes, 107
    "position of function," 104
    reduce swelling first, 110
    remove for night, 110
    rolled-up elastic bandage, 105, 106
    temporary, 110
    thumb or index finger, 106
    upper joints, 107–108
    yarn ball, elastic bandage, 105
Sprain:
    term, 85
    what to do, 88
State agencies, 228–233
State Department of Vocational Rehabilitation, 24
Stiff weak limb syndrome:
    amputation, 157
    arthritis, 138–146
    double trouble, 154–155
    physiotherapy, principles, 148–151
    sand, 155–157
    stroke, 144–154
    water, 157–158
Stomach, 163
Stones, kidney, 169
Strain:
    dealing with, 86
    term, 85
Stress:
    alcohol, 75
    arthritis, 70–71
    biofeedback, 81–82
    breeds frustration, 82–84
    counteract, 76–78
        avoid potent medicines, 78
        avoid self-pity, 78
        avoid tranquilizers, 78
        death of loved one, 77

Stress *(continued)*
    exercise routine, 76
    get away from stress, 76
    meditation, 76
    reduce effects, 77
    gouty arthritis, 71, 75–76
    low back pain, 82–84
    lumbago, 78
    many forms, 76–78
    osteoarthritis, 71, 78–81
    rheumatoid arthritis, 71, 72–75
    role, 72–81
    traumatic arthritis, 71
Stroke, 24, 52, 59, 144–154, 154–155
Surgery:
    bone graft for ununited fractures, 63–64
    disc, 217
    elbow joints, 61
    fusion of joints, 63
    heart, 154
    hip joints, 61
    joints replaced, 61
    knee joints, 61
    less formidable, 63–65
    muscle tendon transfer, 64
    osteotomy, 63
    release of tethered tendons and ligaments, 63
    severe distress and deformity, 62
    when it will help, 61–63
Swallowing apparatus, 162–163
Sway back, 224–225
Swine flu, 201

T

Teeth, 160–162
Tendons, 15, 63
Tethered tendons and ligaments, 63
Thighs, 247
Toes, care, 192
Tone, 33, 58–61, 177–181, 206–208, 224–225
Tranquilizers, 78
Traumatic arthritis, 71
Treatment, 17
Tumors, 189, 208

U

Urinary stones, 169–170
Urinary tract, 41, 167–170
U.S. Department of Labor, 234

V

Vertebrae, 210
Veterans Administration, 233
Veterans Reemployment Rights Commission, 233
Visiting Nurse Service, 24
Vocational Rehabilitation, 24, 228–232

W

Walking devices, 115–121
Water, benefits, 157–158
Weak stiff limb syndrome, 138–159 (see also Stiff weak limb syndrome)
Weight, 18, 19, 20, 58, 258–264
Welfare department, 232–233
Whiplash, 17, 220–223
Work, getting back, 228–235
Wrist, care, 189